Perinatal Genetics

Perinatal Genetics

MARY E. NORTON, MD

Professor
Obstetrics, Gynecology, and Reproductive Sciences and Center for
    Maternal-Fetal Precision Medicine
Division of Maternal-Fetal Medicine
University of California
San Francisco, CA, United States

JEFFREY A. KULLER, MD

Professor
Obstetrics and Gynecology
Division of Maternal-Fetal Medicine
Duke University
Durham, NC, United States

LORRAINE DUGOFF, MD

Professor
Obstetrics and Gynecology
Divisions of Reproductive Genetics and Maternal-Fetal Medicine
University of Pennsylvania
Philadelphia, PA, United States

ELSEVIER

Publisher: Mica Haley
Acquisition Editor: Sarah Barth
Editorial Project Manager: Jennifer Horigan
Project Manager: Kiruthika Govindaraju
Cover Designer: Alan Studholme

ELSEVIER

3251 Riverport Lane
St. Louis, Missouri 63043

  Working together
to grow libraries in
developing countries

www.elsevier.com • www.bookaid.org

List of Contributors

Joseph R. Biggio Jr., MD, MS
System Chair for Women's Services
System Chair Maternal Fetal Medicine
Ochsner Health System
New Orleans, LA, United States

Bryann Bromley, MD
Professor
Obstetrics, Gynecology and Reproductive Biology
Massachusetts General Hospital
Harvard Medical School
Boston, MA, United States

Lorraine Dugoff, MD
Professor
Obstetrics and Gynecology
Divisions of Reproductive Genetics and
    Maternal-Fetal Medicine
University of Pennsylvania
Philadelphia, PA, United States

P. Kaitlyn Edelson, MD
Clinical Research Fellow
Department of Obstetrics and Gynecology
Massachusetts General Hospital
Boston, MA, United States

Jessica L. Giordano, MS, CGC
Program Manager
Reproductive Genomic Study
Department of Obstetrics and Gynecology and
    Institute of Genomic Medicine
Columbia University Medical Center
New York, NY, United States

Anthony R. Gregg, MD, MBA
Chair, Obstetrics and Gynecology
Director, Maternal-Fetal Medicine
Baylor University Medical Center at Dallas
Dallas, TX, United States

Michael H. Guo, MD, PhD
Program in Medical and Population Genetics
Broad Institute of Harvard and MIT
Cambridge, MA, United States

Stephanie Guseh, MD
Clinical Fellow
Maternal Fetal Medicine and Clinical Genetics
Brigham and Women's Hospital and Boston
    Children's Hospital
Harvard Medical School
Boston, MA, United States

Susan Klugman, MD
Director
Reproductive and Medical Genetics
Professor
Obstetrics & Gynecology and Women's Health
Albert Einstein College of Medicine/Montefiore
    Medical Center
Bronx, NY, United States

Jeffrey A. Kuller, MD
Professor
Obstetrics and Gynecology
Division of Maternal-Fetal Medicine
Duke University
Durham, NC, United States

Brynn Levy, PhD
Department of Pathology and Cell Biology
Columbia University Medical Center
New York, NY, United States

Lauren Lichten, MS, CGC
Licensed Genetic Counselor
Associate Professor of the Practice
Associate Director, Genetic Counseling Program
Brandeis University
Waltham, MA, United States

Tippi C. MacKenzie, MD
The Center for Maternal-Fetal Precision Medicine
University of California
San Francisco, CA, United States

Department of Surgery
University of California
San Francisco, CA, United States

Michael T. Mennuti, MD
Professor Emeritus
Obstetrics and Gynecology
University of Pennsylvania
Perelman School of Medicine
Philadelphia, PA, United States

Quoc-Hung L. Nguyen, MD
Resident Physician
Surgery
University of California, San Francisco
San Francisco, CA, United States

Mary E. Norton, MD
Professor
Obstetrics, Gynecology, and Reproductive Sciences
    and Center for Maternal-Fetal Precision Medicine
Division of Maternal-Fetal Medicine
University of California
San Francisco, CA, United States

Barbara M. O'Brien, MD
Associate Professor
Obstetrics, Gynecology, and Reproductive Biology
Beth Israel Deaconess Medical Center
Harvard Medical School
Boston, MA, United States

Soha S. Patel, MD, MS, MSPH
Assistant Professor
Vanderbilt University Medical Center
Department of Obstetrics and Gynecology
Division of Maternal-Fetal Medicine
Nasheville, TN, United States

Malavika Prabhu, MD
Department of Obstetrics and Gynecology
Harvard Medical School, Massachusetts General
    Hospital
Boston, MA, United States

Department of Obstetrics and Gynecology
Warren Alpert Medical School at Brown University
Women and Infants Hospital of Rhode Island
Providence, RI, United States

Sara Schonfeld Rabin-Havt, MD
Clinical Instructor
Obstetrics & Gynecology and Women's Health
Albert Einstein College of Medicine/Montefiore
    Medical Center
Bronx, NY, United States

Aleksandar Rajkovic, MD, PhD
Professor
Department of Pathology
Department of Obstetrics, Gynecology and
    Reproductive Sciences
University of California, San Francisco
San Francisco, CA, United States

Rebecca Reimers, MD, MPH
Clinical Fellow
Maternal Fetal Medicine and Clinical Genetics
Brigham and Women's Hospital and Boston
    Children's Hospital
Harvard Medical School
Boston, MA, United States

Britton D. Rink, MD, MS
Director of Medical Genetics
Mount Carmel Health Systems
Columbus, OH, United States

Melissa Stosic, MS, CGC
Associate Director
Reproductive Genetics
Department of Obstetrics and Gynecology and
    Institute of Genomic Medicine
Columbia University Medical Center
New York, NY, United States

Ignatia B. Van den Veyver, MD
Professor
Department of Obstetrics and Gynecology
Baylor College of Medicine
Houston, TX, United States

Ronald Wapner, MD
Professor
Department of Obstetrics and Gynecology
Columbia University Medical Center
New York, NY, United States

Louise Wilkins-Haug, MD, PhD
Professor
Harvard Medical School
Division Director
Maternal Fetal Medicine and Reproductive Genetics
Obstetrics and Gynecology
Brigham and Women's Hospital
Boston, MA, United States

Russell G. Witt, MD
Department of Surgery
The Center for Maternal-Fetal Precision Medicine
University of California
San Francisco, CA, United States

Svetlana A. Yatsenko, MD
Associate Professor
Department of Pathology
Department of Obstetrics, Gynecology & Reproductive
  Sciences
University of Pittsburgh
School of Medicine
Pittsburgh, PA, United States

The Rapidly Evolving World of Perinatal Genetics

The field of medical genetics has advanced more rapidly than any other in medicine. The obstetrician-gynecologist and maternal–fetal medicine specialist must be able to keep abreast of this complex and changing field. The three of us were approached to write and edit a textbook to provide information on prenatal genetics that covers the depth and breadth of this evolving specialty.

Our 16 chapters are written by leaders in reproductive genetics, prenatal diagnosis and treatment, and fetal ultrasound. Many, including the three editors, are trained and boarded in both maternal–fetal medicine and clinical genetics. We begin with chapters on genetic counseling, and Mendelian and non-Mendelian genetics. Nontraditional forms of inheritance, including uniparental disomy and mitochondrial disorders are explained. The principles of cytogenetics and how they can be practically applied are detailed in two chapters. We then discuss the various approaches to genetic screening including ethnicity-based, pan-ethnic, and expanded carrier screening. Several chapters are devoted to prenatal screening for aneuploidy using first and second trimester ultrasound, serum screening, and cell-free DNA. Much of the rest of the textbook is devoted to prenatal diagnosis, including procedures as well as laboratory techniques and considerations. These have significantly evolved from the days when a simple karyotype was the mainstay of diagnostic testing. Fetal testing using the evolving technologies of chromosomal microarray and exome and genome sequencing is explained. These techniques have expanded our ability to test for genetic abnormalities, especially in the fetus with structural anomalies. And finally, chapters on preimplantation genetic testing and fetal treatment discuss how genetic abnormalities can be screened and tested prior to implantation and treated during the fetal period.

Editors

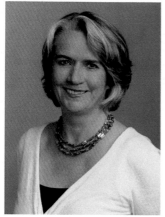

Mary E. Norton, MD
Professor
Obstetrics, Gynecology, and
Reproductive Sciences
and Center for Maternal-Fetal
Precision Medicine
Division of Maternal-Fetal
Medicine
University of California
San Francisco, CA, United States

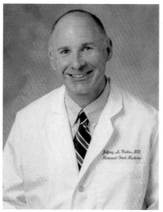

Jeffrey A. Kuller, MD
Professor
Obstetrics and Gynecology
Division of Maternal-Fetal
Medicine
Duke University
Durham, NC, United States

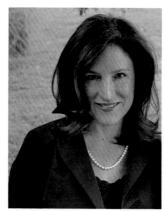

Lorraine Dugoff, MD
Professor
Obstetrics and Gynecology
Divisions of Reproductive Genetics
and
Maternal-Fetal Medicine
University of Pennsylvania
Philadelphia, PA, United States

Acknowledgements

The editors wish to thank our outstanding contributors to this text. We are indebted to our editors at Elsevier, Jennifer Horigan and Sarah Barth. We are forever thankful to our spouses, Tom, Susan, and Bill for their love, patience, and faith in us, and to our children who continue to keep us grounded.

Contents

1 **Principles of Genetics and Genomics,** *1*
Joseph R. Biggio Jr., MD, MS

2 **Non-Mendelian Genetics,** *11*
Susan Klugman, MD and Sara Schonfeld
Rabin-Havt, MD

3 **Principles of Genetic Counseling,** *21*
Britton D. Rink, MD, MS

4 **Cytogenetics: Part 1, General
Concepts and Aneuploid
Conditions,** *27*
Michael T. Mennuti, MD

5 **Cytogenetics: Part 2, Structural
Chromosome Rearrangements and
Reproductive Impact,** *39*
Michael T. Mennuti, MD

6 **Molecular Genetics,** *49*
Stephanie Guseh, MD, Rebecca Reimers, MD,
MPH, and Louise Wilkins-Haug, MD, PhD

7 **Carrier Screening for Genetic
Conditions,** *63*
Michael H. Guo, MD, PhD and Anthony R.
Gregg, MD, MBA

8 **Serum and Ultrasound Based
Screening Tests for Aneuploidy,** *75*
Barbara M. O'Brien, MD and Lauren Lichten,
MS, CGC

9 **Cell-Free DNA Screening,** *85*
Soha S. Patel, MD, MS, MSPH and Lorraine
Dugoff, MD

10 **Ultrasound Markers for Aneuploidy
in the Second Trimester,** *95*
Malavika Prabhu, MD, Jeffrey A. Kuller, MD, and
Joseph R. Biggio Jr., MD, MS

11 **Genetic Evaluation of Fetal
Sonographic Abnormalities,** *105*
P. Kaitlyn Edelson, MD, Lorraine Dugoff, MD, and
Bryann Bromley, MD

12 **Chromosomal Microarray Analysis,** *125*
Jessica L. Giordano, MS, CGC, Melissa
Stosic, MS, CGC, Brynn Levy, PhD, and
Ronald Wapner, MD

13 **Exome and Genome Sequencing,** *137*
Ignatia B. Van den Veyver, MD

14 **Prenatal Diagnostic Testing,** *149*
Mary E. Norton, MD

15 **Preimplantation Genetic Testing,** *161*
Svetlana A. Yatsenko, MD and Aleksandar
Rajkovic, MD, PhD

16 **Fetal Treatment of Genetic
Disorders,** *175*
Quoc-Hung L. Nguyen, MD, Russell G. Witt, MD,
and Tippi C. MacKenzie, MD

INDEX, *187*

CHAPTER 1

Principles of Genetics and Genomics

JOSEPH R. BIGGIO JR., MD, MS

INTRODUCTION

Few areas in medicine have seen such rapid and dramatic advances in knowledge and technology as the field of genetics has over the past two decades. Breakthroughs such as the mapping of the human genome and technological advancements enabling rapid gene sequencing have not only greatly enhanced our understanding of common and uncommon disorders but also changed the way the medical profession approaches the diagnosis, prevention, and treatment of disease. In the field of obstetrics and gynecology, the ability to map fragments of cell-free placental DNA to specific chromosomes has led to highly accurate screening tests for common aneuploidies. Similarly, the use of genomic hybridization techniques has enabled the detection of small variations in genomic composition below the resolution of conventional karyotype that are now known to be responsible for a variety of genomic disorders. The impact of precision medicine remains fledgling in the field of perinatal medicine, but with its growing utility in other areas of medicine, especially with regard to targeted pharmacologic therapy, it is very likely that we will see similar application of precision medicine to perinatal medicine in the coming years.

Genetics is no longer a field of rare diseases that only a few need to understand. With our rapidly growing understanding of the human genome, it is clear that there is a genetic underpinning to almost all medical conditions, structural abnormalities, and functional disorders. Modern genetics and genomics provide the medical professional deeper insight and more information into medical disorders with far less material and less invasive approaches than ever before. With the increasingly commonplace application of genetic and genomic principles to the diagnosis and management of many disorders, it is essential that all providers develop an understanding of the basic principles underlying the field of genetics.

WHAT IS THE DIFFERENCE BETWEEN "GENETICS" AND "GENOMICS"?

The field of medical genetics focuses on the contribution of changes (or "variants") in individual genes to human variation and disease. In contrast, genomics focuses on all of the genes, called the genome, and how multiple genes interact and function to result in either a state of health or disease. The study of genomics has only become possible recently with advances in DNA sequencing technology.

HOW DOES THE STRUCTURE AND ORGANIZATION OF GENES AFFECT THE REGULATION OF GENE FUNCTION?

The cell nucleus and the mitochondria contain all of the genes in humans. The 46 nuclear chromosomes—22 paired autosomes and 2 sex chromosomes—contain the majority of this genetic material. Although the Y chromosome contains only a few genes in addition to those responsible for male sexual differentiation and development, the X chromosome has a number of genes that are integral to normal development and physiologic function for both sexes.

There are approximately 3 billion base pairs of DNA per human genome, and DNA length is normally measured in kilobases (1000 bases, kb) or megabases (1,000,000 bases, Mb). Humans have between 20,000 and 23,000 genes—fewer than the 40,000 postulated before the completion of the Human Genome project; this represents only approximately 10%–15% of the total complement of the DNA.

Each gene contains the information necessary for production of an intact protein and is composed of sequences of DNA that contain regulatory elements and coding regions (Fig. 1.1). Four purine and pyrimidine bases are the building blocks for each gene and ultimately determine the protein sequence produced. Exons are the segments of coding DNA that

Perinatal Genetics. https://doi.org/10.1016/B978-0-323-53094-1.00001-1

are transcribed into messenger RNA (mRNA), which then serves as the template from which the amino acid sequence, and ultimately the protein structure, is determined. A series of three nucleotide base pairs, termed a codon, determines the amino acid to be added to the building protein chain as the mRNA is translated. Because there are 64 possible codons and only 20 amino acids, there is redundancy with many amino acids coded for by multiple codons.

Introns are noncoding regions within the gene that separate exons. Although introns were once thought to be "junk" DNA, it is now known that DNA sequences within the introns play a role in gene regulation and expression. For example, some genes may encode multiple proteins with the ultimate protein product determined by how the exons are spliced together, a process controlled by the DNA sequences within the introns. Other noncoding regulatory regions are located outside the coding region of the gene in the upstream 5′ untranslated region and the downstream 3′ untranslated region. In addition to these DNA segments that are actually transcribed into the initial mRNA transcript, a number of other DNA regulatory elements that

allow for binding of molecules involved in control of transcription are located in the 5′ upstream area, e.g., promoter region, or TATA box.

The complexity of these regulatory processes is far more involved than previously thought, and the role of genetic variation in these regulatory elements and in the molecules they bind in human disease is only beginning to be understood. In addition to changes in the DNA sequence affecting gene transcription, other modifiable processes can also alter gene expression. Epigenetic changes, such as DNA methylation and histone acetylation, control gene transcription by preventing or facilitating binding of key molecules involved in DNA transcription. Such changes appear to play a role in tissue-specific and time-specific gene expression.

WHAT ARE THE TYPES OF DNA SEQUENCE VARIATION THAT CAN OCCUR?

Although greater than 99% of DNA is identical from one individual to the next, genetic variation occurs at various sites throughout the genome. The different variants that exist at any one site or locus are termed *alleles*.

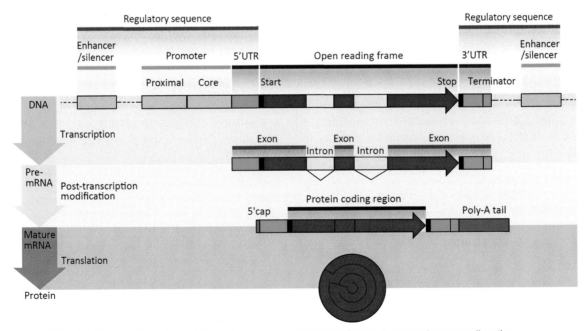

FIG. 1.1 The structure of a protein-coding gene demonstrating the regulatory regions as well as the protein-coding regions with the introns and exons that are transcribed into mRNA. The mRNA molecule undergoes modification to a mature molecule, which is then translated to create a protein. (Retrieved from WikiMedia Commons at https://commons.wikimedia.org/wiki/File:Gene_structure_eukaryote_2_annotated. svg on March 4, 2018. Shafee T, Lowe R. Eukaryotic and prokaryotic gene structure. *WikiJ Med.* 2017; 4(1). ISSN 20024436. https://doi.org/10.15347/wjm/2017.002. posted on April 9, 2015.)

Polymorphisms are differences in DNA that occur in the population throughout the genome and can consist of single nucleotide changes or duplications or deletions of larger segments of DNA. Most polymorphisms are benign and do not result in alteration of protein function, although some polymorphisms have been associated with altered protein function (e.g., factor V Leiden). *Mutations* are changes in DNA sequence that result in altered protein production, structure, or function.

Single nucleotide polymorphisms (SNPs) are the replacement of a single base for another in the DNA sequence. SNPs are the most common form of genetic variation and occur approximately every 200–300 base pairs. Such substitutions typically have no significant effect on gene function, but depending on the location, significant effects on protein production or function can be seen. The distinction between a polymorphism and a mutation is to some degree a matter of semantics, but historically polymorphisms have largely been viewed as benign genetic changes that are found in the population more commonly than mutations are thought to occur.

Nonsense mutations result when the base substitution results in a change that alters the codon for an amino acid to one for a stop codon, leading to premature termination of protein synthesis from the mRNA molecule. *Missense mutations* occur when the SNP changes the codon for one amino acid to that for another amino acid; depending on the amino acid change, the structure and function of the protein may be changed. *Splice site mutations* are those that occur at an intron-exon boundary and affect the normal splicing of mRNA such that an intron is retained or an exon skipped in the mature mRNA molecule. *Silent mutations* occur when there is no change in the amino acid sequence because although the DNA sequence changed, the amino acid coded for by the mRNA codon did not change because of redundancy in the genetic code. In addition to point mutations, which retain the same number of nucleotides, insertions or deletions of bases can also occur. Most commonly involving one or two bases, such insertions or deletions cause *frameshift mutations* and alter the reading frame of the codons in the mRNA. The amino acid sequence downstream from the insertion is typically altered substantially.

In addition to intragenic changes, polymorphisms can also occur in regulatory regions. These *regulatory polymorphisms* may alter the binding of transcription factors, enhancers, silencers, or similar molecules. The protein sequence remains intact, but protein expression can be substantially altered.

WHAT ARE THE CLASSIC PATTERNS OF GENETIC INHERITANCE? WHAT ARE THE RECURRENCE RISK FOR DISORDERS INHERITED IN EACH FASHION?

Classic Mendelian genetics is based on the principle that a specific disease or phenotype is determined by a single gene. Although the phenotype of an individual with a specific disorder is largely due to the specific mutations present at the genetic locus, in many disorders not all individuals with the same genotype manifest the identical phenotype because of the potential effects of a number of modifying genes that also contribute to the phenotype. Nonetheless, when considering the occurrence of genetic disease, the original framework of Mendelian genetics remains an important foundation upon which to build an understanding of the inheritance of genetic disease.

Autosomal Dominant

All genes located on the autosomes (chromosomes 1–22) are inherited in a biallelic (two copies) fashion. If one of the alleles at a specific locus is expressed in preference to the other, and hence defines a specific disorder or phenotype, that condition is considered to be inherited in an *autosomal dominant* fashion. Autosomal dominant inheritance is characterized by transmission of the associated allele to 50% of offspring, the presence of the disorder in both sexes, and the possibility of male-to-male transmission (Fig. 1.2). In addition, the phenotype of individuals who inherit an autosomal dominant disorder is also influenced by the *penetrance* and *expressivity* of the associated allele.

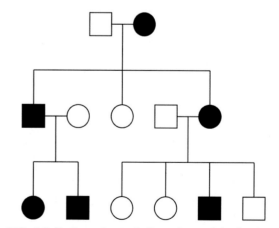

FIG. 1.2 Pedigree demonstrating autosomal dominant inheritance. Male-to-male transmission as well as male-to-female transmission is seen. Approximately 50% of offspring inherit the disorder.

Penetrance reflects whether the mutant allele is expressed or not. For an individual, the gene is either penetrant or nonpenetrant, but when all individuals with the mutant gene are considered, the gene is considered to have either *complete penetrance*, meaning that all individuals who inherit the allele will express the disorder, or *incomplete penetrance*, when only a portion with the mutated gene express the disorder. Although incomplete penetrance may account for the appearance that some disorders will skip a generation, some autosomal dominant disorders have age-related penetrance and do not manifest until later in life (e.g., some forms of Alzheimer disease). In the case of tumor suppressor genes (e.g., *BRCA1*), some require a second hit to result in clinical disease. *Expressivity* describes the variation in the phenotype from mild to severe that is seen in individuals who inherit a mutation at a disease locus. Variable expressivity can be related not only to the specific mutant allele inherited and its effect on protein function and production but also to the effect of other modifying genes. Many disorders have *allelic heterogeneity* in which many different mutant alleles have been described and are responsible for clinical disease. This can be a potential explanation for variable expressivity. The same phenomenon of allelic heterogeneity occurs in autosomal recessive disorders as well.

In some cases, both alleles of a gene are different from each other but are equally expressed and affect the phenotype produced. Although not often considered in the classic pattern of inheritance, this type of inheritance and gene expression is termed *codominant*. Examples of this type of inheritance include the ABO blood group antigens (e.g., A on one gene and B on the other resulting in AB blood group) and the β-globin gene (e.g., hemoglobin S allele on one gene and hemoglobin A allele on the other, resulting in sickle trait).

Autosomal Recessive

In *autosomal recessive* conditions, a mutation is required in each copy of the gene to result in the condition being expressed. Individuals who inherit two identical mutations and express the trait or condition are *homozygous* for that gene or are *homozygotes*. In some cases, individuals may inherit two different mutations—one in each copy of the gene—each of which affect protein function or production, resulting in disease. Such individuals are *compound heterozygotes* for this gene but typically express the disease phenotype as if they were homozygotes. An example of this is cystic fibrosis, where there are thousands of known mutations in the CFTR gene. If only one gene has a mutation, the individual is a *heterozygote* or a *heterozygous carrier* for that gene.

Typically, carriers do not manifest a specific phenotype for autosomal recessive conditions; however, biochemical testing may reveal changes in amount or function at the protein level in some conditions (as many autosomal recessive conditions are associated with enzyme function). In most disorders, however, no such changes can be noted. Because carriers are asymptomatic, carrier status for autosomal recessive conditions is often unknown until an affected offspring is diagnosed or until genetic carrier screening is performed as part of a preconception or antenatal genetic screening program. Because of the overall rarity of autosomal recessive conditions, family history alone is of limited utility in identifying carriers of autosomal recessive conditions as most families who have an affected child have an otherwise negative family history (Fig. 1.3).

To produce an affected offspring, both parents must be carriers of a mutation in the specific gene (Fig. 1.4). If both parents are carriers of a mutation in the same gene, the chance of an affected offspring is 25%. Of the offspring a carrier couple can produce, 25% will be affected, 50% will be unaffected carriers, and 25% will be noncarriers. However, a more clinically useful approach to estimating carrier risk in a family is to consider that any unaffected sibling of an affected individual has a 2/3 chance of being a carrier and a 1/3 chance of having two normal alleles. In such cases, the other possibility of having two mutations and being affected has been excluded.

Sex-Linked Inheritance

In addition to genes that play a role in sexual development, the X chromosome carries a number of genes that are important for normal physiologic function in both males and females. Because females carry two X chromosomes, one X chromosome is randomly inactivated in each cell to achieve the correct balance of genetic material. Therefore, although females have two copies of each X chromosome gene, only one copy is expressed from any given cell. Males have only a single X chromosome and hence have only one copy of the X chromosome genes; they are *hemizygous* for any gene on the X chromosome.

X-linked inheritance can be either dominant or recessive, but recessive is more common. Many *X-linked dominant* conditions are lethal in males (e.g., incontinentia pigmenti) because the only copy of the gene present will carry the mutation. In contrast, females have two copies of the gene, only one of which carries the mutation. X-chromosome inactivation is variable, independent, and random in each cell. This results in some cells expressing the mutated gene and some

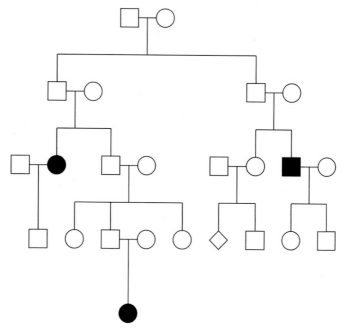

FIG. 1.3 Pedigree demonstrating autosomal recessive inheritance reflecting the overall infrequent occurrence of disease even in affected families.

	A	a
A	**AA** Unaffected Non-carrier	**Aa** Unaffected Carrier
a	**Aa** Unaffected Carrier	**aa** Affected

FIG. 1.4 Punnet square representing the possible genetic outcomes when two carriers of an autosomal recessive condition produce offspring. 25% will be noncarriers and unaffected, 50% will be carriers and unaffected, and 25% will be affected. Of the unaffected offspring, two of the three will be carriers.

expressing the normal allele. In the case of X-linked dominant disorders that are not lethal in males (e.g., vitamin D–resistant rickets), all of the daughters of an affected male will have the disorder, whereas none of his sons will (Fig. 1.5). *X-linked recessive* conditions primarily affect males, although females may also manifest a phenotype that is typically milder, depending on the X chromosome inactivation. Common X-linked recessive conditions include hemophilia A and Duchenne muscular dystrophy. Female carriers of X-linked

conditions will pass the mutation to 50% of their offspring; 50% of daughters will be carriers (and likely unaffected), whereas 50% of sons will be affected. A male with an X-linked recessive condition will pass the mutation to 50% of his daughters, but because he does not transmit his X chromosome to his sons, none of them will inherit the mutated gene (Fig. 1.6).

WHAT ARE GENOMIC DISORDERS?

A variety of phenotypes historically identified based on physical and other clinical findings are known to have characteristic deletions or duplications of chromosome segments. A number of common conditions associated with specific chromosome areas have been described, suggesting a predilection for abnormalities in these areas, e.g., DiGeorge syndrome associated with a 22q11 deletion. With our enhanced knowledge of the sequence and structure of the human genome, it is now understood that these disorders characterized by recurrent deletions or duplications of similar chromosome regions are due to the presence of repetitive elements in these areas of the genome. The repetitive nature of these elements at these "hot spots" predisposes to misalignment during meiosis, resulting in uneven exchange of genetic material between sister chromatids because of

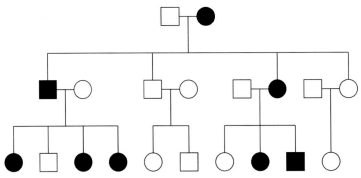

FIG. 1.5 Pedigree demonstrating X-linked dominant inheritance with predominantly affected females, and all female offspring of affected males are affected.

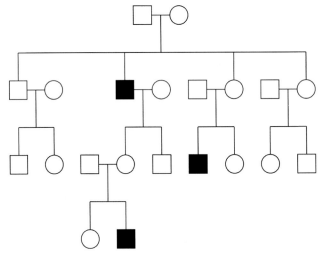

FIG. 1.6 Pedigree demonstrating X-linked recessive inheritance. Females are typically unaffected, 50% of male offspring of carrier females are affected, and 50% of daughters of affected males are carriers at risk to have affected sons.

nonallelic homologous recombination. This results in one chromosome with a duplicated amount of genetic material and another chromosome with a missing amount of genetic material.

Terminal deletions and duplications can also occur due to chromosome breakage with either loss or gain of genetic material in these areas because of areas of repetitive DNA elements in the terminal portions (*telomeres*) of the arm of each chromosome. These disorders are typically characterized by abnormalities in the chromosomes too small to be visualized on conventional karyotype but can be identified with techniques focused on molecular level assessment, including fluorescence in situ hybridization (FISH) or chromosomal microarray (see Chapter 12). Because these disorders are caused by structural elements within the genome, as opposed to single gene mutations or absence of an entire chromosome, these disorders are now often classified as *genomic disorders*.

The size of the repetitive elements and the extent of the misalignment can vary from one individual to another; hence the breakpoints of the involved region can be variable. Deletion or duplication syndromes typically involve several genes colocated in the same chromosome region, but the number of genes involved can vary from one individual to another. Microdeletion syndromes are among the most well-characterized of this type of disorder and are a prototype of these *contiguous gene deletion syndromes*. Examples include Cri du chat and DiGeorge syndrome.

WHAT OTHER GENETIC MECHANISMS ARE IMPLICATED IN GENETIC DISEASE OCCURRENCE?

Although the classic models of inheritance play a key role in the transmission of genetic traits and disorders from one generation to the next, there are a number of other genetic mechanisms that contribute to disease transmission. The complexity of these models can complicate counseling regarding recurrence risk for offspring or the likelihood of disease in a given individual. For this reason, it is important that obstetric care providers understand how these mechanisms affect inheritance patterns.

Hereditary Unstable DNA

A number of genes have been found to contain intragenic repetitive elements that expand, or increase the number of repeats, during the process of meiosis. Classically, these disorders were thought to be characterized by triplet or *trinucleotide repeats* (e.g., CGG), but genes with repetitive elements of four or five nucleotides have also been identified. As the number of repeats increases, gene expression may be decreased through methylation or protein function may be altered through other mechanisms. Many of the disorders that demonstrate this pattern of inheritance are characterized by abnormal neurologic or neuromuscular function, including fragile X, Huntington disease, myotonic dystrophy, and ataxia telangiectasia. The number of repeats can change from one generation to the next—either increasing via a process called *anticipation* or contracting in size. In general, for each condition, there is a range of repeat number that varies within normal individuals, as well as a premutation range in which there is a risk of expansion, and a full mutation threshold above which a phenotype is usually present. For patients with the number of repeats in the full mutation range, as the number of repeats increases, typically, the severity of the disorder increases and its age of onset decreases. In addition to this mechanism of unstable DNA inheritance, each disorder is also inherited according to classic Mendelian inheritance patterns. For example, fragile X follows X-linked inheritance, whereas Huntington disease is autosomal dominant.

Imprinting and Epigenetic Modification

Although it was once thought that gene function depended solely on the inherited DNA sequence, as we learned more about the sequence of the human genome, it became clear that the expression and function of certain genes could be affected by modifications to DNA that were reversible and did not affect the actual sequence of the DNA. *Epigenetic modification* is a reversible process whereby changes, such as DNA methylation or histone acetylation of the chromatin molecules responsible for packaging DNA, can be made that affect the expression of the particular gene through inactivation or blocking of the promoter region. Epigenetic modification of DNA typically involves methylation of the promoter region, whereas epigenetic modification of histones involves acetylation or deacetylation, which then controls whether the promoter region of the DNA molecule is accessible for transcription factor and RNA polymerase binding.

A number of genes have been identified throughout the genome whose expression and function is determined by the parent from whom the gene is inherited, and is different when inherited from the mother versus the father. *Imprinting* is the epigenetic control of gene expression based on the parental origin of the specific copy of the inherited gene. For some imprinted genes, the paternal copy of the gene is inherited in a methylated/inactivated state, whereas for other genes, the maternal copy is inactivated.

There are a number of imprinted areas throughout the genome that contain genes with the potential to result in phenotypic abnormalities if imprinting is abnormal. However, the proportion of the genome that is imprinted is quite small, and the phenotypes are highly variable depending on the specific genes involved. From a clinical standpoint, imprinting has been implicated in some cases of Prader-Willi and Angelman syndrome with deletion of the 15q11-13 region. Paternal deletion results in Prader-Willi syndrome, whereas maternal deletion results in Angelman syndrome (see Chapter 2).

Uniparental disomy is a scenario in which both chromosomes of a particular pair are inherited from the same parent. In most cases, this occurs in a zygote or embryo that is trisomic for the particular chromosome and then, during the process of cell division, one of the extra copies is lost. This phenomenon of trisomic rescue is random with regard to which two chromosomes are retained, and therefore, two copies from the same parent could be retained. If the implicated chromosome contains imprinted genes, e.g., chromosome 15, the potential for a clinical phenotype should be considered. Although chorionic villus sampling traditionally has been associated with a 1% incidence of placental mosaicism and a potential for trisomy, cell-free DNA screening has the potential to identify placental mosaicism for trisomies that may be important if imprinted chromosomes are present.

Mitochondrial Inheritance

The mitochondria play a key role in energy metabolism, and most mitochondrial disorders involve tissues with high energy requirements such as the central nervous system, heart, and skeletal muscles. Each cell contains hundreds of mitochondria. Each mitochondrion has its own circular double-stranded DNA molecule containing 37 genes. The genetic sequence of each mitochondrion is independent and is replicated in a process separate from that of nuclear DNA. Because few mitochondria are present in sperm, but tens of thousands are present in the oocyte, all of the mitochondria, and the mitochondrial DNA, inherited by the zygote are maternal in origin. If a mutation is present in the DNA of a mitochondrion, it can be promulgated with each replication of the mitochondrion. Thus, within each cell, there is a mix of mitochondria with different genetic composition—some with and some without the mutation—a condition called *heteroplasmy*. The number of mitochondria with the mutation differs in each cell with some trending toward normal and others toward predominantly mutated. Moreover, the proportion of mutant and normal mitochondria can vary by tissue type; prenatal diagnosis of mitochondrial disorders is possible but challenging. Mitochondrial inheritance is characterized by maternal transmission to both male and female offspring in equal proportions and no paternal transmission (Fig. 1.7).

Germline and Somatic Mosaicism

With increases in the ability to obtain genomic sequences on a variety of tissue types, both healthy and those affected by cancer, the occurrence of genetic mosaicism has become better recognized. This genetic variation is due to postzygotic mutation that typically occurs in developing cells and then is passed on through cell replication in the developing embryo. The cells derived from the original cell in which the mutation occurred will all carry the genetic variant, whereas those derived from other cells will not. The significance of the mutation depends on the gene involved as well as the cell type and tissue affected. If this process occurs in cells that are destined to give rise to the gonads, *gonadal mosaicism* can develop with the potential that the mutation will be transmitted to all cells of offspring who inherit the mutation.[1] Such a phenomenon is thought to explain some cases of recurrent autosomal dominant disorders in families with unaffected parents (e.g., achondroplasia or type 2 osteogenesis imperfecta). Unfortunately, with current capabilities, it is not possible to determine whether a new autosomal dominant disorder in a family is due to a spontaneous mutation in a single gamete or due to gonadal mosaicism. In cancer, postzygotic mutation occurs, often due to some types of environmental exposure, in a gene with a role in cell cycle control (e.g., a tumor suppressor gene), and results in the uncontrolled cell replication or failure of cell senescence in a particular organ. The refinements of genetic sequencing technologies are only now beginning to uncover the immense genetic variation within each of us and our tissues. The longstanding belief of a single identical genome in all of our cells is no longer true, especially as genetic variation accumulates with generations of cell replication associated with aging.

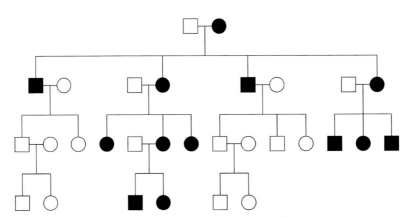

FIG. 1.7 Pedigree demonstrating mitochondrial inheritance with matrilineal inheritance because of transmission of mitochondrial DNA in the oocyte. Because of heteroplasmy, the offspring of affected individuals may all be affected although the severity of the disorder can vary from one sibling to the next based on the proportion of mutant:normal mitochondria inherited.

Digenic Inheritance

Although classic thought about the inheritance of genetic disease has focused on the role of single genes, with increasing knowledge of the human genetic sequence, several exceptions to this rule have been noted. A number of disorders have now been found in which mutations in two or more genes are necessary to express the phenotype.[2] In retinitis pigmentosa, digenic inheritance has now been implicated in other disorders including facioscapulohumeral muscular dystrophy, Bardet-Biedl syndrome, some forms of hereditary deafness, and Hirschsprung disease.[3] The requirement of two mutations reflects the gene-gene (*epistatic*) interactions that occur between a number of genes affecting gene expression, protein function, and phenotype expression. Although digenic inheritance may reflect a simpler level of polygenic inheritance in which multiple genes interact, in the future, it is likely that the number of disease phenotypes influenced by epistatic effects will grow as we learn more about gene sequences, gene expression, and protein-protein interactions.

Multifactorial or Complex Inheritance

Multifactorial inheritance refers to disorders and genetic traits that occur and are determined by the interaction of environmental factors and multiple genes. In many cases, the specific genes involved in these disorders are unknown or their role is poorly characterized. Multifactorial inheritance, generally, is thought to encompass *threshold traits, qualitative traits, and complex disorders of adulthood,* such as diabetes and heart disease. A number of common birth defects are believed to be inherited in a multifactorial fashion as threshold traits. *Threshold traits* are present only if a certain level of the combination of genetic liability and environmental exposure is reached. Neural tube defects, congenital heart defects, cleft lip, and club foot are all most commonly due to multifactorial genetic inheritance, although some may be due to monogenic or chromosome disorders. In contrast, for *qualitative traits* that result from the interaction of multiple genes and the environment, the distribution and phenotype of the trait follows a normal, bell-shaped distribution. Many human traits (e.g., height, weight, blood pressure, intelligence) are inherited in this manner. Although it is clear that many disorders of adulthood have genetic and environmental interactions, with clear clustering in families and strong environmental influences, the underlying genes and genetic mechanisms are poorly characterized for most of these conditions.

Birth defects due to multifactorial inheritance are often seen to occur in a family at a higher incidence than that in the general population; however, the inheritance pattern does not follow that of classic Mendelian inheritance. A number of basic principles govern counseling on recurrence risk of multifactorial disorders or birth defects. First, the risk is highest in first-degree relatives of an affected individual, and the risk decreases substantially for more distant relatives. For many multifactorial disorders, if a parent or sibling (first-degree relative) is affected, the recurrence risk in future offspring is estimated to be 3%–5%. In third-degree relatives (e.g., first cousins), the recurrence risk approaches that of the general population. Second, the more family members affected, the greater the risk of recurrence because this reflects a greater genetic contribution to the phenotype. Third, the more severe the disorder, the higher the recurrence risk. If a parent was born with a bilateral cleft lip and palate, the recurrence risk in his offspring is higher than if he had only a unilateral cleft. Similarly, hypoplastic left heart is in the same spectrum of disorders as bicuspid aortic valve. A woman who has had a prior child with hypoplastic left heart is at higher risk to have a child with any type of left-sided flow–related cardiac defect compared with a woman with an isolated bicuspid valve. Fourth, many multifactorial disorders demonstrate a sex predilection. If the affected individual is of the less frequently affected sex, the recurrence risk in future offspring is higher. For example, pyloric stenosis is more common in males than females. If a female is affected, the recurrence risk is increased in future male and female offspring. The male sibling of an affected female has a 10% risk of having pyloric stenosis, whereas the male sibling of an affected male has a risk of approximately 4%.

HOW HAVE ADVANCES IN GENOMIC MEDICINE CHANGED SCREENING AND DIAGNOSTIC TESTS TYPICALLY USED IN THE ASSESSMENT OF GENETIC DISEASE IN PERINATAL MEDICINE?

Advances in molecular diagnostics have greatly changed the approach to screening and diagnosis of genetic disease in perinatal medicine. Conventional karyotype analysis relies on the appearance of Giemsa-banded (G-banded) chromosomes to detect numeric and structural abnormalities. The ability to detect structural abnormalities is limited to the resolution visible under the microscope, approximately 5–7 megabases. Molecular cytogenetic testing first became available using fluorescent oligonucleotide probes capable of bonding to unique sequences of DNA in the genome to perform fluorescent in situ hybridization (FISH). This methodology can be used to determine numerical abnormalities as well as submicroscopic deletions and duplications. When used in the setting of prenatal diagnosis, FISH can be used as a rapid assessment of chromosome numbers in interphase cells to exclude the common aneuploidies and in metaphase cells to assess for targeted submicroscopic deletions or duplications of concern. Further advances in molecular techniques allowed the development of microarray analysis. Genomic sequences representative of all the chromosomes are fixed to a slide and allow interrogation of a sample of interest for the amount of genetic material present in all of the chromosomes. With comparative genomic hybridization (CGH), the sample of interest is labeled with one fluorescent probe and a reference DNA sample with another probe. The relative amount of DNA binding of each probe at a particular locus is assessed and can be used to assess the DNA content of the sample of interest at sites throughout the genome. CGH microarray analysis has become standard of care in the evaluation of fetuses and infants with congenital anomalies because of the increased yield compared with conventional karyotype as well as in the evaluation of stillbirth.[4,5]

Advances in DNA mutation detection and DNA sequencing have also had a profound impact on the approach to screening and diagnosis of single-gene disorders. Next-generation sequencing technologies have greatly increased the speed with which gene sequencing can be performed and reduced the cost. These advances have led to the development and feasibility of cell-free DNA screening for aneuploidy, expanded carrier screening for genetic disease, and genome sequencing, all of which are discussed elsewhere in this issue.

Although these technologies are able to identify more variants in the genome than ever before, the significance of some of these variants may be unclear. Any variant in the genetic sequence may represent a benign variant, a pathologic variant, or a *variant of uncertain significance (VUS)*. This applies to point mutations identified through genomic sequencing as well as to copy number variation identified via CGH. Although the significance of some genomic variants can be estimated or predicted based on an extrapolated effect on gene function or dose, for a number of genetic variants, such prediction is not possible. The clinical significance of a VUS is only able to be determined based on the correlation of the genetic variant with the phenotype produced. Accrual of sufficient experience and information in the genomic catalogs is continually evolving, and as our experience with advanced molecular techniques and sequences grows, the number of VUS will decrease even further than it already has.

CONCLUSION

Few fields have demonstrated as dramatic of changes in technology and application to medical care as has the field of perinatal genetics in the past 20 years. As technology continues to advance, the use of genetic techniques in providing routine medical care and improving pregnancy outcomes will continue to grow. An understanding of the principles of genetics and genomics is imperative for providers of perinatal care.

REFERENCES

1. Forsberg LA, Gisselsson D, Dumanski JP. Mosaicism in health and disease -clones picking up speed. *Nat Rev Genet.* 2017;18(2):128–142. https://doi.org/10.1038/nrg.2016.145. PubMed PMID: 27941868.
2. Lupski JR. Digenic inheritance and Mendelian disease. *Nat Genet.* 2012;44(12):1291–1292. https://doi.org/10.1038/ng.2479.
3. Schäffer AA. Digenic inheritance in medical genetics. *J Med Genet.* 2013;50(10):641–652. https://doi.org/10.1136/jmedgenet-2013-101713.
4. Wapner RJ, Martin CL, Levy B, et al. Chromosomal microarray versus karyotyping for prenatal diagnosis. *N Engl J Med.* 2012;367(23):2175–2184. https://doi.org/10.1056/NEJMoa1203382. PubMed PMID: 23215555; PubMed Central PMCID: PMC3549418.
5. Reddy UM, Page GP, Saade GR, et al. NICHD Stillbirth Collaborative Research Network. Karyotype versus microarray testing for genetic abnormalities after stillbirth. *N Engl J Med.* 2012;367(23):2185–2193. https://doi.org/10.1056/NEJMoa1201569. PubMed PMID: 23215556; PubMed Central PMCID: PMC4295117.

CHAPTER 2

Non-Mendelian Genetics

SUSAN KLUGMAN, MD • SARA SCHONFELD RABIN-HAVT, MD

INTRODUCTION

Mendel wrote in 1865 that when crossing plants, "numerous experiments have demonstrated that the common characters are transmitted unchanged to the hybrids and their progeny."[1] Mendel described that "common characters," or genes, are passed unchanged from the parent to the offspring, and therefore Mendelian patterns of inheritance are very predictable.[1] Classically, these include single-gene disorders that follow autosomal dominant, autosomal recessive, and X-linked inheritance patterns. Non-Mendelian patterns of inheritance are seen with disorders that occur due to hereditary unstable DNA repeats, parent-of-origin specific disorders, mitochondrial disorders, mosaicism, and a broad category of disorders with complex, multifactorial patterns of inheritance. It is important to remember, however, that even with Mendelian disorders, while the genes may be transmitted unchanged, the disease phenotype may not follow a predictable pattern because of variable expressivity and/or reduced penetrance.

WHAT ARE HEREDITARY UNSTABLE DNA REPEAT DISORDERS?

Variants that follow Mendelian patterns of inheritance are, in most cases, unchanged when passed from parent to offspring. Diseases that occur due to hereditary unstable DNA repeat expansions do not follow this rule. These conditions are a group of approximately 20 neurodevelopmental disorders that include fragile X syndrome, Huntington disease, Friedreich ataxia, and myotonic dystrophy (DM1 and DM2)[2] (Table 2.1). For some disorders, the unstable repeat sequence is within the transcribed region of the gene, and for others, the expansion is in the noncoding region. The inheritance pattern of these disorders is characterized by unstable transmission and so-called *genetic anticipation*, in which the length of the segment including the repeats increases in size with subsequent generations. Expansion of the repeats, which are in most (but not all) cases trinucleotide repeats, can disrupt gene function and result

in a variety of largely neurologic conditions. Typically, the age of onset is earlier and/or the symptoms are more severe with increasing number of repeats.

WHAT ARE EXAMPLES OF DISORDERS DUE TO HEREDITARY UNSTABLE DNA REPEATS?

Fragile X Syndrome

Fragile X syndrome is the most common inherited form of intellectual disability, with a prevalence of approximately 16–25/100,000 in males and half of that for females.[3,4] Clinical characteristics can be variable and include intellectual disability, which is typically moderate for males and more mild for females. Males with fragile X syndrome have characteristic facial features, connective tissue findings such as lax joints, and macroorchidism, although some have few or no physical findings. About 25% of individuals with fragile X syndrome also meet criteria for autism spectrum disorder (ASD).

Fragile X syndrome is a trinucleotide repeat disorder that results from expansion of a trinucleotide cytosine-guanine-guanine (CGG) segment of DNA of the *fragile X mental retardation 1 (FMR1)* gene on the long arm of the X chromosome (Xq27.3). If the region expands to include greater than 200 CGG repeats, this leads to hypermethylation and inactivation of the gene product (fragile X mental retardation protein), which is expressed in many tissues but most abundantly in neurons.[2]

Normally, noncarrier individuals have fewer than 45 CGG repeats in this gene; the average is approximately 29 repeats. Individuals with 55–200 repeats are referred to as "premutation carriers" and are at risk of expansion to a full mutation (more than 200 repeats) in their offspring (Fig. 2.1). Although premutation carriers have a 50% chance of passing on the abnormal allele, whether it expands to a full mutation and results in a child with fragile X syndrome depends on the size of the premutation. The chance of expansion of the gene, if it is passed on, ranges from about 3% with premutations that are 55–65 repeats, to nearly 100% if the premutation is larger than 100 repeats. Although premutation size alleles can be present in either parent, they only expand when passed

Perinatal Genetics. https://doi.org/10.1016/B978-0-323-53094-1.00002-3

TABLE 2.1
Examples of Unstable DNA Repeat Disorders

Disorder	Symptoms	Repeats (Gene)	Effect of Repeats
Fragile X syndrome	ID, ASD, dysmorphic facial features	CGG n ≥ 200 (FMR1)	Methylation and silencing of gene
Myotonic Dystrophy 1 Myotonic Dystrophy 2	Muscle weakness and wasting	CTG n ≥ 50 (DMPK) CCTG n ≥ 75 (CNBP)	Repeats bind to RNA-binding proteins
Huntington Disease	Neurodegenerative disorder, chorea, death	CAG n ≥ 40 (HTT)	Repeats lead to mutant protein
Spinocerebellar ataxia Type 1 (SCA1)	Ataxia, dysarthria, bulbar dysfunction	CAG ≥ 39 in (ATXN1)	Repeats lead to abnormal protein

ASD, atrial septal defect; *DNA*, deoxyribonucleic acid; *RNA*, ribonucleic acid.

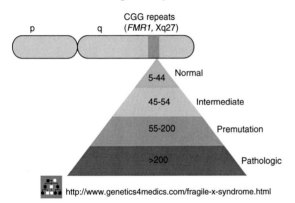

http://www.genetics4medics.com/fragile-x-syndrome.html

FIG. 2.1 Fragile X syndrome (http://www.genetics4me dics.com/fragile-x-sydrome.html). Clinical significance of increasing number of CGG repeats in the fragile X mental retardation 1 (FMR1) gene. Individuals with 6–44 repeats are unaffected, those with 45–54 are in an intermediate range, 55–200 are premutation carriers, and >200 repeats is a full mutation and is associated with the syndrome.

on by the mother and are stable in size when passed on by the father.[5] Individuals with 45–54 repeats are referred to as intermediate or "gray zone" carriers, as their gene may expand to the carrier or premutation size range but will not expand to a full mutation. Therefore, they are at risk to have grandchildren with fragile X syndrome, but not children. Expansion of less than 55 repeats to a full mutation has not been reported in a single generation. In families affected by fragile X syndrome, it is common to see more affected family members in subsequent generations due to genetic anticipation.

Unlike most autosomal recessive diseases, there are risks associated with being a premutation carrier in both men and women. Female premutation carriers are at risk for premature ovarian insufficiency (POI), defined as menopause earlier than 40 years old.[6] Male, and sometimes female, premutation carriers are also at risk for fragile X–associated tremor/ataxia syndrome (FXTAS), a progressive, neurodegenerative disease that can lead to cerebellar symptoms and memory loss, as well as other neurologic deficits that increase with age.[2] Individuals who have fragile X syndrome do not develop ataxia—it only affects premutation carriers.

Testing for fragile X syndrome can be performed on DNA from blood (to identify female carriers or affected individuals) or on amniotic fluid or chorionic villi (to identify affected fetuses) through a combination of polymerase chain reaction (PCR) and Southern blot analysis.[7] Ideally, carrier screening for fragile X syndrome should be done in the preconception period, although it can also be performed during pregnancy. The American College of Obstetricians and Gynecologists (ACOG) recommends carrier screening for fragile X syndrome for women who are pregnant or considering pregnancy who have a family history of a fragile X–related disorder or of intellectual disability.[8] ACOG also recommends testing for fragile X syndrome for women with unexplained premature ovarian failure or insufficiency, but at the present time, ACOG does not recommend universal screening for fragile X syndrome.[8]

Myotonic Dystrophy

Myotonic dystrophy 1 (DM1) is a neuromuscular condition with symptoms that include muscle spasm (myotonia) and muscle weakness. It affects a variety of organ systems, leading to cardiac conduction defects, testicular atrophy, insulin resistance, cataracts, and in the congenital form, intellectual disability. The pathogenesis of DM1 is expansion (to 50 repeats or greater) of a cytosine-thymine-guanine (CTG) repeat in the 3′ untranslated region of the *DMPK* gene. DM1 has a severe, lethal congenital form that includes severe neonatal hypotonia and weakness, respiratory failure, death, and intellectual disability in those that survive the neonatal period.

Myotonic dystrophy 2 (DM2) shares many of the clinical features of DM1 but occurs due to a tetranucleotide (CCTG) repeat expansion in the gene *CNBP*. Clinically, the presentations of DM1 and DM2 are very similar, except that DM2 does not have a congenital form. With both forms of myotonic dystrophy, the chance of passing on the abnormal allele is 50%, so the genetics are similar to classical autosomal dominant inheritance. However, the expansion demonstrates anticipation and increased severity of symptoms with repeat size and through generations, as is seen with other trinucleotide repeat disorders. The congenital form of myotonic dystrophy results from anticipation and expansion to greater than 1000 repeats. There is also a mild, late onset adult form, a more classical adult form, as well as a childhood form.

Huntington Disease

Huntington disease is a neurodegenerative disorder that follows an autosomal dominant pattern of inheritance, leading to chorea, uncontrolled limb writhing movements, psychiatric abnormalities, dementia, and death usually by age 60 years.[9] In this disorder, the expanding repeat sequence is a cytosine-adenine-glycine (CAG) repeat (to greater than or equal to 40 repeats) in the *HTT* gene. When this expansion occurs, it results in formation of an abnormal form of a protein called huntingtin that becomes toxic to neurons. As with other trinucleotide repeat disorders, Huntington disease demonstrates anticipation, with increasing number of repeats seen in subsequent generations and associated with younger age of onset. Inheritance through the father can lead to greater repeat expansion and earlier onset of symptoms.

Huntington disease is 100% penetrant, and essentially all affected individuals develop symptoms, usually at the same age or somewhat earlier than their affected parent. In most cases, individuals do not become symptomatic until age 40 years or older, generally after they have had children. Many patients wish to have unaffected children but prefer not to learn their own status given that treatment is not available. In such situations, a form of nondisclosure preimplantation genetic testing can be performed, in which only unaffected embryos are implanted, but the parents are not informed as to whether any of the embryos are affected. It is also possible in some cases to perform prenatal diagnosis through linkage analysis without revealing the status of the parent.

WHAT ARE IMPRINTING DISORDERS AND UNIPARENTAL DISOMY?

Genomic imprinting and uniparental disomy (UPD) refer to the genetic parent-of-origin and are relevant to a specific group of genes that have different function depending on whether they were inherited from the mother or the father. Mendelian patterns of inheritance typically dictate that we receive one copy of each of our genes from each of our parents and, usually, that they are both equally active or functional. However, there are times when only the maternal or paternal copy is active (because of genomic imprinting). A number of different genetic conditions result from situations in which the normal active gene is not present, because of either a deletion of the active gene or the presence of two copies of the inactive form of the gene.

Genomic imprinting is a process whereby methylation (the addition of methyl groups to DNA during oogenesis or spermatogenesis) deactivates one copy of a gene. It is not entirely understood why some genes function differently when they are paternally or maternally inherited.[10] However, for a number of genes, only the maternal or paternal copy is active because of genomic imprinting. Many imprinted genes affect fetal and/or postnatal growth. For example, macrosomia is seen in Beckwith-Wiedemann syndrome and fetal growth restriction seen in Russell-Silver syndrome. Approximately 80% of imprinted genes are found in clusters on specific regions of chromosomes, and about 75 imprinted genes have been identified in humans.[10]

Uniparental disomy occurs when both copies of the same chromosome are inherited from one parent. UPD can happen due to trisomic rescue, when a zygote with trisomy loses the extra chromosome. Although the embryo is no longer trisomic, if the two remaining chromosomes were inherited from the same parent, UPD will result. In many cases, UPD has no effect because most genes do not undergo genomic imprinting (i.e., both copies are active and there is no consequence if both copies come from the same parent). However, in cases of an imprinted gene, UPD may lead to loss of function of a gene. For example, if imprinting normally deactivates the maternal copy of the gene and the embryo is left with two copies of the maternal gene, there will be no active copies,[12] and therefore, no functional gene. UPD can also result in unmasking of an autosomal recessive disorder if, for example, the mother carries a recessive condition (such as cystic fibrosis) and the fetus has UPD for the chromosome carrying that gene. Even if the father is not a carrier, if

TABLE 2.2
Imprinting Disorders

Disorder	Symptoms	Region	Parent-of-Origin Defect
Prader-Will syndrome	Mild ID, obesity, hypogonadism	15q11-13	Paternal
Angelman syndrome	Severe ID, seizures, developmental delay	15q11-13	Maternal
Beckwith-Wiedemann syndrome	Macrosomia, macroglossia, omphalocele, predisposition to embryonic tumors	11p15	Maternal
Russell-Silver syndrome	Intrauterine growth restriction, poor postnatal growth, triangular faces, developmental delay, learning disabilities	11p15.5	Paternal

both copies of the gene are inherited from the mother and she is a carrier, the fetus may be affected.

A classic example of UPD that obstetrician-gynecologists encounter is complete hydatidiform mole, which affects about 1 in 1500 pregnancies.[11] Hydatidiform moles have 46 chromosomes, all of paternal origin. Partial moles, in contrast, demonstrate triploidy and have 69 chromosomes (typically 23 of maternal and 46 of paternal origin).

WHAT ARE EXAMPLES OF DISORDERS THAT OCCUR DUE TO IMPRINTING AND UNIPARENTAL DISOMY?

Prader-Willi Syndrome

Prader-Willi syndrome affects approximately 1 in 10,000–30,000 individuals.[13] It is characterized by hypotonia and failure to thrive in infancy, progressing to developmental delay, short stature, rapid weight gain and obesity due to hyperphagia (excessive appetite), and intellectual disability. Prader-Willi syndrome is caused by loss of function of specific paternally derived genes on chromosome 15. Several different mechanisms can lead to the loss of the paternal copy of these genes. Most cases (70%) are due to a deletion of a segment of paternal chromosome 15. In 30% of cases, there are no paternal genes because of maternal uniparental disomy, in which two maternal copies, and no paternal copies, of chromosome 15 are present. In rare cases, Prader-Willi syndrome can be caused by a chromosomal translocation, an imprinting defect or even a single gene mutation. Patients with a family history of Prader-Willi syndrome can be reassured that there is usually no increased risk to their children given that in most cases this condition is caused by a random error of oogenesis or spermatogenesis (see Fig. 2.2; Table 2.3).

Prader-Willi syndrome : Genetic mechanisms

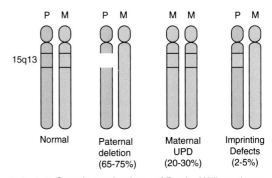

FIG. 2.2 Genetic mechanisms of Prader-Willi syndrome (http://www.genetics4medics.com/prader-willi-sydrome.html). Schematic depiction of the chromosomal basis of Prader-Willi syndrome (PWS). Different mechanisms can lead to lack of expression of the paternal chromosome 15q11-q13 and cause PWS. *M*, maternal; *P*, paternal. http://www.genetics4medics.com/prader-willi-sydrome.html.

Angelman Syndrome

Angelman syndrome has a prevalence of 1 in 12,000–24,000 and is characterized by severe intellectual disability, developmental delay, seizures, and difficulty with balance and walking.[14] Angelman syndrome results from abnormalities in the same gene region as Prader-Willi syndrome but occurs due to loss of the maternal contribution, with only the paternal genes present. This can occur from multiple genetic mechanisms that lead to lack of the maternally derived active gene, including a deletion, paternal UPD, an imprinting error, or a single-gene mutation of the maternal copy of the gene[2] (Table 2.3). In contrast to the mild intellectual disability seen with Prader-Willi syndrome, patients with Angelman syndrome have severe

TABLE 2.3
Genomic Mechanisms Causing Prader-Willi and
Angelman Syndrome

Mechanism	Prader-Willi Syndrome	Angelman Syndrome
15q11.2-q13 deletion	~70% (paternal)	~70% (maternal)
Uniparental disomy	~20–30% (maternal)	~7% (paternal)
Imprinting center mutation	~2.5%	~3%
Gene mutations	Rare	~10% (UBE3A mutations)
Unidentified	<1%	~10%

Data from Cassidy SB, Schwartz S, Miller JL, et al. Prader-Willi syndrome. *Genet Med*. 2012;14:10–26; Dagli AI, Williams CA. Angelman syndrome. In: Pagon RA, Adam MP, Bird TD, et al, eds. *GeneReviews [Internet]*. University of Washington, Seattle: Seattle; 1993–2013. http://www.ncbi.nlm.nih.gov/books/NBK1144/.

developmental delay, intellectual disability, and speech impairment. Patients with Angelman syndrome also exhibit a characteristic behavioral pattern of inappropriate laughing, smiling, and excitability.[14]

Beckwith-Wiedemann Syndrome

Beckwith-Wiedemann syndrome is characterized by overgrowth due to excess *IGF2* expression (which regulates growth). It is associated with macrosomia, an enlarged placenta, macroglossia, cardiomyopathy, and a predisposition to development of embryonal tumors (including Wilms tumor and hepatoblastoma). An increased risk for Beckwith-Wiedemann syndrome, as well as for Angelman syndrome, both of which can arise due to a maternal imprinting defect, has been observed after use of assisted reproductive technology (ART), specifically IVF and intracytoplasmic sperm injection.[15] In one study of nearly 380,000 live births, the risk of Beckwith-Wiedemann was 10-fold higher in patients conceived through ART.[16] It is thought that there is no increased risk of Prader-Willi syndrome with IVF given that paternal imprinting takes place well before IVF.[2] As the use of ART advances, more research is needed to clarify the cause and magnitude of these risks.

Russell-Silver Syndrome

Russell-Silver syndrome has a prevalence of approximately 1:100,000[17] and is characterized by fetal growth restriction, postnatal growth restriction, and dysmorphism. The genetics of Russell-Silver syndrome are complex,

and it is thought to result from abnormal regulation in certain genes that control growth. In most cases, it is caused by either an imprinting defect at 11p15.5 or maternal UPD of chromosome 7.

WHAT IS MULTIFACTORIAL INHERITANCE?

Multifactorial inheritance refers to disorders caused by multiple genes and environmental factors. This group of disorders includes a broad range of medical (cardiac disease and diabetes), congenital (birth defects including cardiac malformations, neural tube defects, and cleft lip and/or palate), and neuropsychiatric (ASD, schizophrenia, bipolar disorder) diseases. Family and twin studies have shown that these diseases have a genetic component; however, it is also clear that there are environmental contributors. Sometimes, gender can affect inheritance. For example, research has shown that a male sibling is more likely to be diagnosed with ASD if a sibling has been diagnosed.[18] Many neuropsychiatric diseases and birth defects demonstrate complex multifactorial inheritance (Table 2.4; Reprinted with permission, originally Box 1 in ACOG Technology Assessment in Obstetrics and Gynecology No. 11: Genetics and Molecular Diagnostic Testing [Reference #7])

WHAT ARE EXAMPLES OF DISORDERS THAT EXHIBIT MULTIFACTORIAL INHERITANCE?

Neuropsychiatric Disorders

Neuropsychiatric disorders, although common (with a prevalence of 4%), present a challenge for counseling on recurrence risk because of their multifactorial etiology.[2] Major depressive disorder, bipolar disorder, and schizophrenia are examples of diseases that commonly affect reproductive-age women, and therefore OB/GYN providers will often be involved in their diagnosis and management. Twin and family studies have shown that there is a genetic component to schizophrenia, as monozygotic twins are four to six times more likely to be affected than dizygotic twins. First- and second-degree relatives of individuals with schizophrenia are more likely to be affected, with a recurrence risk of 8%–46% for first-degree relatives and 1%–8% for second-degree relatives[2] (see Table 2.4).

Prenatal diagnosis for most multifactorial diseases is not available, and the same is true for neuropsychiatric diseases. At this time, a few specific genes that contribute to neuropsychiatric diseases have been identified,[2] for example, genetic deletions such as the 22q11 deletion syndrome. 22q11 deletion syndrome can be detected prenatally by chromosomal microarray

TABLE 2.4
Characteristics of Multifactorial Inheritance

- Disorder is familial, but pattern of inheritance is not apparent
- Risk to first-degree relatives is the square root of the population risk
- Risk is significantly decreased for second-degree relatives
- Recurrence risk is increased if more than one family member is affected
- Risk is increased if the defect is more severe (e.g., recurrence risk for bilateral cleft lip is higher than unilateral cleft lip)
- If the defect is more common in one sex than in the other sex, the recurrence risk is higher if the affected individual is of the less commonly affected sex

Reprinted with permission from Genetics and Molecular Diagnostic Testing. Technology assessment in obstetrics and gynecology. No. 11. American College of Obstetricians and Gynecologists. *Obslet Gynecol.* 2014;123(2):394–413. https://doi.org/10.1097/01.AOG.0000443280.91145.4f.

(CMA) or fluorescence in situ hybridization (FISH) through chorionic villus sampling or amniocentesis. Although 22q11 deletion accounts for less than 2% of schizophrenia, 25% of patients with 22q11 deletion syndrome develop schizophrenia. Other deletions and duplications that are detectable with CMA have also been associated with a variety of psychiatric disorders.

Birth Defects

Birth defects (congenital anomalies) are abnormalities in the development of organs or structures that are present at birth.[2] Structural birth defects represent a common yet complex multifactorial group of disorders that obstetrical providers often encounter. They are a major cause of infant morbidity and mortality, and 20% of infant deaths are due to birth defects and genetic disorders.[19] Congenital disorders also contribute to both physical and intellectual disability and morbidity.[2] Counseling regarding recurrence risk of birth defects is challenging because of the varied etiologies (genetic, environmental, or a combination).

Birth defects can be grouped into three classes based on their etiology: malformations, deformations, and disruptions. Malformations are due to intrinsic genetic mutations and are therefore often associated with other malformations (due to an intrinsic abnormality of a developmental pathway). One example is congenital heart malformations in association with aneuploidy such as trisomies 21, 18, and 13. Deformations and disruptions, by

contrast, are typically not caused by genetic intrinsic factors but by physical constraints (such as contractures due to preterm premature rupture of membranes [PPROM] or oligohydramnios) or destruction of normal tissue (such as an amputation due to amniotic bands). Deformations, as opposed to malformations or disruptions, can sometimes resolve after birth.

There are multiple genetic contributors to birth defects. Approximately one-quarter of all birth defects are due to aneuploidy, 10% are due to copy number variants identifiable by CMA, and 20% are due to mutations in single genes (such as in achondroplasia or Smith-Lemli-Opitz syndrome)[2] (Fig. 2.3). The other 40% of birth defects are multifactorial—there is no obvious genetic etiology, but recurrence risk is higher in families than would be expected in the general population. Some examples of this include cleft lip with or without cleft palate, congenital heart defects, and neural tube defects (Table 2.5). For most multifactorial disorders, the risk to a sibling is about 3%–4% (10% with two affected siblings), the risk to a second-degree relative (uncle, aunt, nephew, or niece) is about 0.5%, and the risk to a third-degree relative (first cousin) is about 0.17%.[20,21]

WHAT IS MITOCHONDRIAL INHERITANCE?

Mitochondrial diseases, although rare, have a unique inheritance pattern and can present in a wide range of organ systems and diseases. Mitochondria are the organelles in each of the body's cells that are responsible for energy production and aerobic respiration. Although the majority of human DNA is contained in the nucleus of the cell, mitochondria contain their own DNA, which encodes 37 genes. Mitochondrial disorders can present at any age but often present in infancy with hypotonia, failure to thrive, and neurodegeneration.

According to the Society for Inherited Metabolic Disorders, mitochondrial diseases can present with any symptom, in any organ system, and at any age. Mitochondria, and therefore mitochondrial defects, are inherited maternally. Each human oocyte contains approximately 100,000 mitochondria, whereas the 100 mitochondria found in sperm are eliminated during fertilization.[5] This is referred to as matrilineal inheritance. Mitochondrial diseases can develop if an oocyte that contains mutated mitochondrial DNA is fertilized. Although both male and female offspring of an affected female will inherit the disease, in general, the offspring of an affected male will not inherit the disease as the male does not contribute mitochondria to his offspring.

Because mitochondria play a key role in energy production, mitochondrial diseases primarily affect

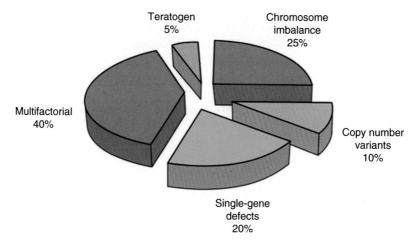

FIG. 2.3 The relative contribution of single-gene defects, chromosome abnormalities, copy number variants, multifactorial traits, and teratogens to birth defects. (Reprinted from Nussbaum RL, McInnes RR, Huntington FW. *Thompson & Thompson Genetics in Medicine;* 2016. https://doi.org/10.1001/jama.1992.03480150121052. Thompson and Thompson 2016 (Reference #7), originally Figure 14-4 on page 285.)

TABLE 2.5
Common Birth Defects

	Genetic Causes	Other Causes
Congenital heart disease	22q11 microdeletion syndrome, aneuploidy	Congenital rubella, maternal DM, teratogens
Neural tube defects	Aneuploidy, 22q11 microdeletion syndrome, Waardenburg syndrome	Folic acid deficiency, teratogens
Cleft lip with or without cleft palate	Trisomy 13, other rare syndromes	Pierre-Robin sequence, teratogenic medications (Accutane, antiepileptics), maternal DM, maternal smoking
Club foot	Single-gene mutations, aneuploidy, rare syndromes	Bone or connective tissue disease, oligohydramnios

Adapted from Nussbaum RL, McInnes RR, Huntington FW. *Thompson & Thompson Genetics in Medicine;* 2016. https://doi.org/10.1001/jama.1992.03480150121052.

organ systems with high energy requirements, such as the brain and nervous system, heart, and musculoskeletal system. Unlike the 46 nuclear chromosomes, which divide in a highly predictable way, mitochondrial DNA (mtDNA) are replicated and then sort randomly to daughter cells. Therefore, daughter cells can have variable amounts of normal mtDNA and mutant mtDNA, which explains why mitochondrial disorders have variable phenotypes and reduced penetrance.[2] These features of mitochondrial diseases also make prenatal testing challenging. In addition, testing of family members may be of limited value, because at times, the mutation is not found in blood. Patients who have a family of history of mitochondrial disorders should be referred for genetic consultation (Table 2.6).

WHAT IS MOSAICISM?

Mosaicism is the presence of two or more different cell lines in an individual, tissue, or organ.[2] Mosaicism can result from an error of mitosis or meiosis (depending on when it occurs), and there are several different types of mosaicism that can affect an embryo. Confined placental mosaicism (CPM) occurs when mosaicism is detected in the cytotrophoblast (developing placenta) but not the embryo. Confined placental mosaicism can complicate the interpretation of invasive prenatal testing, more commonly CVS testing. In CVS samples, 1%–2% show a discrepancy between the placenta and the fetus (as determined by amniocentesis or cord blood at birth). When mosaicism is identified by CVS, amniocentesis is generally recommended to evaluate the fetus more directly and to rule out CPM.

TABLE 2.6
Examples of Mitochondrial Diseases

Disorder	Phenotype
Mitochondrial DNA depletion syndrome	Infantile muscle weakness, hypotonia, poor growth, respiratory failure, death
Leigh syndrome	Infantile neurodegeneration, hypotonia, developmental delay, optic atrophy, respiratory abnormalities
MELAS (mitochondrial encephalopathy with lactic acidosis and strokelike episodes)	Myopathy, encephalomyopathy, lactic acidosis, diabetes, deafness
MERRF (myoclonic epilepsy with ragged-red fibers)	Epilepsy, myopathy, ataxia, sensorineural deafness, dementia
LHON (Leber hereditary optic neuropathy)	Optic nerve atrophy leading to rapid onset of blindness, affects males > females
NARP (neuropathy, ataxia, retinitis pigmentosa)	Neuropathy, ataxia, retinitis pigmentosa
Kearns-Sayre syndrome	Ophthalmoplegia (eye muscle weakness), cardiomyopathy, heart block, ptosis, retinal pigmentation, ataxia, diabetes

Adapted from Nussbaum RL, McInnes RR, Huntington FW. *Thompson & Thompson Genetics in Medicine;* 2016. https://doi.org/10.1001/jama.1992.03480150121052.

Somatic mosaicism occurs when mosaicism is present in some (segmental) or all of the tissues of the embryo but is not present in the gametes. Germline mosaicism is present in the gametes and can result in a phenotypically unaffected individual who has the potential to pass on a pathogenic variant to offspring.

Germline mosaicism may be the cause of genetic conditions that did not seem to be present in the family previously. The possibility of germline mosaicism should be considered in families with two or more affected siblings and no previous family history. If a child is diagnosed with an autosomal dominant or X-linked disorder, and the parents are not affected, there is a possibility that this is due to germline mosaicism and not a de novo mutation. There are certain disorders that have a higher incidence of germline mosaicism, such as osteogenesis imperfecta and Duchenne muscular dystrophy (DMD). In all, up to 14% of cases of DMD are likely due to germline mosaicism, which significantly increases the recurrence risk to future siblings[2].

CONCLUSION

Non-Mendelian genetic conditions comprise a broad category of disorders that have complex inheritance. Obstetrical providers should be generally familiar with these conditions and appropriate situations in which referral for genetic counseling is indicated. Knowledge of inheritance patterns, screening and testing options, and ability to reassure and refer are essential parts of providing obstetrical care in a rapidly changing perinatal genetic environment.

REFERENCES

1. Mendel G. Experiments on plant hybridization. *Proc Nat Hist Soc Brünn.* 1865.
2. Nussbaum RL, McInnes RR, Huntington FW. *Thompson & Thompson Genetics in Medicine;* 2016. https://doi.org/10.1001/jama.1992.03480150121052.
3. Saul RA, Tarleton JC. FMR1-Related disorders. *Gene Rev.* University of Washington, Seattle. 1998. http://www.ncbi.nlm.nih.gov/pubmed/20301558.
4. de Vries BB, van den Ouweland AM, Mohkamsing S, et al. Screening and diagnosis for the fragile X syndrome among the mentally retarded: an epidemiological and psychological survey. Collaborative Fragile X Study Group. *Am J Hum Genet.* 1997;61(3):660–667.
5. Nolin SL, Sah S, Glicksman A, et al. Fragile X AGG analysis provides new risk predictions for 45-69 repeat alleles. *Am J Med Genet.* 2013;161A(4):771–778. https://doi.org/10.1002/ajmg.a.35833.
6. Sherman SL. Premature ovarian failure among fragile X premutation carriers: parent-of-origin effect? *Am J Hum Genet.* 2000;67(1):11–13. https://doi.org/10.1086/302985.
7. Genetics and Molecular Diagnostic Testing. Technology assessment in obstetrics and gynecology. No. 11. American College of Obstetricians and Gynecologists. *Obslet Gynecol.* 2014;123(2):394–413. https://doi.org/10.1097/01.AOG.0000443280.91145.4f.

8. Carrier Screening for Genetic Conditions. Committee opinion No. 691. American College of Obstetricians and Gynecologists. *Obslet Gynecol.* 2017;129:e41–e55. https://www.acog.org/-/media/Committee-Opinions/Committee-on-Genetics/co691.pdf?dmc=1&ts=2018011 5T1421598478.

9. Warby SC, Graham RK, Hayden MR. *Huntington Dis.* 2010;58. http://www.ncbi.nlm.nih.gov/books/NBK1305/.

10. Peters J. The role of genomic imprinting in biology and disease: an expanding view. *Nat Rev Genet.* 2014;15(8):517–530. https://doi.org/10.1038/nrg3766.

11. Diagnosis and Treatment of Gestational Trophoblastic Disease. Practice Bulletin No. 53. American College of Obstetricians and Gynecologists. Obstet *Gynecol.* 2004;103:1365–1377.

12. National Institute of Health: Genetics Home Reference. *What Are Genomic Imprinting and Uniparental Disomy? - Genetics Home Reference*; 2018. https://ghr.nlm.nih.gov/p rimer/inheritance/updimprinting.

13. Driscoll DJ, Miller JL, Schwartz S, Cassidy SB. Prader-Willi syndrome. *Gene Rev.* 1998. http://www.ncbi.nlm.nih.gov/pubmed/20301505.

14. Dagli AI, Mueller J, Williams CA. Angelman syndrome. *Gene Rev.* 2018. University of Washington, Seattle http://www.ncbi.nlm.nih.gov/pubmed/20301323.

15. Hiura H, Okae H, Chiba H, et al. Imprinting methylation errors in ART. *Reprod Med Biol.* 2014;13(4):193–202. https://doi.org/10.1007/s12522-014-0183-3.

16. Hormone Therapy in Primary Ovarian Insufficiency. Committee opinion No. 698. American College of Obstetricians and Gynecologists. Obstet *Gynecol.* 2017;129:e134–e141.

17. Saal HM. *Russell-silver Syndrome.* Seattle: University of Washington; 1993. http://www.ncbi.nlm.nih.gov/pubm ed/20301499.

18. Palmer N, Beam A, Agniel D, et al. Association of sex with recurrence of autism spectrum disorder among siblings. *JAMA Pediatr.* 2017;171(11):1107. https://doi.org/10.1001/jamapediatrics.2017.2832.

19. Christianson A, Howson CP, Modell B. *March of Dimes Global Report on Birth Defects. White Plains, NY;* 2006.

20. Neural Tube Defects. Practice Bulletin No. 187. American College of Obstetricians and Gynecoloists. Obstet *Gynecol.* 2017;130(44):e279–e290.

21. Toriello HV, Higgins JV, Opitz JM. Occurrence of neural tube defects among first-, second-, and third-degree relatives of probands: results of a United States study. *Am J Med Genet.* 1983;15(4):601–606. https://doi.org/10.1002/ajmg.1320150409.

CHAPTER 3

Principles of Genetic Counseling

BRITTON D. RINK, MD, MS

OVERVIEW

Genetic counseling is a process of evaluating family history and medical information to advise patients of the risk of a genetic condition. This can have both a diagnostic and supportive element. The National Society of Genetic Counselors officially defines genetic counseling as, "the process of helping people understand and adapt to the medical, psychological and familial implications of genetic contributions to disease. This process integrates the following: 1) interpretation of family and medical histories to assess the chance of disease occurrence or recurrence; 2) education about inheritance, testing, management, prevention resources and research; and 3) counseling to promote informed choices and adaptation to the risk or condition."[1] Genetic counseling should include a discussion of available genetic screening and testing and informed consent with limitations, risks, and benefits associated with a genetic test. The patient should be made aware of the risk to develop disease and should be educated on the natural history of the condition and impact on the patient and at-risk family members, as well as potential interventions, research, and treatment.[2]

Rapidly advancing genetic technology and decreased cost of genetic testing has led to increased patient demands and expectations. Although new genetic technologies afford increased information, the issues of genetic heterogeneity, such as variable penetrance and expressivity, variants of uncertain significance, and uncertain phenotype and unanticipated information, highlight the need and value of genetic counseling. The current climate of advanced prenatal genetic technologies to screen and diagnose genetic abnormalities in the fetus is also rapidly evolving. The complexity of genetic information available before birth has increased such that obstetric providers are challenged to have the time and expertise to discuss genetic testing options with patients. The obstetric provider should apply professional judgment to the specific clinical circumstance presented by the patient when determining whether the patient would benefit from consultation with a genetic specialist. Indications for genetic counseling in the obstetric patient include the following[3,4]:

- A known or suspected genetic diagnosis in the patient or family member
- Suspected fetal anomaly
- Abnormal or unanticipated result from a screening test
- Abnormal or unanticipated result from a diagnostic test
- Advanced parental age during pregnancy
- Teratogenic exposure
- Patient's reported ethnicity associated with an increased prevalence of a genetic diagnosis
- Recurrent pregnancy loss
- Consanguinity
- Any patient who wishes detailed information about carrier and/or aneuploidy testing beyond what the obstetric provider can deliver

Advances in genetic and genomic technologies offer new opportunities in prenatal testing and may empower families with knowledge about reproductive risk and support reproductive autonomy. These testing strategies, however, must be implemented in an ethically responsible manner and studied to determine best practice. Providing nondirective, comprehensive genetic counseling to obstetric patients is a critical component of this goal.

WHAT IS THE ROLE OF A GENETIC COUNSELOR?

Genetic counselors are medical professionals with specialized graduate degrees in medical genetics, genomics, and counseling. In the clinical setting, a genetic counselor works to integrate genetic technologies into clinical practice, providing comprehensive genetic services to patients. Genetic counselors often are members of a healthcare team, but their training and expertise allow

Perinatal Genetics. https://doi.org/10.1016/B978-0-323-53094-1.00003-5

independent interaction with patients. The role of a genetic counselor includes the collection and evaluation of a medical and family history, providing guidance to the healthcare team on available genetic screening and testing, educating the patient about complex genetic principles, discussing benefits and limitations of genetic screening and testing in the process of informed consent, coordinating sample collection, promoting communication among medical professionals, interpreting and communicating genetic test results to the medical team and to the patient, advocating for patient needs as a result of a genetic diagnosis, and presenting risk-reduction strategies, management, or treatment options based on a genetic diagnosis.[1] Providing these services, and others, allows the physician or allied health professional to be more efficient, enhance patient knowledge and satisfaction, as well as decrease liability and cost given their knowledge and role in the provision of care.[5] Beyond direct clinical care, genetic counselors may work in a laboratory, have a role in genetic research, government, and legal affairs, or work for industry.

The American Board of Genetic Counseling (ABGC), through an examination process, certifies genetic counselors. In several states, a license is required to practice as a Certified Genetic Counselor (CGC) with the goal of ensuring competency. Licensure also allows genetic counselors to work in a more independent fashion. It also provides the credentials that many hospitals need to approve billing and reimbursement for these services and affords flexibility in the delivery of services.

WHAT ARE THE CHARACTERISTICS OF A PATIENT WHO MAY BENEFIT FROM REFERRAL TO A PROVIDER WITH GENETICS EXPERTISE?

Referrals to a provider with genetics expertise should be considered if a patient is at risk for or affected with a genetic disorder.[4] This may include a genetic counselor, medical geneticist, maternal fetal medicine specialist, or practitioner with specialized training in genetics. A provider with genetics expertise can obtain and critically evaluate the family history, identify the appropriate tests to order, provide pre- and posttest counseling related to genetic testing, and provide information about the treatment prognosis for patients or family members diagnosed with a genetic disorder. They may also recommend referrals to other medical specialists as indicated. Genetic counseling is also critical for helping patients understand implications of genetic test results and risk assessment for other family members.

Specific elements of a family history that should be considered for referral include one or more members with intellectual disability, structural birth defect, or the diagnosis of a genetic condition. Other family history elements that should prompt referral include one or more family members with sudden or early death of unknown origin and adult-onset health conditions such as cardiovascular disease or cancer, particularly if the cancer diagnosis was made in early adulthood. Patients who have experienced recurrent pregnancy loss, have a pregnancy at risk for or identified to have a health complication or birth defect, or are pregnant and are concerned about an exposure to medication should be offered a referral to a provider with genetics expertise. Other patients who may benefit from genetic counseling include patients in a consanguineous relationship or those patients who would like information and testing for genetic conditions that occur within their ethnic group.[4]

WHAT ARE THE NECESSARY COMPONENTS OF PRE- AND POSTTEST COUNSELING TO CONSIDER WHEN COUNSELING PATIENTS ON CARRIER SCREENING?

Obstetric care providers are faced with many decisions when offering genetic screening and testing in an effort to meet the needs of their patient population and workflow. Pre- and posttest counseling are essential to the process of carrier testing in clinical practice. The global goals of pretest counseling are to provide education and personalized and nondirective information about testing options and facilitate informed consent. Many professional organizations have published components of pretest counseling that providers should be aware of when offering genetic testing[6-9] (Table 3.1). An obstetric care provider should identify those women with risk factors including advanced maternal age, family history of a genetic condition, or individual with features that may constitute a genetic diagnosis including intellectual disabilities, multiple miscarriages or birth defects, underlying maternal medical conditions (e.g., maternal phenylketonuria or cystic fibrosis), and/or teratogenic exposures that should prompt referral to a provider with genetics expertise. Any discussion of testing should include a review of the baseline risk to have a child born with a birth defect or intellectual disability, which is 3%–4% in the general population.[10] Patients should also be informed at the beginning of the discussion that genetic testing is optional. Specific to carrier screening, using neutral and nonjudgmental language, the provider should broadly describe the types of conditions for which carrier screening

TABLE 3.1
Components of Prenatal Pretest Counseling

- Genetic testing is optional
- Assess risk for genetic disorders based on age, family history, maternal health, or exposures (medication, virus, etc.) to ensure appropriate test offered
- Consider risks and benefits of screening versus diagnostic tests available to all women regardless of a risk status
- Review clinical features of genetic conditions for which testing may be available
- Describe performance of testing options, which may include sensitivity/specificity, positive/negative predictive value, concept of residual risk when applicable
- Describe how chosen test is performed
- Negative or low risk screening result does not guarantee a healthy child
- Positive or high risk screening result does not mean fetus is affected
- Discuss cost of testing
- Review potential for unanticipated information, variant of uncertain significance, incidental finding if applicable
- Discuss plan for disclosure of results

is available and explain that some conditions may have poorly defined phenotypes. In addition, the provider should review the risks and benefits as well as the possibility for variants of unknown clinical significance. The concept of residual risk should be explained. A "negative" carrier screen result, for most conditions, only reduces the likelihood of the patient to be a carrier. There usually remains, however, a residual risk that may or may not be quantifiable based on the prevalence or mutation frequency of the condition. A plan for how and when results will be confidentially disclosed should be outlined. The patient should be informed that results of carrier screening are confidential. Providers are obligated to follow all Health Insurance Portability and Accountability Act (HIPAA) regulations. As cost may be an important factor in the decision-making process for an individual patient, the provider should be prepared to address this issue before testing, so a patient may obtain the necessary information.

Posttest counseling should also be conveyed in a nondirective and objective manner by the process that was outlined with the patient during pretest

counseling.[6,11] A discussion of low risk or negative test results from carrier screening should again include a discussion of negative predictive value and residual risk. With an increased risk or positive carrier screen result, the significance of the result including information about the specific condition and options for ongoing management should be reviewed. Discussion of partner testing is essential. If both partners are identified to be carriers, genetic counseling by a certified genetics professional is indicated. For a currently pregnant patient, prenatal diagnosis should be offered. The patient should also be made aware of the potential risk for other family members and given written information as requested.[6,11]

WHAT ARE THE NECESSARY COMPONENTS OF PRE- AND POSTTEST COUNSELING TO CONSIDER WHEN COUNSELING PATIENTS ON ANEUPLOIDY SCREENING?

Current prenatal screening technologies for chromosomal aneuploidy present a challenge to obstetric providers. Whereas traditional prenatal aneuploidy testing was largely based on maternal risk factors, biochemical markers, and/or ultrasound findings associated with a genetic diagnosis, aneuploidy risk assessment is now available by next-generation sequencing of circulating cell-free fetal DNA.[12,13] Although new technologies have changed the landscape of prenatal testing, the foundation of prenatal screening and diagnosis remains the same. It is the acknowledgement that all women, regardless of age or a priori risk, should have access to screening and diagnostic testing options in pregnancy and subsequent autonomy to make reproductive choices based on the results. Pretest counseling with informed decision-making and posttest counseling, both done in an objective and nondirective manner, are the underpinnings of this fundamental principle. There are no current "best practice" guidelines or consensus statements on the recommended approach to informed consent for patients considering aneuploidy screening. There are, however, several recognized components of genetic counseling that should be incorporated into pre- and posttest counseling for aneuploidy screening[6] (Table 3.1). As the expertise and education necessary to offer genetic testing is critical to the provision of care, referral to a provider with genetics expertise should be considered if the obstetric provider does not have the necessary knowledge or time to counsel a patient.

Pretest counseling for aneuploidy testing should include a discussion of the test performance, limitations, risks, and alternatives of various methods of prenatal screening and diagnostic testing, including the option of no testing. Parallel or synchronous screening for aneuploidy by multiple different modalities should not be performed, as these will increase the false-positive rates.[12] The patient should be made aware of the potential for unanticipated information as a result of a genetic test, including the diagnosis of a chromosomal abnormality in the patient or a test result indicating an increased risk for an underlying maternal medical condition including cancer. Family history should be reviewed to determine whether the patient should be offered other forms of screening, referral to a specialist with genetics expertise (such as a cancer geneticist or a medical geneticist), or prenatal diagnosis for a particular disorder. After a screening test for aneuploidy is identified, the patient should be made aware of the chromosomal conditions that are evaluated by the chosen screening test. The provider should be prepared to discuss cost or direct the patient to the appropriate entity who could answer questions about the financial obligation. Patients' concerns regarding privacy and discrimination should be addressed. A plan for disclosure of results should be established.

Posttest counseling with any screening test is critical to explain the results and residual risk for the condition(s) in question in a nondirective and unbiased manner. This may include a discussion of the positive and negative predictive value of a test result. The patient should be made aware that a negative screening test does not ensure an unaffected pregnancy. A positive or increased result from a screening test does not mean the fetus is affected. All patients who receive an abnormal result or an uninterpretable result from a screening test should receive further genetic counseling and be offered diagnostic testing.[12]

WHAT IS THE DUTY OF THE PROVIDER TO DISCLOSE GENETIC TEST RESULTS TO OTHER FAMILY MEMBERS?

Genetic information may have considerable impact on people's self-image and identity. Disclosure of genetic test results evokes several important principles of biomedical ethics, including autonomy, justice, and beneficence. There are also important medical-legal ideologies relative to disclosure of genetic information. This type of testing is complicated by the influence of genetic information extending past the individual by definition of the shared genetic material within family members.

Communicating genetic information to at-risk family members has been the subject of an extensive debate, particularly with the expansion of genetic technologies, lowered cost, and increased access (with some testing available directly to the consumer). There are significant ethical and legal aspects to consider, and it is incumbent on any provider who offers genetic testing to understand and be prepared to deal with these issues. Investigating familial relationships and the level of communication among its members may assist the obstetric provider in identifying an acceptable path forward. The provider and patient may arrive at a decision not to disclose genetic test results, following serious consideration of the moral, psychologic, legal and social implications of such a decision. However, when a patient refuses to inform relatives of their risk for genetic disease, the healthcare professional may be faced with conflicting moral obligations to the patient and at-risk family members. On one side of the issue is the obligation to respect and protect patients' right to privacy. On the other side is the obligation to prevent harm and promote the welfare of the family members, despite the directive of the patient.

Organizations that promulgate guidelines for genetic care and counseling have proposed different approaches to the disclosure of genetic information. There is some consensus among organizations that the provider has an obligation to disclose genetic test results if serious harm would occur if the disclosure were not made. However, there is no clear definition of "serious" or further guidance on immediacy of risk.[14-16] If a provider has any question about the parameters of legal obligation for disclosure, counsel from professionals with expertise in ethics and the law is recommended.[6] This may be done within the scope of patient privacy through consultation with qualified professionals or ethics committee.

HOW SHOULD GENETIC RISK ASSESSMENT BE ADDRESSED IN A PATIENT WITH REPORTED CONSANGUINITY?

There is limited information to guide a practitioner on genetic counseling for consanguineous couples. The terms inbreeding and consanguinity may be used interchangeably to describe a couple who share at least one common ancestor. In many cultures, marriages between relatives are preferred and are common. It is important to differentiate these terms from incest, which has a different connotation in both biologic and legal settings. Incest may include unions between nonbiologic relatives (e.g., between stepfather and stepchild) or biologic relatives (e.g. parent and child or siblings), which impacts genetic risk assessment. Providers should be aware of the legal obligation to report incest according to state law. Psychosocial counseling regarding consanguineous unions is important to provide and should be performed in a manner without bias, demonstrating respect for different belief systems or cultural practices.

Pregnancies from consanguineous unions may be at increased risk for genetic disorders because of recessive gene mutations inherited from a common ancestor. The closer the biologic relationship, the greater the risk for a fetus to inherit a mutated allele. There are mathematic formulas including coefficient of inbreeding to determine the probability of an individual inheriting both alleles of a pair from an identical ancestor. For example, first cousins are expected to share 1/8 or 12.5% of their genes. For a first-cousin union, theoretic calculation predict that each pregnancy will be identical or homozygous at 6.25% or 1/16 of the entire genome. There is no clear evidence that consanguinity increases risk for multifactorial disorders.[17]

There is no absolute number used to predict an adverse outcome including structural anomalies or intellectual disability in the offspring of consanguineous union as compared with a nonconsanguineous union. Data obtained on consanguineous couples and their offspring vary by population, ascertainment bias, and underreporting. In available studies of first-cousin unions, the increased risk for a major structural abnormality in offspring of a first-cousin union ranged between 1.7% and 2.8% above the baseline population risk.[17] Nonetheless, individualized risk assessment for a consanguineous couple should include consideration of the family history, baseline population risk, and degree of consanguinity. Referral to a healthcare provider with genetics expertise may be indicated to evaluate each of these factors. This is particularly relevant with the identification of an individual affected with a genetic condition or inborn error of metabolism. Should a personal medical and family history of a couple with shared ancestor be unrevealing, there is no indication to offer genetic screening on the basis of their relatedness alone.[15] Within certain ethic populations, there may be a higher prevalence of heritable disorders for which screening may be indicated (e.g., Tay-Sachs in individuals of Eastern or Central European Jewish, French Canadian, or Cajun descent). Also, current guidelines from academic organizations, including ACOG, ACMG, SMFM, and NSGC, recommend carrier screening for all patients of reproductive capacity, including cystic fibrosis, hemoglobinopathies, and spinal muscular atrophy.[9] Expanded carrier screening is also a consideration for all couples regardless of race, ethnicity, or relatedness. Screening and diagnostic testing for common aneuploidy should be offered to all obstetric patients. The risk for aneuploidy does not appear to be increased above age-related or influenced by consanguinity.[18] Fetal anatomic survey is indicated, given the higher risk for structural anomalies in the consanguineous couple.

WHAT ADDITIONAL RESOURCES ARE AVAILABLE TO EDUCATE A PATIENT CONSIDERING REPRODUCTIVE GENETIC TESTING?

Patient education is the foundation necessary for shared decision-making, informed consent, and optimization of outcomes. It is a critical component of modern healthcare. Patient education resources have the ability to enhance the patient-physician relationship and increase motivation, empowerment, and satisfaction.[19] In reproductive genetics, patient education by a variety of modalities has been demonstrated to enhance decision-making, improve knowledge, and improve patient satisfaction.[19-22] There are a number of educational tools an obstetric provider may consider, including printed information, videos or podcasts, computer programs, Internet-based resources, group classes, or trained peer educators. There is no single type of resource that is appropriate for all patients but should include factors such as literacy, education level, culture, or health status.

REFERENCES

1. National Society of Genetic Counselors' Definition Task Force, Resta R, Biesecker BB, Bennett RL, et al. A new definition of genetic counseling: National Society of genetic counselors' task force report. *J Genet Couns.* 2006;15(2): 77–83.
2. Baker DL, Schuette JL, Uhlmann WR. *A Guide to Genetic Counseling.* New York: Wiley-Liss; 1998.
3. Bernhardt BA, Haunstetter CM, Roter D, Gellar G. How do obstetric providers discuss referrals for prenatal genetic counseling? *J Genet Couns.* 2005;14:190.
4. Pletcher BA, Toriello HV, Noblin SJ, et al. Indication for genetic referral: a guide for healthcare professionals. *Genet Med.* 2007;9(6):385–389.
5. National Society of Genetic Counselors. About Genetic Counselors: How Do Genetic Counselors Benefit the Healthcare Team? https://www.nsgc.org/page/experience thebenefits.
6. Counseling about genetic testing and communication of genetic test results. Committee opinion No. 693. American College of Obstetricians and Gynecologists. *Obstet Gynecol.* 2017;129:e96–e101.
7. Carrier screening in the age of genomic medicine. Committee opinion No. 690. American College of Obstetricians and Gynecologists. *Obstet Gynecol.* 2017;129:e35–e40.

8. Carrier screening for genetic conditions. Committee opinion No. 691. American College of Obstetricians and Gynecologists. *Obstet Gynecol.* 2017;129:e41–e55.

9. Edwards JG, Feldman G, Goldberg J, et al. Expanded carrier screening in reproductive medicine—points to consider: a joint statement of the American College of Medical Genetics and Genomics, American College of Obstetricians and Gynecologists, National Society of Genetic Counselors, Perinatal Quality Foundation, and Society for Maternal-Fetal Medicine. *Obstet Gynecol.* 2015;125(3):653–662.

10. Hoyert DL, Mathews TJ, Menacker F, et al. Annual summary of vital statistics. *Pediatrics.* 2004;2006(117):168–183.

11. Tracking and reminder systems. Committee opinion No. 546. American College of Obstetricians and Gynecologists. *Obstet Gynecol.* 2012;120:1535–1537.

12. Screening for fetal aneuploidy. Practice bulletin No. 163. American College of Obstetricians and Gynecologists. *Obstet Gynecol.* 2016;127(5):979–981.

13. Cell free DNA screening for fetal aneuploidy. Committee opinion No. 640. American College of Obstetricians and Gynecologists. *Obstet Gynecol.* 2015;126(3):e31–e37.

14. Professional disclosure of familial genetic information. ASHG statement. The American Society of Human genetics social issues subcommittee on familial disclosure. *Am J Hum Genet.* 1998;62:474–483.

15. President's Commission for the Study of Ethical Problems in Medicine and Biomedical and Behavioral Research. *Screening and Counseling for Genetic Conditions: A Report on the Ethical, Social, and Legal Implications of Genetic Screening, Counseling, and Education Programs.* Washington, DC: U.S. Government Printing Office; 1983.

16. Ethical issues in genetic testing. Committee opinion 410. *Obstet Gynecol.* 2008;111(6):1495–1502.

17. Bennett RL, Motulsky AG, Bittles A, et al. Genetic counseling and screening of consanguineous couples and their offspring: recommendations of the National Society of genetic counselors. *J Genet Couns.* 2002;11(2):97–119.

18. Sayee R, Thomas IM. Consanguinity, non-disjunction, parental age and Down's syndrome. *J Indian Med Assoc.* 1998;96:335–337.

19. Knutzen DM, Stoll KA, McClellan MW, Deering SH, Foglia LM. Improving knowledge about prenatal screening options: can group education make a difference? *J Matern Fetal Neonatal Med.* 2013;26(18):1799–1803.

20. Skjoth MM, Draborg E, Pedersen CD, et al. Providing information about prenatal screening for Down syndrome: a systematic review. *Acta Obstet Gynecol Scand.* 2015;94(2):125–132.

21. Kupperman M, Pena S, Bishop JT, et al. Effect of enhanced information, values clarification and removal of financial barriers on use of prenatal genetic testing: a randomized clinical trial. *J Am Med Assoc.* 2014;312(12):1210–1217.

22. Kuppermann M, Norton ME, Gates E, et al. Computerized prenatal genetic testing decision-assisting tool: a randomized controlled trial. *Obstet Gynecol.* 2009;113(1):53–63.

CHAPTER 4

Cytogenetics: Part 1, General Concepts and Aneuploid Conditions

MICHAEL T. MENNUTI, MD

WHAT IS CYTOGENETICS?

Cytogenetics is the study of chromosomes and the clinical application of chromosome analysis for diagnostic purposes. This chapter will deal with traditional cytogenetics, which involves examination of metaphase chromosomes.

The normal euploid or diploid chromosome constitution in human cells is 46. These are present in the nucleus of the cell as 23 pairs. Germ cells in the gonads with the normal diploid chromosome constitution produce haploid gametes with 23 chromosomes; one member from each pair is contributed to the gamete, as a result of meiotic division. The diploid number of chromosomes is reconstituted at fertilization, and as a result of this process, the members of each chromosome pair are biparentally inherited. Twenty two of the pairs, known as autosomes, are numbered based on size and position of a primary constriction termed a centromere. The location of the centromere is used to classify chromosomes as metacentric (centromere at or near the middle of the chromosome), submetacentric (centromere dividing the chromosome into a short arm and long arm that are unequal in size), or acrocentric (centromere at or near one end of the chromosome). The 23rd pair is the sex chromosomes that are usually XX in females or XY in males (Fig. 4.1). Chromosomes containing the nuclear DNA may be subject to partial or complete copy number variations, resulting in aneuploidy with phenotypic changes of clinical importance. In contrast to nuclear chromosomes, maternally inherited DNA in the mitochondria is not visualized by cytogenetic testing but is studied by molecular methods. Similar to nuclear DNA, mitochondrial DNA is subject to copy number variation and mutations that may be associated with phenotypic effects and diseases (see Chapters 2 and 15).

WHY AND HOW IS CHROMOSOME TESTING PERFORMED?

Chromosome testing is performed to ascertain whether there is the normal number of chromosomes in the somatic cells of an individual or fetus and to detect abnormalities of chromosome structure that may have clinical or reproductive consequences.

In the cytogenetic laboratory, chromosomes are examined microscopically after staining and fixing cells on a glass slide. A standard cytogenetic test usually includes examination of clusters of chromosomes in 20 cells undergoing metaphase division. Chromosomes are physically spread on a slide by several different methods; ideally, spreading is sufficient to minimize overlapping of chromosomes but controlled to the extent that intact metaphases can be identified by electronic scanning and evaluated by experienced laboratory staff. This minimizes preparation artifact because of loss of chromosomes from one metaphase or gain of chromosomes from nearby metaphases.

WHAT IS "CHROMOSOME BANDING"?

Methods to differentially stain areas of chromosomes are referred to as banding. These staining methods enable identification of individual chromosomes by creating internal patterns in the members of the chromosome pairs that are common in the general population. Pretreatment with trypsin before staining with Giemsa solution results in typical staining patterns known as G-bands. G-banding is the most commonly performed banding method and produces a recognizable pattern of alternating dark and clear (light) bands, which distinguishes each chromosome pair. Some variation in size and/or staining of certain chromosome regions is observed with sufficient frequency in the general population to be categorized as normal variants or heteromorphisms. A number of staining methods other than G-banding result in patterns that may provide information about specific chromosome regions. However, these are rarely used since the advent of newer molecular methods such as microarray.

HOW AND WHEN IS FISH TESTING USED?

FISH uses fluorescent DNA probes that bind to regions of a chromosome that have a high degree of sequence complementarity with the probe. Upon binding, the FISH

Perinatal Genetics. https://doi.org/10.1016/B978-0-323-53094-1.00004-7

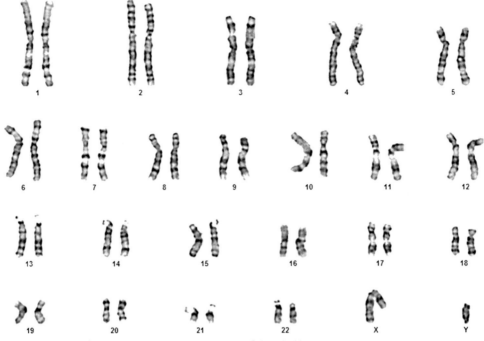

FIG. 4.1 Normal male G-banded karyotype.

probe for a particular chromosome region will emit specific color fluorescence. Fluorescence microscopy is used to identify binding of the probe to the nucleus of interphase cells or to the metaphase chromosomes in cells undergoing mitosis. FISH on interphase nuclei may be used for rapid detection of copy number of chromosomes in cells from amniotic or chorionic villus samples when a specific trisomy is suspected. FISH probes can also be used to detect duplications, deletions, or structural rearrangement of chromosome regions, such as balanced or unbalanced reciprocal translocations, based on the locations of signals in the metaphase chromosomes (see Fig. 4.2).

WHAT TISSUES ARE USED FOR CLINICAL CHROMOSOME ANALYSES?

Clinical chromosome analysis is performed on cells that are at the metaphase stage of mitotic division when there is compaction of the chromosomes into microscopically visible structures. The testing is most commonly performed on peripheral blood samples. Following addition of a mitogen to induce division of lymphocytes, exposure to an agent that arrests metaphase (e.g., colcemid) enables analysis of chromosomes in peripheral lymphocytes. Chromosomes may also be examined from cells undergoing tissue culture that have been established from biopsies of skin or other organs, including

placental fragments from chorionic villus samples and desquamated cells in amniotic fluid sampling.

Tissue biopsies obtained at the time of early pregnancy loss, after stillbirth or postmortem, can often be successfully grown in tissue culture. The outer limit of time for possible growth of biopsies in tissue culture following pregnancy loss or fetal death in utero has not been defined. Chromosomal microarray (CMA) on DNA extracted from fetal tissue is recommended as the first-line test in cases of fetal death, in part because avoiding tissue culture eliminates culture failures and maternal cell contamination (see Chapter 12). When traditional chromosome analysis is performed tissue culture success is maximized by obtaining samples under sterile conditions and placing them in sterile containers with tissue culture media or balanced salt solution to prevent drying. When in doubt regarding the viability of the cells, it is appropriate to submit samples rather than forego indicated testing.

WHAT TISSUE CULTURE METHODS ARE PREFERRED FOR PRENATAL DIAGNOSIS OF CHROMOSOME ANEUPLOIDY?

Short-term growth of amniotic cells or fragments of placental villi is preferred for prenatal diagnosis of chromosome abnormalities to obtain results as rapidly as

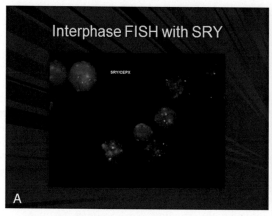
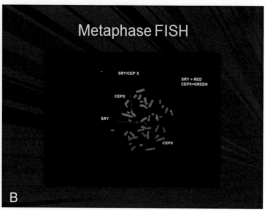

FIG. 4.2 **(A)** SRY translocation to Xpter. Image on the left demonstrates interphase nuclei with one SRY signal (red) and two X chromosome centromeres (green). **(B)** Image on the right demonstrates metaphase chromosomes with two centromeres (green) of X chromosomes and SRY signal (red) hybridized to tip of short arm of one X.

possible and to minimize abnormalities or artifacts that arise in cell division during tissue culture. Laboratory standards are available regarding the processing and methods for tissue culture of samples.[1] Counting and examining individual chromosomes in a total of 20 cells from two different tissue culture flasks or examination of chromosomes in 15 patches of cells grown on coverslips in petri dishes is recommended for prenatal diagnosis. The short-term nature of the tissue culture process on coverslips also means that there are fewer cell divisions before harvesting and consequently, less opportunity for introduction of in vitro chromosome errors.

IS DIRECT CHROMOSOME ANALYSIS OF VALUE IN PRENATAL DIAGNOSIS?

Some tissues, such as first-trimester placenta, are growing so rapidly that there are sufficient spontaneous mitoses that can be arrested in metaphase division without initiating tissue culture. Chromosome analysis on these unstimulated samples is referred to as "direct chromosome analysis." As maternal cells are not spontaneously dividing in placental biopsies, in addition to the rapid availability of the result, direct chromosome analysis on chorionic villus fragments excludes error introduced by maternal cell contamination. Direct chromosome analysis is not used routinely because the number and quality of complete metaphases suitable for analysis are less consistent than obtained from tissue culture. In addition, the accuracy when compared with cultured preparations is less, in part because of an increased rate of confined placental mosaicism in direct preparations.

HOW SHOULD A CLINICIAN INTERPRET A REPORT FROM THE CYTOGENETIC LABORATORY?

Standard laboratory reports will indicate the source of material studied, and the number of cells examined, usually 20, and the type of staining or banding performed. The report may also describe the banding level by subjectively estimating the number of bands in a haploid set of chromosomes. The expected sensitivity of standard G-banding for detection of copy number variants is 5–10 Mb.

The report should provide a karyotype designation, which indicates the number of chromosomes in the cells and the sex chromosome pattern observed. If abnormalities or structural rearrangements are present or when multiple different cell lines are observed, these should be described according to standard karyotype designations described in the International System for Human Cytogenetic Nomenclature (ISCN).[2]

The number of cells examined enables estimation of the confidence intervals for detection of mosaicism at certain percentages of a cell line.[3] See Table 4.1 for estimates of detection of mosaicism by examination of 20 or more cells by diagnostic testing. Additional cells may be examined if there is concern about the initial findings or when there is concern for low-percentage mosaicism or maternal cell contamination.

If the karyotype is other than normal, a narrative may follow that provides a more understandable description of the findings for the clinician who is not likely to be familiar with complex karyotype nomenclature and abbreviations. The report may also describe

TABLE 4.1
% Mosaicism by Number of Cells Examined With the Identical Karyotype*

	LEVEL OF MOSAICISM CONFIDENCE INTERVAL	
No. of cells (n)	**0.95**	**0.99**
20	14%	21%
40	8%	11%
50–55	6%	9%
99–112	3%	5%
299–458	1%	2%
>459	1%	1%

*Ref. 3.

clinical implications of unusual or abnormal findings and recommend additional cytogenetic analysis, including testing of the parents, other diagnostic tests, and/or genetic counseling.

WHAT ARE THE CONSEQUENCES OF ANEUPLOIDY?

Conditions in which there are extra or missing chromosomes in the cells of an individual or a fetus are collectively referred to as aneuploidies. Detection of a duplication or deletion of a portion of a chromosome is referred to as partial aneuploidies. When there is complete or partial aneuploidy, the loss or gain of copies of the genes may result in a constellation of phenotypic features that describe a syndrome, e.g., 22q11.2 deletion syndrome. In some instances, a phenotypic feature may be attributable to a specific gene or to several contiguous genes, and in other situations, the phenotype may be due to the collective effect of many genes present in a single copy or three copies.

Reports of large series of individuals with the same aneuploidy have enabled description of the features of syndromes associated with the aneuploidy and the frequency at which the features of the syndrome occur. Discrete features such as a structural malformation are most often seen in only a percentage of individuals with the same aneuploidy. Continuous variables, such as height or I.Q., occur as a range that differs from but may overlap, with the range in the general population. Information in case series about structural malformations and continuous variables is useful in counseling and for planning care.

WHAT ARE THE MOST COMMON ANEUPLOIDIES SEEN IN CHILDREN?

The nonmosaic aneuploidies that occur most frequently in newborns are trisomy 21, 18, and 13 and sex chromosome aneuploidies (45,X; 47,XXX; 47,XXY and 47,XYY). When encountered, trisomies for other chromosomes are often of midsized chromosomes and are mosaic (e.g., mosaicism for trisomy 8 or trisomy 9 in conjunction with a cell line with a normal chromosome complement). Partial duplications or deletions of chromosome regions, and low-percentage mosaicism for trisomies of other chromosomes, may be compatible with prolonged survival in some cases.

Rare reports of autosomal monosomy usually involve the smallest chromosomes (#21, #22) and are either mosaic or involve only a partial deletion or duplication of chromosome regions. Before the advent of microarray, there were only a few rare partial monosomy syndromes detected by traditional cytogenetic testing, e.g., a small deletion in the short arm of a #4 chromosome (4p-) as a cause of Wolf-Hirschhorn syndrome and a small deletion in the short arm of a #5 chromosome (5p-) as a cause of cri-du-chat syndrome. Although many of these cases are due to de novo terminal deletions, others are the result of unbalanced translocations inherited from a parent with a balanced translocation. More recently, a number of recurrent clinically important microdeletions and microduplications with clinically described phenotypes have been identified by microarray (see Chapter 12).

HOW FREQUENTLY ARE CHROMOSOME ABNORMALITIES SEEN IN NEWBORN CHILDREN?

Chromosome abnormalities contribute to birth defects, neonatal mortality, early childhood deaths, and major disabilities. In a study of almost 35,000 live births over 13 years, Nielsen and Wohlert reported a frequency of autosomal abnormalities of 1 in 164 births and the combined frequency of autosomal and sex chromosome abnormalities was 1 in 118.[4] It should be noted that this survey also included a small number of pregnancies terminated for abnormal chromosome findings on prenatal testing. Estimates of the frequency of trisomy 13 and trisomy 18 vary widely in the literature and for that reason are presented in Table 4.2 as a range.

More current data are not likely to become available, as this would depend on observational studies performed by systematic testing of very large numbers of consecutive live born children. In such a study, the detection of mosaicism would be dependent on the

TABLE 4.2 Incidence of Aneuploidy in Newborn Infants*		
All sex chromosomes Aneuploidy	1:426	
	47,XXY	1:576
	47,XYY	1:851
	47,XXX	1:947
	Turner syndrome	1:1893
All autosomal abnormalities (includes trisomies and rearrangements)	1:164	
	Down syndrome	1:592
Combined incidence for sex chromosomes and autosomes	1:118	
	Trisomy 13	1:6500–1:15,000
	Trisomy 18	1:3500–1:5000

*Ref. 4. Aggregated data and individual frequencies for sex chromosome aneuploidy and Down syndrome from study of 34,910 newborns.[4] Estimates of trisomy 13 and 18 from various sources.

number of cells examined and partial deletions or duplications of chromosomes would depend on the quality of banding and the addition of microarray testing. Furthermore, results obtained over a long period of time would be influenced by trends in factors such as maternal age distribution, introduction of more sensitive early prenatal screening, and changing attitudes regarding termination of affected pregnancies.

WHAT IS THE FREQUENCY OF CHROMOSOME ABNORMALITIES IN LATE PREGNANCY LOSS?

Compared with live births, chromosome abnormalities are overrepresented in late pregnancy losses and in most instances the presence of a chromosome abnormality is assumed to be causally related to the loss. It has been estimated that 6%–12% of stillbirths after 20 weeks' gestation are associated with chromosome abnormalities.[5] The type of autosomal abnormalities

observed in these cases is similar to those encountered in live births. Because of failure to successfully obtain chromosome results from fetal tissue, and the potential for maternal cell contamination of placental cultures, it is commonly accepted that the frequency of chromosome abnormalities in stillbirths is underestimated. Report of microarray studies of late losses confirms incremental success in obtaining results and exclusion of maternal cell contamination, resulting in improved detection of abnormalities.[6]

HOW COMMON ARE CHROMOSOME ABNORMALITIES IN EARLY PREGNANCY LOSS?

Collective data regarding chromosome abnormalities in early pregnancy loss are biased toward the later part of the first trimester and early second trimester. In part, this bias is due to failure to obtain adequate tissue, bacterial or fungal contamination, and maternal cell overgrowth of samples from the earliest losses. Additionally, a lower quality of the band resolution in samples from pregnancy losses compared with lymphocyte chromosome testing also limits detection of structural chromosome abnormalities. Although the observed rate of aneuploidy in successfully tested samples is generally >50%, it has been estimated that the rate of aneuploidy in early losses probably approaches 70%.[7,8] Autosomal trisomies are the most common abnormalities in early pregnancy loss and account for at least one-half of the aneuploidies in these samples. This is followed in frequency by monosomy X (45,X), which is the single most common chromosome abnormality in human conceptions, and then by polyploidy (triploidy with 69 chromosomes per cell and tetraploidy with 92 chromosomes per cell). A small portion of aneuploidies in first trimester losses are associated with double trisomy of two or more different chromosomes, mosaicism, balanced and unbalanced structural abnormalities, and unidentifiable marker chromosomes. In contrast to aneuploidies in newborns and stillbirths, trisomy of every chromosome has been reported in spontaneous early pregnancy losses although autosomal monosomies are not seen with any reported frequency in these surveys.

The gestational age at which pregnancies with any specific aneuploidy are lost is influenced by the size of the chromosomes, the density of genes, and the impact of specific genes on early fetal development. Trisomy of the small and medium-sized chromosomes appears to be overrepresented in early losses, whereas trisomy for the largest chromosomes is much less frequently observed. Trisomy 16 is the most common trisomy detected in first-trimester spontaneous abortions, followed in frequency by trisomy 22. It is not clear if this relates to an increased vulnerability of chromosome 16 to meiotic nondisjunction or to certain critical genes that allow fetal development to a gestational age when tissue might be captured for testing. Pregnancies with trisomy 16 often present with empty sacs and disordered embryonic development. Infrequently, maternal theca lutein cysts and hydatidiform changes in the placenta have been associated with trisomy 16 in the late first trimester and early second trimester. Rare cases of neonates with mosaicism for trisomy 16 and also children with maternal and paternal UPD for chromosome 16 have been reported. The latter suggests that some trisomy 16 conceptions are rescued by loss of the extra chromosome (termed trisomy rescue). This observation is also consistent with cases in which cells with trisomy 16 have been seen in chorionic villus samples but not confirmed by amniocentesis or newborn testing.

Indirect calculations based on the frequency of trisomy 21 and 45,X in live births, stillbirths, and early losses estimate that 80% of trisomy 21 conceptions and >99% of 45,X conceptions are lost before live birth. These indirect calculations are supported by the observation of an increased rate of early and late spontaneous losses of continuing pregnancies after prenatal diagnosis of these chromosome abnormalities. The utility of antenatal fetal testing to decrease the rate of late pregnancy loss has not been systematically studied in pregnancies in which the fetus has diagnosis of an autosomal trisomy or 45,X chromosome constitution.

Studies of preimplantation blastocysts conceived by assisted reproductive technologies vary depending on the technology used for testing but confirm a high frequency of chromosome abnormalities in these pregnancies.[9] In addition to meiotic errors, these observations also include a striking frequency of mitotic errors resulting in mosaicism. The highest rates of chromosome abnormalities are reported in embryos produced by assisted reproductive technologies with early developmental arrest or that fail to implant (see Chapter 15).

WHAT ARE THE MECHANISMS THAT CAUSE ANEUPLOIDY?

Nondisjunction is the most common mechanism resulting in aneuploidy. Nondisjunction is an error in which there is unequal distribution of the members of a single chromosome pair in cell division. After fertilization, this results in daughter cells with either one or three copies of the involved chromosome rather than

the usual two copies. The occurrence of nondisjunction appears to relate to the strength of the attachment of the chromosomes to the spindle fibers that form during cell division and the separation or cohesion of the chromatids. Nondisjunction in meiosis can result in pregnancy loss or birth of a child with an extra chromosome in all cells, whereas nondisjunction in mitosis will result in mosaicism with two or more cell lines.

Aneuploidy may also result from anaphase lag. Anaphase lag occurs when there is delayed movement of a chromosome during anaphase. A chromosome in meiosis or a chromatid in mitosis that fails to migrate or connect to the pole of the spindle apparatus will be lost from the nucleus as division is completed. Anaphase lag with loss of an X or a Y chromosome is thought to be responsible for the aneuploidy in most embryos with a 45,X chromosome constitution.

WHAT IS THE ROLE OF NONDISJUNCTION IN NUMERICAL CHROMOSOME ABNORMALITIES?

Nondisjunction may occur in maternal or paternal gametogenesis at any age. The only factor clearly associated with increase in the frequency of meiotic nondisjunction is advancing maternal age. The frequency of trisomy 21 offspring increases steadily throughout the reproductive years, and there is a steep increase in frequency in women in their mid- to late 30 years of age and older. A similar association of mean maternal age at birth of children with trisomy 13, trisomy 18, 47,XXX, and 47,XXY has also been observed. The prenatal diagnosis of fetal trisomy is also greater earlier in pregnancy because of loss of chromosomally abnormal fetuses over the course of pregnancy. Thus, the number of abnormal amniocentesis results at 16 weeks is higher than the risk projected for term. The chance of Down syndrome and of all chromosome problems for each year of the mother's age at expected delivery date are readily available for counseling of patients (Table 4.3). Year by year chance of trisomy 13 and 18 based on maternal age is not readily available but is included in the cumulative estimated chance for of all chromosome abnormalities at each year of age.[10] A 47,XYY chromosome constitution in the fetus is not related to maternal age, as this occurs due to paternal nondisjunction. Similarly, occurrences of 45,X due to anaphase lag are not associated with maternal or paternal age.

TABLE 4.3
Risk of Chromosome Abnormalities Based on Maternal Age at Term

Age at Term	Risk of Trisomy 21[a]	Risk of Any Chromosome Abnormality[b]
15[c]	1:1578	1:454
16[c]	1:1572	1:475
17[c]	1:1565	1:499
18[c]	1:1556	1:525
19[c]	1:1544	1:555
20	1:1480	1:525
21	1:1460	1:525
22	1:1440	1:499
23	1:1420	1:499
24	1:1380	1:475
25	1:1340	1:475
26	1:1290	1:475
27	1:1220	1:454
28	1:1140	1:434
29	1:1050	1:416
30	1:940	1:384
31	1:820	1:385
32	1:700	1:322
33	1:570	1:285
34	1:456	1:243
35	1:353	1:178
36	1:267	1:148
37	1:199	1:122
38	1:148	1:104
39	1:111	1:80
40	1:85	1:62
41	1:67	1:48
42	01:54	01:38
43	01:45	01:30
44	01:39	01:23
45	01:35	01:18
46	01:31	01:14
47	01:29	01:10
48	01:27	1:8
49	01:26	1:6
50	01:25	d

[a]Morris JK, Wald NJ, Mutton DE, Alberman E. Comparison of models of maternal age-specific risk for Down syndrome live births. *Prenat Diagn.* 2003; 23:252–258.

[b]Risk of any chromosome abnormality includes the risk of trisomy 21 and trisomy 18 in addition to trisomy 13, 47,XXY, 47,XYY, Turner syndrome genotype, and other clinically significant abnormalities, 47,XXX not included. Data from Hook EB. Rates of chromosome abnormalities at different maternal ages. *Obstet Gynecol.* 1981; 58:282–285.

[c]Cuckle HS, Wald NJ, Thompson SG. Estimating a woman's risk of having a pregnancy associated with Down's syndrome using her age and serum alpha-fetoprotein levels. *Br J Obstet Gynecol.* 1987; 94; 387–402.

[d]Data not available.

WHAT ARE THE MECHANISMS THAT RESULT IN POLYPLOIDY AND WHAT IS THE RANGE OF CLINICAL MANIFESTATIONS?

Triploidy is most commonly due to dispermy, an error in which an egg is fertilized by two spermatozoa. A conception with 69 XXX, XXY or XYY chromosome constitution may result. A large portion of these pregnancies are lost in the first trimester. Ultrasonic features often include placental changes consistent with hydatidiform mole or gestational trophoblastic disease. Triploid pregnancies that progress into the second trimester are characterized by severe malformations, disparity between the head circumference and abdominal circumference, molar changes in the placenta, and bilateral ovarian enlargement with theca lutein cysts. The ultrasound findings often raise suspicions of triploidy. Mothers in whom a triploid pregnancy progresses into the second trimester may experience early-onset severe preeclampsia and/or hyperthyroidism. Triploid pregnancies rarely carry to term. Most triploid fetuses that are alive at birth are mosaic, have severe malformations, and do not survive. Termination of pregnancy is recommended when a triploidy pregnancy is diagnosed because of the uniformly poor outcome for the fetus and in the interest of maternal health. Clinically relevant factors leading to a failure of the block to polyspermy have not been described. Persistent trophoblastic disease following a "partial mole" associated with triploidy is so rare that it is difficult to ascertain if persistent trophoblastic disease is increased following removal of a triploid placenta compared with a normal term delivery. Nevertheless, following termination of a triploid pregnancy associated with a partial mole, patients are generally encouraged to use effective contraception and are followed until quantitative hCG levels return to zero for a period of time.

Tetraploidy may be seen in amniotic or chorionic villus tissue culture. It is considered to be due to a failure of chromosome separation into daughter cells during mitosis. There are no reports of children with tetraploidy in all cells and only a few rare case reports of children with severe abnormalities who appear to be mosaic for diploid and tetraploid cell lines.

WHY IS A WIDE RANGE OF OUTCOMES AND PHENOTYPIC SEVERITY SEEN IN 45,X?

The wide range of outcomes in pregnancies with 45,X chromosome constitution has not been explained. In the first trimester, this chromosome constitution is associated with a high rate of loss associated with failed embryonic development, while the late first trimester and early second trimester is characterized by cystic hygroma and hydrops. In stark contrast, neonates with 45,X may not have phenotypic features that result in clinical suspicion of the diagnosis. During childhood, girls with Turner syndrome may only come to attention because of short stature or at the time of delayed menarche. These observations have prompted speculation regarding possible biologic reasons for the severity of the phenotype in early pregnancy compared with the girls with the same chromosome constitution. This has led to a hypothesis that all 45,X survivors are mosaic or cryptic mosaics.[11] This would imply that the mechanism for the abnormality was the result of a mitotic event.

Compared with autosomal aneuploidies, Turner syndrome diagnosis is associated with a relatively high frequency of mosaicism and structural abnormalities of the X chromosome. Mosaicism with more than two cell lines is not unusual. Among women with Turner syndrome who have mosaicism, some have 45,X/46,XX, whereas others have 45,X/46XY. This supports the view that mitotic loss of an X or a Y chromosome resulting in a 45,X cell line may occur with similar frequency. Findings of mosaicism that include cell lines with both 45,X and 47,XXX suggest that at least in some cases, the mechanism might be mitotic nondisjunction rather than anaphase lag.

Amniotic fluid chromosome testing at times detects pregnancies in which the majority of cells have a 46,XY chromosome constitution with a varying percentage of 45,X cells. The majority of the pregnancies that continue result in the birth of normal males.[12] Initial reports noted the very different clinical findings among patients with this chromosome constitution diagnosed by amniocentesis when compared with patients ascertained during childhood, often due to genital abnormalities, features of Turner syndrome, and growth disturbance. Recent long-term follow-up comparing 20 males who were diagnosed prenatally with 20 males who came to attention in childhood has been reported. All of the boys had either no or only mild anomaly of the external genitalia. Although boys diagnosed in childhood had more features of Turner syndrome, mean final height was not significantly different in the two groups, and there was greater similarity between the two groups than previously recognized. The potential benefits of systematic follow-up are apparent from this report.[13]

Because loss of a structurally abnormal Y chromosome predisposes to 45,X/46XY mosaicism, studies of the structural integrity of the Y chromosome should be performed when a 45,X cell line meets criteria for mosaicism. Based on the cytogenetic findings, a combination of FISH and molecular studies should be considered. Cord blood chromosome analysis and tissue culture of foreskin, if circumcision is performed, can provide confirmation of prenatal test results and provide another tissue for assessment of mosaicism.

IS THERE CLINICAL VALUE TO PERFORMING CHROMOSOME TESTING ON PREGNANCY LOSSES?

Cytogenetic studies of early spontaneous losses consistently demonstrate that many are associated with chromosome abnormalities that are due to random events. Studies of consecutive spontaneous abortions have not identified clinically relevant associations other than confirming the maternal age effect. Studies have demonstrated that women with a history of a chromosomally normal early loss who have another early loss have an increased chance that the second loss will also be chromosomally normal.[14] Thus, it is possible that a chromosomally normal early loss may be a useful marker for investigating other potential causes of recurrent losses. Studies of chromosome abnormalities in early loss have not demonstrated an impact on subsequent reproduction. One study of recurrence risk of trisomy by combining data from testing spontaneous early losses and prenatal diagnosis demonstrated small increases in a different trisomy at a level of 1.6-fold increase (90% CI 1.1–2.4). Although the findings demonstrate that a subset of parents may have an increased propensity for nondisjunction, it was noted that these findings are unlikely to have clinical utility as a large portion of women who experience the birth of a child with trisomy and many women with a history of loss of a chromosomally abnormal pregnancy opt for early sensitive screening or diagnostic testing in subsequent pregnancies.[15] Mechanisms with a basis for recurrence, e.g., low percentage mosaicism in a parent, or unbalanced translocation and inversions, are rarely suspected based on the findings of testing tissue from early pregnancy losses.

In spite of these limitations, there are perceived emotional benefits from cytogenetic testing of pregnancy losses. Learning of a chromosome abnormality as an explanation for the loss, and the information that this is most likely due to a nonrecurrent random event, often helps the resolution of grief. This information from the cytogenetic test may also be useful for avoiding extensive testing to determine the cause of the losses.

Evaluation of recurrent pregnancy loss is discussed in Chapter 5.

WHAT CAUSES MOSAICISM?

Mosaicism occurs when there are two or more lines of cells with different numbers of chromosomes in the same fetus or person. Chromosomal mosaicism results from nondisjunction in mitosis of a normal cell or an aneuploid cell. Although nondisjunction in mitosis of euploid cells should result in both monosomic and trisomic daughter cells, a cell line with monosomy is infrequently observed. This may be due to attrition of cells that lack important genetic material. More commonly, following nondisjunction in a euploid cell, only two cell lines are subsequently observed, one of which is euploid and the other is trisomic. Mosaicism may also arise from loss of one of the extra chromosomes in a trisomic cell (trisomy rescue) or from duplication of the remaining single chromosome in a monosomic cell. Clinically, mosaicism appears to be more common in association with sex chromosome abnormalities or situations when one member of a chromosome pair is a small structurally abnormal derivative (e.g., marker chromosome).

In an individual with mosaicism, multiple cell lines may be seen and the distribution of normal and abnormal cell lines may vary in different tissues or organs. Clinical features of mosaicism are generally the same or milder than those seen when all cells have the same aneuploidy. Mosaic cell lines in clinically affected individuals are reported in percentages usually determined by one isolated test from a single tissue source. It is unusual for clinical testing to be performed on multiple tissues and/or to have the relative proportion of cell lines in a single tissue tracked over time, although these differences may influence clinical outcomes.

DOES LOW-LEVEL PARENTAL MOSAICISM EXPLAIN OCCURRENCE OR RECURRENCE OF ANEUPLOID PREGNANCIES?

Low-percentage mosaicism has not been quantitatively defined. Standard chromosome analysis is performed on 20 cells. This has been roughly estimated to detect 20% mosaicism with 99% confidence.

Very-low-percentage mosaicism in lymphocytes, e.g., 1%–3%, may be an acquired finding on chromosome testing because of in vitro errors in mitosis or preparation artifact. For example, the frequency of occasional cells with sex chromosome aneuploidy has been observed, and a number of studies of this phenomenon have been published.[16] This may involve X or Y chromosomes in either males or females. A cell or cells with loss of an X chromosome have been observed more commonly in women and appear to be acquired inasmuch as this phenomenon is more frequent in older women.[17] Distinguishing in vitro errors or preparation artifact from constitutional low-percentage mosaicism may not be possible at these very low levels. The finding of occasional cells with X chromosome aneuploidy has not been associated with clinical features or infertility. If they are observed in a woman who has clinical findings consistent with features of X chromosome aneuploidy, the finding may justify more extensive testing or repeat testing.

Importantly, a low percentage of constitutional mosaicism or mosaicism limited to the gonad (gonadal mosaicism) may result in recurrence of aneuploidy. The observation of a low but increased (1%–2%) recurrence risk for trisomy 21 due to nondisjunction in siblings has been associated with parental low-level constitutional mosaicism.[18] Sensitivity for diagnosis of low-level mosaicism would be expected to increase with examination of chromosomes in more than the usual number of cells. Although increasing the number of metaphases examined may improve sensitivity for detection of low-level mosaicism, this may also increase the likelihood of introducing artifact. Interphase FISH has been used for detection of low-level mosaicism, but this requires the availability of a probe for the area of interest or the specific genetic locus being evaluated. False-positive and false-negative FISH results can occur due to failure of hybridization or artifact due to superimposition of fluorescent signals, respectively. Microarray can also detect mosaicism at certain levels (see Chapter 12). Although the sensitivity for detection of very-low-level mosaicism by microarray is limited, this is likely to improve with advances in technology.

IS THERE CLINICAL VALUE IN TESTING PARENTS FOR LOW-LEVEL MOSAICISM AFTER THE BIRTH OF A CHILD WITH A TRISOMY DUE TO NONDISJUNCTION?

Low-percentage mosaicism for trisomy 21 in parents has been associated with birth of children with 47,XX,+21 or 47,XY,+21 and with recurrence of Down syndrome in siblings. In spite of these observations, parental chromosome analysis is not usually recommended for couples who have a child with trisomy 21. The rationale is that very-low-level constitutional mosaicism or mosaicism confined to the germ cells can never be confidently excluded by blood testing even when a large number of cells are examined. For these reasons,

parental testing is generally not performed in these couples and they are counseled regarding a 1%–2% risk level based on this mechanism, and the options of prenatal diagnostic testing or noninvasive screening using cell-free DNA sequencing should be offered.

HOW SHOULD WOMEN BE COUNSELED AFTER DETECTION OF FETAL MOSAICISM BY PRENATAL CHROMOSOME TESTING?

Prenatal cytogenetic diagnosis relies on the assumption that desquamated cells in amniotic fluid or tissue culture of fragments of placental biopsy will accurately reflect the fetal chromosome constitution. Large worldwide experience over many decades confirms that this testing is highly accurate and that the assumption is usually correct. Nevertheless, when dealing with mosaicism, there are concerns that relate both to limits of the sensitivity and to false-positive rates. Mosaic cells can arise due to mitotic nondisjunction in cells of the fetus, or they may be limited to a focus in the amnion or in the cells from a placental biopsy. There is also a theoretical concern that clinically important mosaicism in the fetus might not be detected by testing these desquamated cells or placental fragments. The percentage of aneuploid cells in amniotic fluid or chorionic villus samples may not accurately reflect the percentage of aneuploid cells in the fetus, and even assessment of mosaicism from fetal blood sampling may not reflect the level of mosaicism in all tissues/organs. Furthermore, the distribution of those aneuploid cells in various tissues and organs may be the most important determinant of phenotype. Although it is clear that children who have mosaicism for a trisomy tend to have less severe phenotypic expression, it should be apparent that there are limitations to the confidence in predicting the phenotype based on findings of mosaicism found in prenatal diagnostic tests.

WHAT MANAGEMENT IS RECOMMENDED WHEN FETAL MOSAICISM IS DETECTED BY CVS?

There is a higher level of mosaicism in chorionic villus samples than in amniocentesis. Although mosaicism is suspected in 3% of chorionic villus samples in many of these cases, it is limited to placental cells, i.e., confined placental mosaicism (CPM). The finding of mosaicism in a chorionic villus sample is usually best resolved by subsequent amniocentesis for mosaic aneuploidy in the fetus and testing for uniparental disomy (UPD) if the involved chromosome has been associated with an imprinted disorder (see Chapter 2).

WHY DOES MOSAICISM RAISE CONCERNS ABOUT IMPRINTING DISORDERS DUE TO UPD?

Most autosomal genes are biparentally inherited and expressed. Imprinted genes are only expressed by one member of a gene pair that is inherited from a specific parent. Absence or loss of the parental contribution from an imprinted gene may be due to a mutation in the gene, a microdeletion that includes the gene, UPD, or an abnormality of the imprinting control region. At this time, a limited number of clinical disorders due to imprinting errors in humans are relevant to prenatal diagnostic testing.

The development of a euploid cell line (46 chromosomes) in a trisomic conception by the very early loss of one of the trisomic chromosomes is referred to as "trisomy rescue." Uniparental disomy (UPD) results when the two remaining chromosomes that are retained in the cells are inherited from the same parent. UPD can be seen in all of the cells of a person with a normal chromosome number, but mosaicism for cells with a trisomy may be the first clue that the euploid cells have UPD as a result of trisomy rescue. Imprinting defects occur when the genetic contribution from the critical parental is absent. Mosaicism for a trisomic cell

line and a euploid cell line during prenatal chromosome testing is a concern when the involved chromosome is the one associated with a clinical disorder due to imprinting errors. At this time, chromosomes associated with imprinted disorders relevant to prenatal diagnosis include 6,7, 11, 14, 15, and 20 (Table 4.4).[19] It is possible that imprinting will be identified as the mechanism of additional disorders in the future.

Other cytogenetic findings involving nonhomologous and homologous Robertsonian translocations, as well as isochromosomes of the long arms of chromosomes 14 and 15, also appear to be associated with an increased frequency of imprinting disorders associated with those chromosomes.

WHEN ARE THERE ADDITIONAL CONCERNS ABOUT AN INCREASED FREQUENCY OF AUTOSOMAL RECESSIVE DISORDERS DUE TO UPD?

In addition to imprinting, when UPD of any chromosome is present, there may be an increased risk of clinical disorders due to homozygosity for recessive mutations on the involved chromosome. When two

TABLE 4.4
Imprinting Disorders in Humans Caused by UPD

Chromosome with UPD	Parent Contributing Both copies	Syndrome	Chromosome Region or Gene Involved
6	Paternal	Transient neonatal diabetes (41%)*	6q24
7	Mother	Russell-Silver syndrome (10%)*—IUGR, growth delay Other 90% complex with several different chromosomes and genes involved	7p11.2-p13 7q31-qter
11	Paternal	Beckwith-Wiedemann (15%)* Other 85% complex epigenetic changes	11p15.5—IGF2; H19
14	Paternal	Temple syndrome—IUGR, developmental delay polyhydramnios, thoracic and abdominal defects	14q32—DLK1 gene
14	Maternal	Milder than paternal UPD syndrome IUGR; hypotonia; developmental delay	14q32—GTL2 gene
15	Paternal	Angelman syndrome (3%–7%)*	15q11.3-q13 UBE3A
15	Maternal	Prader-Willi syndrome (25%)*	15q11.3-q13 Contiguous genes
20	Paternal	Albright hereditary osteodystrophy (AHOD) is autosomal dominant and differs if there is maternal or paternal inheritance. A case with pseudohypoparathyroidism (Php 1b) type due to 20q paternal UPD has been reported.	GNAS gene 20q13.32

*Percentage in parentheses indicates the % of cases attributed to UPD.

entirely different chromosomes are inherited from the same parent, the condition is referred to as "UPD with heterodisomy." This is not a concern if that parent does not have a recessive disorder attributed to a gene on that chromosome.

UPD can also occur in diploid cells when a chromosome is lost, resulting in monosomy and compensatory duplication of the other member of that pair, termed monosomy rescue. This is referred to as "UPD with isodisomy." If there is UPD with isodisomy that harbors a recessive disease causing mutation, then the fetus will be homozygous for that mutation even though the parent is only a carrier and the other parent is not a carrier. Mixed isodisomy and heterodisomy may be seen depending on whether the region of interest did or did not cross over during meiosis. When UPD with isodisomy is found in any chromosome, it becomes important to consider identifying any recessive variants on that chromosome that could result in offspring with that recessive disease. If a pregnancy is identified to have complete or partial isodisomy of any chromosome, then parental or fetal evaluation might be considered for clinically relevant recessive variants.

REFERENCES

1. Standards and Guidelines for Clinical Genetics Laboratories. *American College of Medical Genetics and Genomics (ACMG) 2018 Edition* Revised. ; January 2018:1–20.
2. McGowan-Jordan J, Simons A, Schmid M. *ISCN 2016: An International System for Human Cytogenomic Nomenclature.* Basel, Switzerland: S. Karger; 2016.
3. Hook EB. Exclusion of chromosomal mosaicism: tables of 90%, 95%, and 99% confidence limits and comments on use. *Am J Hum Genet.* 1977;29:94–97.
4. Nielson J, Wohlert M. Chromosome abnormalities found among 34,910 newborn children: results from a 13-year incidence study in Arhus, Denmark. *Hum Genet.* 1991;87(1):81–83.
5. Silver RM, Varner MW, Reddy U, et al. Work-up of stillbirth: a review of the evidence. *Am J Obstet Gynecol.* 2007;196(5):433–444. https://doi.org/10.1016/j.ajog.2006.11.041.
6. Reddy U, Page GP, Saade GR, et al. Karyotype versus microarray testing for genetic abnormalities after stillbirth. *N Engl J Med.* 2012;367(23):2185–2193. https://doi.org/10.1056/NEJMoa1201569.
7. Boué J, Boué A, Lazar P. Retrospective and prospective epidemiological studies of 1500 karyotyped spontaneous human abortions. *Teratology.* 1975;12(1):11–26.
8. Hardy K, Hardy PJ. 1st trimester miscarriage: four decades of study. *Transl Pediatr.* 2015;4(2):189–200.
9. Munné S, Wells D. Detection of mosaicism at blastocyst stage with the use of high-resolution next-generation sequencing. *Fertil Steril.* 2017;107:1085–1091.
10. Screening for fetal aneuploidy. Practice bulletin No. 163. American College of obstetricians and gynecologists. *Obstet Gynecol.* 2016;128:e123–e137.
11. Hook EB, Warburton D. Turner syndrome revisited: review of new data supports the hypothesis that all viable 45,X cases are cryptic mosaics with a rescue cell line, implying an origin by mitotic loss. *Hum Genet.* 2014;133(4):417–424. https://doi.org/10.1007/s00439-014-1420-x.
12. Hsu LY. Prenatal diagnosis of 45,X/46,XY mosaicism-a review and update. *Prenat Diagn.* 1989;9(1):31–48.
13. Dumeige L, Chatelais L, Bouvattier C, et al. Should 45,X/46,XY boys with no or mild anomaly of external genitalia be investigated and followed up. *Eur J Endocrinol.* 2018;179(3):181–190.
14. Warburton D, Kline J, Stein Z, et al. Does the karyotype of a spontaneous abortion predict the karyotype of a subsequent abortion? – evidence from 273 women with two karyotyped spontaneous abortions. *Am J Hum Genet.* 1987;41:465–483.
15. Warburton D, Dallaire L, Thangavelu M. Trisomy recurrence: a reconsideration based on North American data. *Am J Hum Genet.* 2004;75:376–385.
16. Robberecht C, Fryns J-P, Vermeesch JR. Piecing together the problems in diagnosing low-level chromosomal mosaicism. *Genome Med.* 2010;2(7):47. https://doi.org/10.1186/gm168.
17. Russell LM, Strike P, Browne CE, Jacobs PA. X chromosome loss and ageing. *Cytogenet Genome Res.* 2007;116:181–185. https://doi.org/10.1159/000098184.
18. Hultén MA, Jonasson J, Nordgren A, Iwarsson E. Germinal and somatic Trisomy 21 mosaicism: how common is it, what are the implications for individual carriers and how does it come about? *Curr Genom.* 2010;11:409–419.
19. Eggermann T, Soellner L, Buiting K, Kotzot D. Mosaicism and uniparental disomy in prenatal diagnosis. *Trends Mol Med.* 2015;21(2):77–87.

FURTHER READING

1. Hsu LYF, Benn PA. Revised guidelines for the diagnosis of mosiacism in amniocytes. *Prenat Diagn.* 1999;19:1081–1090.

Cytogenetics: Part 2, Structural Chromosome Rearrangements and Reproductive Impact

MICHAEL T. MENNUTI, MD

WHAT ARE STRUCTURAL CHROMOSOME REARRANGEMENTS AND HOW FREQUENTLY ARE THEY SEEN IN THE GENERAL POPULATION?

As part of cytogenetic testing, the structure of each chromosome is assessed for (1) evidence of losses or gains of material; (2) internal rearrangements within the chromosomes; (3) exchange of material between members of the same chromosome pair; or (4) exchange of material between chromosomes of different pairs. Rearrangements are described based on microscopic examination of the chromosomes and the internal banding pattern within the rearranged chromosome(s).

Depending on the population studied and methods used, structural rearrangements of chromosomes are observed in 1:200–1:500 individuals.[1,2] Unexpected rearrangements on prenatal chromosome tests occur at the higher end of this rate estimate.

HOW ARE STRUCTURAL CHROMOSOME REARRANGEMENTS CATEGORIZED AS BALANCED OR UNBALANCED?

G-banded chromosome analysis is used to determine whether structural rearrangements appear balanced, when all of the genetic material is retained, even though a portion of chromosome material may be aligned in a different sequence within that chromosome or may be moved to another chromosome. The determination that a structural rearrangement is balanced is based on high-resolution banding and implies that on clinical evaluation the person with the rearrangement does not have dysmorphic features, structural malformations, or developmental delays consistent with aneuploidy.

Structural rearrangements may occur within a single chromosome, for example, a balanced inversion, or between members of two or more different chromosomes, for example, a balanced translocation. In contrast, unbalanced rearrangements are defined as having a loss or gain of a microscopically visible chromosome segment. Loss or gain of segments smaller than 5–10 Mb requires detection by other methods, particularly chromosomal microarray. Unbalanced rearrangements can occur within a single chromosome, for example, a terminal deletion at or near the tip of one arm of the chromosome or between members of different chromosome pairs in which there are both deleted and duplicated materials as can occur in unbalanced reciprocal translocations. Chromosomal microarray (CMA) offers more precision in delineation of unbalanced structural rearrangements and often enables detection of more complex rearrangements than is evident from traditional cytogenetic testing with high-resolution G-bands.

WHAT ARE DE NOVO STRUCTURAL REARRANGEMENTS?

Balanced structural chromosome changes may be identified as de novo when they are not inherited from a parent. These occur due to breakage of chromosome(s) at one or more locations followed by rejoining of broken ends such that the alignment on the microscopic examination of the chromosome(s) is different than the usual sequence of bands. When portions of chromosome material are lost in the process, the structural rearrangement is unbalanced. It has been estimated that de novo rearrangements occur in approximately 1–2 per 1000 prenatal chromosome tests. Even when they appear balanced, further evaluation by microarray should be performed to identify small imbalances that may not be evident by G-banded karyotype. De novo structural rearrangements that appear to be balanced are sometimes found by microarray to be more

Perinatal Genetics. https://doi.org/10.1016/B978-0-323-53094-1.00005-9

complex than is evident by standard cytogenetics and may harbor clinically significant loss or gain of chromosome material or may result in disruption of a gene or regulatory region. Disruption of a gene or regulatory region may be detected by sequencing in some cases.

WHAT TYPES OF STRUCTURAL REARRANGEMENTS INVOLVE ONLY A SINGLE CHROMOSOME?

Terminal deletions of chromosomes may occur due to a single break in the chromosome with loss of the acentric fragment that is no longer attached to the centromere in subsequent cell division. Terminal deletions or duplications of the end of a chromosome may be recognizable cytogenetically because in addition to a change in banding pattern, they may result in a change in the ratio of the length of the short and long arms of the chromosome. Generally, small deletions are more compatible with survival. Examples of deletion syndromes that have been described based on cytogenetic detection are Wolf-Hirschhorn syndrome (4p deletion) and cri-du-chat syndrome (5p deletion). Cytogenetic diagnosis of deletions is infrequent when compared with detection by microarray.

WHAT ARE RING CHROMOSOMES?

Chromosomes with simultaneous breaks in the short arm and long arm may assume the configuration of a ring upon reunion of the broken ends (Fig. 5.1). The diagnosis of a ring chromosome implies deletion of the acentric fragments that result from the breakage, and the ring typically includes both variable size segments of the terminal short-arm and long-arm material of that chromosome. Rings of the same chromosome present with a wide range of phenotypic findings. During mitosis, rings may be lost, duplicate, contract, or form duplicated interlocking rings. Mosaicism for a ring combined with variations in constitution of the ring in different percentages of cells make prediction of the phenotype difficult when a ring is found on prenatal cytogenetic diagnosis. Prenatal counseling is dependent not only on review of the literature but also on anatomic findings by imaging with ultrasound and/or MRI. Ring chromosomes initially diagnosed by prenatal microarray often result in highly unusual findings that may be best resolved by confirmatory cytogenetic visualization of the ring and the variant forms observed. Rings involve one member of a chromosome pair and are due to de novo events. They are not likely to recur except in the unusual event of gonadal mosaicism for the ring chromosome in one of the parents.

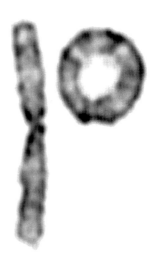

FIG. 5.1 Normal #3 chromosome on left and ring #3 chromosome on right.

WHAT ARE ISOCHROMOSOMES?

Isochromosomes are chromosomes composed of mirror images of one of the arms of the chromosome. As a result, the opposite chromosome arm may be deleted and the cells only have a single copy of the genetic material in the arm present in the normal member of the homologous pair. The other homolog has both the normal short arm and normal long arm (Fig. 5.2). As a result, the cells with an isochromosome have trisomy for the arm that is duplicated in the isochromosome and monosomy for the arm that is not present in the isochromosome. Several mechanisms have been postulated for the formation of isochromosomes, including misdivision of the centromere or sister chromatid breakage and reunion in an area adjacent to the centromere. Many isochromosomes have two centromeres and are dicentric.

An isochromosome of the long arm, the X chromosome, is found in 15%–18% of Turner syndrome cases, and the phenotype is due to having only a single copy of Xp (on the other, normal X). Isochromosomes of Yp are usually dicentric and loss of this structurally abnormal Y may result in mosaicism for a 45,X cell line (see page 34, chapter 4).

Unlike the isochromosome of the long arm of the X and the isodicentric Y, other isochromosomes encountered in prenatal diagnosis are often small supernumerary derivatives that are mosaic. Several of these were initially categorized as marker chromosomes until the source of the genetic material was identified and a syndrome described. Isochromosomes that may be encountered in prenatal diagnosis include (1) cat eye syndrome (CES) due to an isochromosome consisting of a fusion

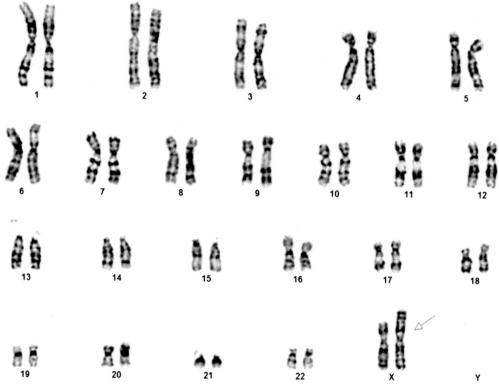

FIG. 5.2 Karyotype from a patient with clinical features of Turner syndrome. The X chromosome on the left is normal and the X chromosome on the right is an isochromosome of the long arm of the X. Arrow points to the mirror image of the long arm that is above the centromere.

of the short-arm centromeres and proximal long arm of chromosome 22; (2) tetrasomy 15q due to an isochromosome consisting of the short arms, centromeres, and proximal long arm of 15q; (3) Pallister-Killian syndrome that is typically due to mosaicism for supernumerary isochromosome of 12p (tetrasomy 12p). Associated diaphragmatic hernia often leads to diagnosis by amniocentesis when the fetus has Pallister-Killian syndrome. An interesting feature of Pallister-Killian is tissue-limited mosaicism in which peripheral blood often does not demonstrate the finding by chromosome analysis.

WHAT ARE PARACENTRIC INVERSIONS ?

Two types of chromosome inversions are seen with very different effects on reproductive potential. Paracentric inversions may occur when there are two breaks on the same chromosome arm (i.e., on one side or the other of the centromere) and reunion occurs after the segment between the breaks flips 180 degrees (Fig. 5.3A). Balanced paracentric inversions may be inherited by familial transmission, and the only phenotypic effect is diminished

reproductive potential. Depending on the size of the inversion, it is difficult for the inverted segment to align and recombine with the noninverted homolog during meiosis. If there are an even number of crossovers on the inverted segment during meiosis, a conception will have a 50% chance of inheriting either the balanced paracentric inversion or the normal homolog that is not inverted. If an odd number (e.g., 1,3,5) of crossovers occur in the inverted segment, daughter cells will inherit either an acentric chromosome derivative that will be lost in subsequent cell divisions or a large dicentric derivative chromosome with deletion of material (Fig. 5.3B). In both instances, participation in fertilization would expect to result in failure of early development or fetal loss.

WHAT ARE PERICENTRIC INVERSIONS?

Pericentric inversions are more common than paracentric inversions and occur when the breaks are on opposite arms or sides of the centromere (Fig. 5.3A). Pairing during meiosis requires the formation of an inversion loop. Similar to paracentric inversions, an even number of exchanges or crossovers in the inversion loop will result in normal gametes, with one-half inheriting the balanced pericentric inversion. In contrast, an odd number of crossovers will result in aneuploid gametes, which will have trisomy for the distal portion of the short arm and monosomy for the distal part of the long arm (Fig. 5.3C), or the derivative chromosomes can have monosomy of the distal portion of the short arm and trisomy of the distal part of the long arm. The combination of a monosomic region and a trisomic region might not

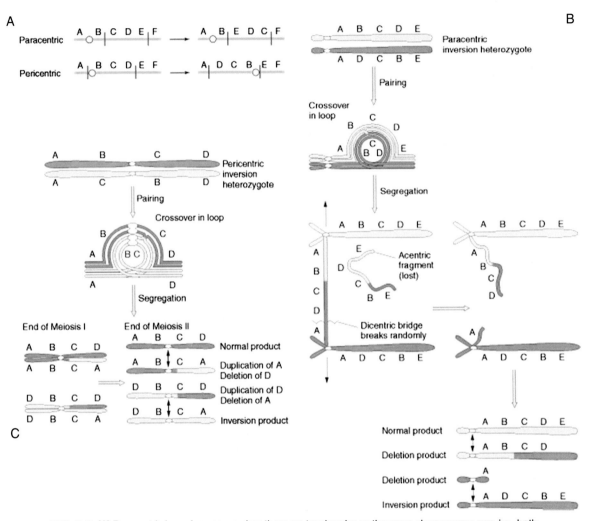

FIG. 5.3 **(A)** Paracentric inversions occur when there are two breaks on the same chromosome arm, i.e., both breaks are on the same side of the centromere. In the example shown above, the breaks occur in the long arm between (B–C) and (E–F). The segment CDE then flips 180 degrees and reunification occurs. The new sequence of segments is A-centromere-BEDCF. Pericentric inversions occur when there is a break on both sides of the centromere. In the example shown above, the break in the short arm occurs between A and the centromere and the break in the long arm occurs between D and E. The segment including the centromere then flips 180 degrees and reunification occurs. The new sequence of segments is ADCB-centromere-EF. **(B)** Heterozygous paracentric inversion. On pairing, in meiosis, a loop is formed. An odd number of crossovers in the loop (one crossover depicted) result in a large dicentric chromosome and smaller acentric fragment. Subsequent breakage of the large dicentric chromosome may result in derivatives with deletions of a portion of the DNA. Fifty percent chance that normal offspring inherit normal homolog or the homolog with the paracentric inversion. **(C)** A pericentric inversion. On pairing, in meiosis, a loop is formed. An odd number of crossovers in the loop (one crossover depicted) result in homologs with duplication of the short arm and deletion of the long arm or deletion of the short arm and duplication of the long arm. Normal offspring has a 50% chance of inheriting the balanced inversion.

be compatible with live birth unless the monosomy is small. The smaller the inverted segment, the larger the partial trisomy and partial monosomy and the higher the likelihood of early spontaneous loss. Thus, large pericentric inversions have a greater chance of resulting in the birth of a child with aneuploidy, whereas some small pericentric inversions are more likely to be associated with recurrent loss due to duplication and/or deletion of large chromosome segments.

IS THERE A CONCERN ABOUT THE COMMON PERICENTRIC INVERSIONS OF CHROMOSOME 9?

A pericentric inversion seen in chromosome 9 is so common as to be classified as a normal variant. It occurs in 1%–2% of the normal population. The breakpoints are commonly designated p11 in the short arm and q12 or q13 in the long arm. This inversion has not been associated with any phenotypic features or adverse reproductive effects, such as an increased frequency of pregnancy loss or unbalanced forms in offspring of carriers. Based on the frequency of this finding in the general population, it is not surprising that individuals who are homozygous for the inverted 9 have been reported and also do not appear to have phenotypic findings or reproductive problems related to the inversion. Similar to other balanced inversions, the pericentric 9 inversion is transmitted in a dominant manner. One-half of the normal offspring of a parent with this inversion are expected to have the inversion. Some laboratories do not report normal variants including the pericentric inversion of 9. If this is reported, the karyotype nomenclature after 46XX or 46XY should indicate (inv9) (p11q12) or (inv9) (p11q13). The common rationale for not reporting a pericentric inversion 9 is that it is not medically actionable. Other normal variants are similarly not usually reported.

WHAT ARE THE TYPES OF BALANCED TRANSLOCATIONS?

Two different types of balanced translocations are distinguished in humans. Robertsonian translocations involve centric fusion of two acrocentric chromosomes and occur in about 1:1000 people, whereas balanced reciprocal translocations involve exchange of material between any of the chromosomes and occur in about 1:700–1:750 people.

Robertsonian translocations occur between two acrocentric chromosomes. The acrocentric chromosomes include chromosomes 13, 14, 15, 21, and 22. By virtue of the fusion of two acrocentric chromosomes,

balanced carriers only have 45 distinctly separate chromosomes in their cells. The breaks resulting in the translocation generally occur in the short arms. When the fusion occurs, the short-arm material is lost in subsequent divisions, but this does not have clinical implications. The most common Robertsonian translocation in humans is a 13/14 fusion chromosome. The cytogenetic designation of a balanced carrier is either 45,XY,rob(13;14) (q10;q10) or 45,XY,der(13;14) (q10;q10). This nomenclature means that there are 45 chromosomes in the cells with a normal male sex chromosome complement and a Robertsonian translocation with a derivative chromosome that is composed of a 13 and 14 chromosome with the breakpoints at q10, which is just at the centromere. Some Robertsonian translocation chromosomes have only one visible centromere, whereas others are dicentric.

Based on the difference in chromosome number, Robertsonian translocations are readily detected by standard cytogenetic analysis and most are familial. The fusion of these two chromosomes does not affect function or have any associated phenotypic features. The short-arm material above the centromere is generally lost in subsequent cell divisions.

WHAT ARE THE REPRODUCTIVE RISKS ASSOCIATED WITH ROBERTSONIAN TRANSLOCATIONS?

There are six potential combinations of the three chromosomes that can go to the gametes, but these do not occur with equal frequency (see Fig. 5.4). Segregation of the two independent chromosomes with normal structure (e.g., in the case of a 13/14 translocation, the single 13 and 14) will result in a gamete that will have a normal chromosome constitution and result in a conception of a pregnancy with either 46,XY or 46,XX, provided the other partner contributed a normal chromosome complement. If the fusion chromosome goes to a gamete, the conception will have the same balanced rearrangement as the parent. Thus, individuals with a balanced translocation can be assured that they can have normal offspring and should be told that one-half of their normal children will be carriers of the translocation.

Sometimes the fusion chromosome and one of the independent homologs will segregate to the gamete. In that case, when fertilization occurs, the conception will inherit three copies of that chromosome, i.e., one from each parent and one in the fusion chromosome. In the example of a 13/14 translocation, this would result in trisomy 13 or trisomy 14. The pregnancies with two independent copies of chromosome 14 and a third copy in the fusion chromosome would result in early miscarriage.

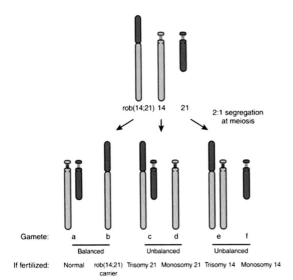

rob(14;21) 14   21

2:1 segregation at meiosis

Gamete: a   b   c   d   e   f

Balanced   Unbalanced   Unbalanced

If fertilized: Normal   rob(14;21) Trisomy 21 Monosomy 21 Trisomy 14 Monosomy 14
                  carrier

FIG. 5.4 Meiotic segregation in a robertsonian t(14;21) (q10;q10) carrier. Of six possible gametes after 2:1 segregation, two (a and b) will be balanced and four (c, d, e, and f) will be unbalanced. Of the unbalanced gametes, only one (c) has the potential to result in a liveborn offspring. (From Yen and Jaffe's Reproductive Endocrinology, by Jerome F Strauss, Robert L. Barbieri, Sixth Edition, Elsevier.)

A majority, but not all, of the conceptions with three copies of chromosome 13 will also be lost spontaneously in the first trimester. A portion of the continuing pregnancies will have trisomy 13 syndrome due to an unbalanced 13/14 translocation. Ultrasound examination during the late first trimester and early second trimester is highly sensitive to detect trisomy 13 syndrome. Even though many pregnancies with trisomy 13 syndrome are spontaneously lost, the chance of pregnancies of individual carriers continuing well into the second trimester is sufficient to recommend diagnostic testing if the couple wishes to avoid the late spontaneous loss or birth of child with trisomy 13 syndrome. Of the remaining two of the six combinations, one would have monosomy for 13 and the other would have monosomy for 14. Both would end very early, possibly before diagnosis of pregnancy.

WHICH UNBALANCED ROBERTSONIAN TRANSLOCATIONS MAY CAUSE DOWN SYNDROME?

About 3%–4% of Down syndrome occurs because of an unbalanced translocation. Any Robertsonian translocation involving a translocation of 21 can result in offspring with Down syndrome. This includes 13/21, 14/21, 15/21, 21/21, and 21/22. A 21/21 translocation is a special situation that will be discussed separately

below. A balanced or unbalanced Robertsonian translocation in a pregnancy or newborn is often inherited because of a parental balanced translocation, but occasionally, de novo Robertsonian translocations are seen.

The risk of having a child with chromosome imbalance is determined by empirical studies and varies depending on the chromosomes involved. A 14/21 Robertsonian fusion chromosome is the most common translocation leading to Down syndrome. Children with Down syndrome on this basis have two separate 21 chromosomes and a third copy of a 21 attached to the short arm of one of their #14 chromosomes. By count, they have 46 chromosomes in their cells, one is a separate 14, another is a 14 with a 21 attached, and there are two separate 21's. This is in contrast to the balanced carriers who have 45 chromosomes in their cells, only one 14, one 21, and the fusion chromosome with a 14 and 21 attached to each other. Children with Down syndrome due to an unbalanced Robertsonian translocation are clinically indistinguishable from children with Down syndrome due to 47 chromosomes with three separate copies of #21 chromosomes in all of their cells. If the mother carries a 14/21 translocation, it has been observed that the chance of amniocentesis resulting in a diagnosis of Down syndrome is 10%–15%. If the father is the carrier of the translocation, it has been observed that the risk of Down syndrome is lower and is often estimated to be 2%.[3] The reason for this difference has not been explained. It has been speculated that sperm with unbalanced chromosome content may be less effective at fertilization.

Cell-free DNA screening for Down syndrome is based on the quantity of cell-free DNA from the #21 chromosomes in the cells. Trisomy 21 with three separate #21 and unbalanced translocations with three copies of #21 in the cells are indistinguishable by cell-free DNA testing and presumably the sensitivity of the testing is the same. Similarly, confirmation of the diagnosis of Down syndrome by microarray does not distinguish between Down syndrome due to three separate 21 chromosomes and an unbalanced translocation. Understanding the mechanism and projecting recurrence risks require cytogenetic evaluation.

WHAT IS DIFFERENT ABOUT HOMOLOGOUS ROBERTSONIAN TRANSLOCATIONS (E.G., 21/21 OR 13/13)?

Rare cases of Down syndrome occur due to 21/21 Robertsonian translocations. Also, 13/13 translocations have been reported in cases of trisomy 13 syndrome. Many cases appear to be de novo events, but a balanced parental translocation 21/21 has serious

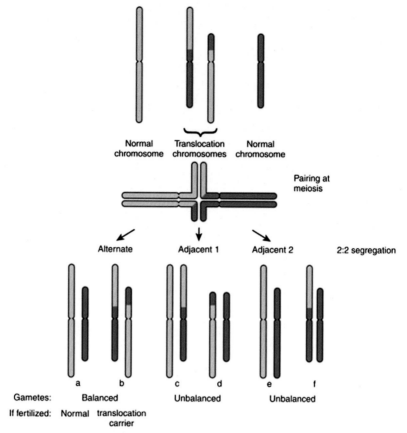

FIG. 5.5 Meiotic segregation with a reciprocal translocation. Of six possible gametes after 2:2 segregation, two will be balanced (a and b) and four will be unbalanced (c, d, e, and f). After fertilization with anormal haploid gamete, gamete a will produce a chromosomally normal conceptus and gamete b will producea balanced carrier of the translocation. (From Yen and Jaffe's Reproductive Endocrinology, by JeromeF Strauss, Robert L. Barbieri, Sixth Edition, Elsevier.)

implications for reproduction. A parent with this finding would have 45 chromosomes by count with two copies of 21 fused. At gametogenesis, they would contribute either the 21q21q fusion chromosome resulting in a Down syndrome conception or if they did not contribute the 21q21q fusion chromosome, a conception would be lost due to monosomy 21; therefore, a euploid conception is impossible for such a carrier. Couples who have a loss or Down syndrome offspring on this basis should have chromosome studies. The risk of recurrence to parents who conceive a pregnancy with a de novo homologous Robertsonian translocation would be limited to the risk associated with low-percentage parental mosaicism or to gonadal mosaicism.

The concerns about imprinting disorders are also relevant to nonhomologous and homologous Robertsonian translocations that involve chromosome 14 or 15 (see Chapter 2) and warrant offering fetal UPD testing when one parent is a balanced carrier, including when the fetus has inherited either the balanced translocation and when the fetus has inherited the normal homologs.[4]

WHAT ARE THE REPRODUCTIVE RISKS DUE TO RECIPROCAL TRANSLOCATIONS?

All of the chromosomes, including the acrocentric chromosomes and the sex chromosomes, can participate in reciprocal translocations. For example, an acrocentric chromosome may participate in a reciprocal translocation by having an exchange between the long arm of the acrocentric and another chromosome. Translocation may occur between the X and Y or between the X or Y and any autosome. Translocation between the X and Y chromosomes may occur when their pseudoautosomal regions pair in meiosis.

Assessing the reproductive risk of translocations can be difficult. Most reciprocal translocations encountered in practice are unique and case reports of individuals with exactly the same break points resulting in both duplication and deletion are usually not available. Case reports of duplications or deletions of the regions involved often only have one but not the other or involve a different chromosome. Factors to consider are the size of the duplicated and/or deleted material that may result, the genes in those segments, and the different segregation patterns discussed below that may occur. Family history can be helpful when there is an affected relative, but a family history may only confirm that the derivatives are consistent with surviving offspring with aneuploidy but not enable numerical estimation of risk. In that case, an empiric risk of 10%–15% is often estimated based on collective experience. When both of the exchanged segments are large, there are often not reported cases of children with those imbalances and it is likely that the translocation will result in early loss rather than newborns with partial aneuploidy. On the other hand, unbalanced translocations that duplicate material from 13, 18, and 21 with very small reciprocal deletions may be more likely to result in newborns with partial aneuploidy.

WHAT ARE THE DIFFERENT TYPES OF SEGREGATION OF RECIPROCAL TRANSLOCATIONS IN MEIOSIS?

Reciprocal translocations require formation of a quadrivalent in meiosis to allow pairing and exchanges between homologs. At the conclusion of meiosis, there are six possible combinations for 2:2 segregation (Fig. 5.5). The two that are most common are alternate segregation resulting in balanced gametes with 50% inheriting the normal homologs and the other 50% inheriting the balanced translocation. The remaining 2:2 segregation patterns are adjacent type I and adjacent type II. With adjacent type I segregation, the centromeres of translocated derivative and the normal chromosome go to opposite poles. After fertilization with a normal gamete, different duplications and deletions are observed. Adjacent type II segregation is very uncommon, probably because it requires that the homologous centromeres of both chromosomes migrate to the same pole of the spindle apparatus. Adjacent Type II derivatives are very infrequently seen in children with aneuploidy.

WHAT FACTORS MAY INFLUENCE THE OCCURRENCE OF 3:1 SEGREGATION OF A RECIPROCAL TRANSLOCATION?

It is observed that 3:1 rather than 2:2 segregation may occur when there is small derivative, particularly when that derivative is an acrocentric chromosome. In general, 3:1 segregation is thought to occur because the small derivative may be dragged along with two other chromosomes during meiosis; such 3:1 segregation results in trisomy for portions of two chromosomes. Depending on the chromosomes and the sizes of the duplicated fragments, they may be consistent with survival of children with aneuploidy or partial aneuploidy. An 11/22 chromosome translocation is the most common recurrent constitutional reciprocal translocation in humans. The distal long arm of a #11 chromosome and that of a #22 chromosome are exchanged. During meiosis, the quadrivalent is formed, and the normal 11, normal 22, and the small derivative segregate to the gamete. The 3:1 segregation results in a small 47th chromosome composed of the short arm-centromere-proximal long arm of chromosome 22 with the attached distal long arm of chromosome 11. This cytogenetic abnormality results in combined trisomy for the proximal long arm of 22 and the distal long arm of the 11 and is associated with Emanuel syndrome. The translocation is sufficiently common to assess the reproductive outcomes of carriers. The risk for 3:1 segregation if the mother is a carrier is about 6% and is 2%–5% if the father is the carrier. One-half of the normal offspring are balanced carriers. Involvement of acrocentric chromosomes is not required for 3:1 segregation. Other examples of reciprocal translocations have been reported to have 3:1 segregation when one derivative is the entire short arm and centromere of a midsized chromosome. These small derivatives may also be dragged along in meiosis; cases of trisomy 9p and trisomy 12p have been reported on this basis.

ARE THERE OTHER TYPES OF TRANSLOCATIONS AND STRUCTURAL REARRANGEMENTS?

Other rearrangements not discussed above, such as insertions and tandem duplications, are rarely encountered in prenatal diagnosis. Translocations involving three chromosomes and more than three breaks are rare and are referred to as complex chromosome rearrangements (CCRs). In a collaborative study of 246 de novo balanced chromosome rearrangements in a prenatal diagnostic laboratory, only 3% were classified as CCRs.[5] Definition of the chromosome structure in these cases may require a combination of cytogenetic, FISH, microarray, and sequencing technology.[6]

WHAT ARE MARKER CHROMOSOMES?

Occasionally, small extra structural abnormal (ESAC) or supernumerary chromosomes are seen in cells during a cytogenetic test. These most likely arise as a result of structural rearrangements and may be retained through cell divisions because of the presence of a centromere. Some very small markers appear to have a ring configuration. The term "marker" is used to signify that these fragments of chromatin are not otherwise cytogenetically identifiable. Supernumerary marker chromosomes are presumably subject to loss in mitosis and are often seen as a mosaic cell line. They may be inherited in a family, and instances of familial mosaicism for the marker have been observed. Often, small familial markers are not associated with any consistent clinical finding or phenotype. This is particularly true when very small markers in a low percentage of cells. Prenatal detection of a marker is problematic because it is difficult to predict whether there will be phenotypic abnormalities as a result of the marker.

Estimates of frequency in live born children and in adults suggest that markers occur in about 1:10,000 individuals. Those detected in children seem to have a higher frequency of phenotypic effects when compared with those diagnosed prenatally. All or part of this difference may be due to ascertainment bias. In contrast, the frequency of prenatal detection of markers has been reported in approximately 1:1000 amniocenteses.[7] About one-third of these are familial. Parental studies, outcome, and follow-up are not consistently available from the reports of marker chromosomes. The possibility of adverse outcomes, even with normal ultrasound findings, has been estimated to range between 5% and 18%.[8]

The evaluation of marker chromosomes should include parental chromosome analysis. In some instances, concern for mosaicism may require examination of more than 20 cells. If a marker is familial, any family members with potentially phenotypic effects should be considered for testing to determine whether the marker may be associated with a phenotype. Identification of the marker should be discussed with the laboratory. Identification of the chromosome of origin and the gene content of the marker should be evaluated using FISH and/or chromosomal microarray, which can often identify the additional genetic material composing the marker chromosome.

WHEN IS CHROMOSOME EVALUATION RECOMMENDED FOR PARENTS OF A PREGNANCY OR FOR COUPLES CONSIDERING A FUTURE PREGNANCY?

Parental chromosome tests should be performed when unanticipated structural chromosome rearrangements are encountered in prenatal genetic diagnosis. In many instances, finding a balanced structural rearrangement in a parent provides reassurance that the fetus has the same balanced rearrangement. In other cases, parental testing may identify that a rearrangement is de novo, and although it may appear balanced, a fetal microarray should be recommended to determine whether there is extra or missing genetic material not visible by karyotype.

Parental chromosome testing may be requested if there is a family history of a chromosome disorder that may be due to a familial rearrangement or if there are family members who have a constellation of malformations, dysmorphic features, or developmental delay that may be associated with an aneuploidy.

Chromosome testing is often performed in males with infertility. Several studies of men with infertility have observed a high frequency of numerical and structural chromosome abnormalities compared with the general population. For example, in one such study, a genetic basis was found in approximately one-half of men with azoospermia or oligospermia. In addition to detection of 47,XXY or structural abnormalities involving the Y chromosome, the frequency of balanced structural chromosome abnormalities was increased compared with the expected rate. These included Robertsonian and reciprocal translocations, as well as inversions.[9] It is not clear why some men with balanced translocations have azoospermia, whereas others appear to have normal fertility. The detection of translocations or inversions in male partners of infertile couples may be useful in deliberations regarding testicular sperm aspiration, preimplantation genetic screening or testing, and for prenatal diagnosis.

IS THERE VALUE IN TESTING COUPLES WITH RECURRENT PREGNANCY LOSS?

A number of studies of couples with two or more pregnancy losses have demonstrated translocations or clinically relevant inversions in one partner in 3%–5% of these couples.[10] Unbalanced translocations or inversions may cause loss at any gestational age and are also associated with births of abnormal offspring. Couples in whom one parent has a translocation or inversion would be expected to experience an increased frequency of early pregnancy loss.

Although a structural rearrangement cannot be changed or corrected, knowledge of the reason for repeated loss is valuable. In addition to providing a probable chromosomal basis for the previous losses, the detection of a translocation or inversion may provide a rationale for reducing risk by using preimplantation testing or donor gametes. It may also help define the management strategy for prenatal screening or diagnosis. As many structural rearrangements are familial, reviewing which family members might benefit from the information and suggestions about how to approach them is an important part of the counseling.

It is generally recommended that testing of normal offspring of translocation or inversion carriers should not be initiated until they reach reproductive age. Similarly, when there has been prenatal diagnosis of an inherited balanced structural rearrangement, delaying disclosure until reproductive age has been recommended. This is done not only to avoid emotional impact of the information, which may be poorly understood in childhood or adolescence, but also because the impact and options for reducing risk may be quite different when they reach reproductive age.

REFERENCES

1. Van Dyke DL, Weiss L, Roberson JR, Babu VR. The frequency and mutation rate of balanced autosomal rearrangements in man estimated from prenatal genetic studies for advanced maternal age. *Am J Hum Genet.* 1983;35:301–308.
2. Hook EB, Schreinemachers DM, Willey AM, Cross PK. Inherited structural cytogenetic abnormalities detected incidentally in fetuses diagnosed prenatally: frequency, parental-age associations, sex-ratio trends, and comparisons with rates of mutants. *Am J Hum Genet.* 1984;36:422–443.
3. Boué A, Gallano P. A collaborative study of the segregation of inherited chromosome structural rearrangements in 1356 prenatal diagnoses. *Prenat Diagn.* 1984;4:45–67.
4. Yip M-Y. Uniparental disomy in Robertsonian translocations: strategies for uniparental disomy testing. *Transl Pedatr.* 2014;3(2):98–107.
5. Giardino D, Corti C, Ballarati L, et al. *De novo* balanced chromosome rearrangements in prenatal diagnosis. *Prenat Diagn.* 2009;29:257–265.
6. Macera MJ, Sobrino A, Levy B, et al. Prenatal diagnosis of chromothripsis, with nine breaks characterized by karyotyping, FISH, microarray and whole-genome sequencing. *Prenat Diagn.* 2015;35(3):299–301.
7. Liehr T, Weise A. Frequency of small supernumerary marker chromosomes in prenatal, newborn, developmentally retarded and infertility diagnostics. *Int J Mol Med.* 2007;19:719–731.
8. Graf MD, Christ L, Mascarello JT, et al. Redefining the risks of prenatally ascertained supernumerary marker chromosomes: a collaborative study. *J Med Genet.* 2006;43:660–664. https://doi.org/10.1136/jmg2005.037887.
9. Yatsenko AN, Yatsenko SA, Weedin JW, et al. Comprehensive 5-year study of cytogenetic aberrations in 668 infertile men. *J Urol.* 2010;183(4):1636–1642. https://doi.org/10.1016/j.juro.2009.12.004.
10. Campana M, Serra A, Neri G. Role of chromosome aberrations in recurrent abortion: a study of 269 balanced translocations. *Am J Med Genet.* 1986;24:341–356.

CHAPTER 6

Molecular Genetics

STEPHANIE GUSEH, MD • REBECCA REIMERS, MD, MPH •
LOUISE WILKINS-HAUG, MD, PHD

INTRODUCTION

In 2003, the sequencing of the human genome propelled the field of genetics in two important directions. Firstly, the concept of "genomics" emerged, which includes both the DNA sequence itself (the blueprint letters that direct genetic contributions to health, variation, and disease) and the response of the DNA to modifiers that alter gene expression (such as the environment or other genes). Additionally, genomics encompasses the genetic applications used for diagnostic and therapeutic medical decision-making and the role of genetics in policy development. Secondly, advances in molecular technologies also arose from the sequencing of the human genome. These tools continue to develop with refinements that expand their application, provide faster time to results, and require diminishing amounts of DNA at a dramatically reduced cost. These molecular tools increase our knowledge of basic biology as well as contribute to the identification and treatment of genetic diseases.

As genetic investigation accelerates, a previously unappreciated degree of DNA sequence variability between humans is being recognized. This variation modulates an individual's response to his/her environment such as the differential responses to medications, susceptibility to adult onset disease (such as diabetes and hypertension), and the likelihood of cancer. Even among recognized Mendelian disorders, gene sequencing continues to document extensive individual variability. For example, the gene responsible for classic cystic fibrosis (CF), the cystic fibrosis transmembrane conductance regulator (CFTR) gene, has more than 1000 different variations. In the prenatal arena, examining genes with sequence variations of unknown significance for the developing fetus is an active area of research.

As of 2018, a number of laboratories offer sequencing of an individual's DNA for less than $1500 and with completion within several months. This is in stark contrast to the $2.7 billion dollars and more than 10 years required to sequence the first human genome. However, although the sequence of nucleotide base pairs within an individual's DNA can now be determined relatively quickly

and inexpensively, an unfathomable amount of information regarding the 3 billion base pairs in an individual's genome is returned. Any one person's unique DNA sequence, if written in 12.0-point font, would span from New York to California. Obtaining the DNA sequence is only one part of a much larger endeavor to understand how the person's genome, or blueprint, impacts cell functioning and ultimately the individual's appearance and function of various organs (phenotype). The study of DNA has evolved from a bird's-eye view of the number of chromosomes (karyotype) to the ability to study a specific gene (genotype), to a more granular level of analysis of the entire genome (whole genome sequencing [WGS]). This chapter will review the various single gene alterations that occur, the technologies in use today, and help the reader develop a framework for understanding genetic disease and human variation in the context of genomics.

WHAT ARE THE MOLECULAR CHANGES THAT OCCUR IN SINGLE GENES?

The ability to examine a specific segment of DNA for changes in the nucleic acid base sequence has rapidly evolved over the past 10 years. With lower costs and faster time to results, the detection of single gene disorders has accelerated (Fig. 6.1).[1] As importantly, a growing understanding of the complexity of the path from nucleotide base sequence to RNA to protein to disease is emerging.

An individual's DNA sequence provides instructions for the orderly development of proteins. Proteins play key roles in the development and function of cells and tissues, maintaining system functions and interacting with the environment. Changes in protein function or quantity can affect these systems. Protein production starts with the molecular reading of the DNA nucleotide bases that contain the genetic line-up (or sequence) that will direct protein development (the exon) as well as the spacing DNA segments that are not incorporated into the protein instructions (the introns). The introns are ultimately removed, leaving the exons and the

Perinatal Genetics. https://doi.org/10.1016/B978-0-323-53094-1.00006-0

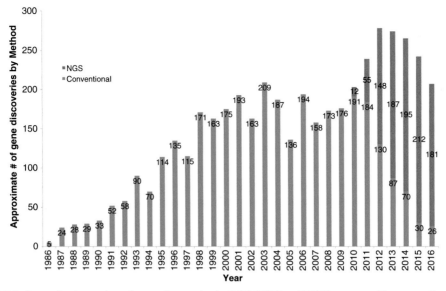

FIG. 6.1 Approximate number of gene discoveries by NGS (WES and WGS) compared to conventional approaches (from Boycott K, 2017).

final template for the protein. This final template then directs the order of the amino acids that together construct a unique protein. Further modifications to the proteins are then sometime incorporated, with changes to the final protein product in ways that impact health, disease, and interaction with the environment.

WHAT ARE THE DIFFERENT TYPES OF PATHOGENIC VARIANTS?

Several types of DNA changes can occur, some of which mean that the protein is absent or no longer functions in the typical fashion. As noted in Table 6.1, the specifics of an alteration, such as the location and size, can have profoundly different effects. In some cases, small changes such as a single nucleic acid base substitution can result in significant disease if the protein produced is damaged. A "point mutation" is a change in a single base pair that can cause a substitution, deletion, or insertion that leads to a heritable change in the quality and quantity of protein produced. A "nonsense" variant can prematurely stop the template and the protein from developing. Frameshift variants are insertions or deletions in the genome that are not in multiples of three nucleotides and therefore result in a change in the gene's reading frame. Variants can also be "silent" if they do not produce a change in

TABLE 6.1
Types of DNA sequence variants and examples of diseases

Variant	Overview	Example
Missense	Variant leading to a different amino acid in translation	Sickle cell anemia
Nonsense	Variant leading to a stop codon, where there is premature termination of translation	Hemophilia A
Frameshift	Base pair insertion or deletion that alters the reading frame of translation	Tay-Sachs
Splice site	Base pair change that leads to errors in post-translation modifications	Adenosine Deaminase deficiency
Transition	Variant that changes a purine base for a purine (A and G), or a pyrimidine for a pyrimidine (C and T)	Beta thalassemia
Transver-sion	Variant that changes a purine base (A or G) for a pyrimidine (C or T), or vice versa	Beta thalassemia

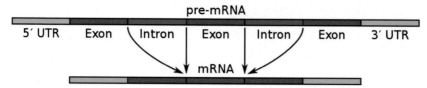

FIG. 6.2 DNA segments code for both introns and exons. A process of maturing occurs by splicing out the introns and connecting the exons as pre-mRNA is converted to mRNA as the template for protein production. Variants can occur in the splice site junctions. "Pre-mRNA to mRNA" By Qef – Own work by uploader, based on the arrangement of a bitmap equivalent by TedE (Public Domain) via Commons Wikimedia

the encoded amino acid. In a large gene, such as the CFTR gene responsible for CF, all three types—missense, nonsense, and frameshift—can occur.

Variants can also occur at the stage of remodeling of the longer template to a shorter version with removal of introns (the nonprotein coding regions) leaving only the exons (protein coding). Splice sites and splice site variants can exist at the sites where the introns are removed. Changes at splice sites can alter the final protein product and in some cases lead to disease.[2] (Fig. 6.2) Introns also play a part in this step and can produce different exon arrangements to make different protein products. In addition, control of the on/off reading of DNA templates is also vulnerable to variation.[3]

The relationship between a genetic variant and the resulting changes in cell development or function, or the "phenotype," is complex. Similar phenotypes can be produced by different types of variants within the same gene (termed allelic heterogeneity) and even by variants in different genes (termed locus heterogeneity). Additionally, the same gene variant may create different phenotypes (polypheny) depending on other modifying genes or the environment.[4,5] One common example of a gene in which variants can cause different disorders is the human beta globin gene. Different variants in this gene can cause beta thalassemia, sickle cell disease, or methemoglobinemia with differing clinical severity and presentation.[5,6]

For a comprehensive description of phenotypes and their genotype correlations, the database Online Mendelian Inheritance in Man (OMIM) is an excellent resource (http://www.omim.org/).

WHAT OTHER CHANGES TO THE DNA CAN PRODUCE VARIATION AND DISEASE?

Control of the onset and duration of transcription of segments of the DNA is essential to the development and function of cells and tissues. This timing can be controlled in several different ways, such as by the configuration of the DNA in its condensed form, by specialized proteins, or by other mechanisms such as methylation. Methylation of designated sites of the DNA to control function is known as "epigenomics." Interaction between the epigenome and the environment plays an important role in the activation or silencing of DNA segments. Methylation and silencing of segments of DNA also plays a role in triplet repeat disorders in which a segment of DNA expands over several generations. Examples include fragile X syndrome and Huntington disease (see Chapter 2).

HOW ARE CHANGES IN THE DNA IDENTIFIED FOR RESEARCH OR IN CLINICAL TESTING?
Genotyping

Genotyping typically evaluates a segment of DNA for previously identified variants. This is in contrast to sequencing, which involves identifying each base pair, or nucleotide, in order, across the length of a gene. Numerous methodologies for genotyping exist. Many of the approaches use indirect means such as altered length of DNA segments, inability to bind to a fluorescently labeled probe, or lack of hybridization to known DNA segments arranged on an array.

The ability to screen large populations of individuals for their carrier status of genetic variants known to cause disease is based largely on genotyping. Genotyping for carrier detection can be useful in homogeneous populations such as the Ashkenazi Jewish (AJ). In this population, because of religious and geographic considerations, genetic variants have traditionally been passed from one generation to the next rather than dispersed across larger populations. This has resulted in a higher carrier frequency for specific autosomal recessive conditions because of a limited number of specific variants. Common examples include Tay-Sachs disease, familial dysautonomia, and Canavan disease (Table 6.2).[7]

TABLE 6.2
Inherited Disorders among the Ashkenazi Jewish Population

Disease	Inheritance	Carrier frequency
LYSOSOMAL STORAGE DISEASES		
Tay-Sachs	AR	1/30
Gaucher Type 1	AR	1/18
Nieman-Pick Type A	AR	1/80
Mucolipidosis Type IV	AR	1/50
NON-LYSOSOMAL STORAGE DISEASES		
Bloom syndrome	AR	1/1,000
Fanconi anemia C	AR	1/90
Canavan	AR	1/59
Familial dysautonimia	AR	1/30
Familial hyperinsulinism	AR	1/89
Familial hypercholesterolemia	AD	1/56
Congenital adrenal hyperplasia	AR	1/10
Familial nonsyndromic deafness	AR	1/25
Glycogen storage disease type 1A	AR	Unknown
Torsion dystonia	AD	1/2000
Factor XI deficiency	AR	1/190

AD, autosomal dominant; *AR*, autosomal recessive.
(Modified from Kedar-Barnes, 2004.)

Genetic screening for Tay-Sachs disease was first initiated among the AJ population, in whom the carrier rate is high (about 1 in 32), and in whom three hexosaminidase A variants are responsible for 98% of the affected cases.[8] This founder effect means that genotyping targeted to these three specific variants is a very sensitive screen for carriers. Among other ethnic groups, different or unknown variants may occur and therefore a biochemical test that measures hexosaminidase enzyme activity may be more effective as this does not depend on knowing the genes that are responsible.[9]

The same principles apply in testing for other genetic disorders in different ethnic and racial populations. For example, screening for cystic fibrosis carriers usually involves testing for 23 known causative variants. These 23 variants are most common in those

of Northern European or AJ heritage, and 90% of CF carriers will be identified by screening for these 23 variants. In more diverse populations, such as among all people in the United States, detection is lower (77%).[10] This decrease in detection reflects the lower ability of the 23-variant panel to identify the more disparate CF variants in a genetically diverse population. For this reason, the detection rate for CF is lower in Hispanic whites, African Americans, and Asian Americans in whom different, often unknown, variants cause more cases of CF.

Limitations exist with genetic carrier testing by genotyping. Genotyping will only detect known variants in a gene and the frequency with which specific known variants cause disease varies by racial and ethnic heritage. For example, delta F508 is the most common cystic fibrosis variant in Northern Europeans (66%), whereas in African Americans, it represents only 48% of the CFTR variants. Overall, 23% of African Americans have CFTR variants not commonly seen in those with Northern European heritage.[11] With increasing cross-cultural heritage, genotyping for a limited number of variants cannot identify all carriers, and there is always a residual risk that an individual is a carrier even after screening. The amount of residual risk will depend on the number of variants genotyped and the gene frequency within the individual's racial/ethnic background (Table 6.3).

Genotyping can be used in prenatal genetic testing with suspected structural fetal anomalies or syndromes. In this setting, the responsible gene and the specific variant must be known to perform the correct test. Some constellations of fetal findings suggest specific genetic conditions, as with common short-limbed dwarfisms including achondroplasia, thanatophoric dysplasia, or campomelic dysplasia. Targeted genotyping panels can assess for the common variants within selected genes that are most often associated with the ultrasound findings. Targeted panels for specific candidate genes can be relatively inexpensive, with a rapid turnaround time, and fewer nonspecific and incidental genetic findings.[12] Although gene panels can be helpful in testing for several different genes associated with a particular ultrasound finding, genotyping panels will test only for the previously recognized genes. In addition, in some cases, gene panels may have been developed based on pediatric findings, and the fetal phenotype may be different as characteristics may differ or appear only later in gestation. Finally, the discovery of new gene alterations and their association with a disease state continues at a rapid pace and targeted gene panels may quickly become outdated.

TABLE 6.3
Cystic Fibrosis carrier screening residual risk after a negative result

Race or Ethnicity	Prevalence of CF	Carrier Frequency	Carrier Testing Detection Rate	Carrier Risk after Negative Result
Northern European	1/2,500	1/25-1/29	85-90%	1/240
Southern European	1/2,500	1/25-1/29	70%	1/80
Ashkenazi Jewish	1/2,800	1/26-1/29	97%	1/833
Hispanic	1/8,100	1/46	57%	1/113
African American	1/14,500	1/60-1/65	72%	1/198
Asian	1/32,000	1/90	30%	1/128

(From Bajaj, 2014.)

Sequencing

Gene sequencing identifies the nucleic acids and their order in a segment of DNA. The introduction of next-generation sequencing (NGS) (Sanger sequencing being first generation) allowed massively parallel sequencing of millions of DNA segments rapidly and relatively inexpensively. However, the amount of data generated can be enormous and represents only the first step of the analysis. The second or bioinformatics step is necessary to interpret the results and uses computer algorithms, public databases, expert opinion, and sometimes functional analysis (detailed below). Following this assessment, each identified DNA sequence change is categorized based on recommendations of The American College of Medical Genetics and Genomics (ACMG); these five categories include the following: (1) pathogenic, (2) likely pathogenic, (3) uncertain significance, (4) likely benign, and (5) benign. The previously used terms "mutation" and "polymorphism" have been largely replaced by the five categories of genetic variant.[13] What was previously referred to as a "mutation" is now most often considered a "pathogenic" or "likely pathogenic" variant, and a polymorphism should be called a "benign variant." NGS can be used to evaluate specific genes, a portion of the genome or the whole genome.[14]

HOW IS NEXT-GENERATION SEQUENCING USED TO STUDY SPECIFIC GENES?

As discussed above, the utility of genotyping is limited by the need for a prior knowledge of the pathogenic variants associated with the suspected anomaly or syndrome, and the differences in variants in different populations. Application of NGS to single genes can overcome some of these obstacles as it does not require prior knowledge of all variants. In some laboratories, genetic carrier screening uses sequencing rather than genotyping of the gene or genes of interest. When an individual is identified as a carrier of a genetic disease, sequencing their partner may be more sensitive than genotyping for only a limited number of variants and can minimize the residual risk by assuring that the partner's gene is thoroughly examined. Sequencing may also be helpful in settings in which an individual is of an ethnicity for which the genotype panel has low detection.

HOW IS NEXT-GENERATION SEQUENCING USED TO STUDY THE EXOME IN WHOLE EXOME SEQUENCING?

The exome consists of only 2% of the total DNA, although it contains at least 22,000 genes and codes for more than 85% of the recognized Mendelian single gene disorders. With whole exome sequencing (WES), the exons of the protein-coding genes are sequenced and compared with a reference human sequence. Variant sequences are selected using algorithms, and their locations within a gene are established. Bioinformatic interpretation is used to determine whether a specific gene variant is benign or pathogenic (disease producing). Unique data-mining strategies are used as well as consultation with geneticists to interpret the WES findings.[13] Although some sequences will be identified as clearly pathogenic or benign, many of the results fall in the middle and are considered variants of uncertain significance (see Chapter 10).

Evaluation of identified DNA sequence variants may include the following four steps:

1. Comparison of the identified sequence to databases cataloging benign and disease-causing variants.

2. "In silico" or computational analysis for prediction of the variant's effect on the encoded protein.
3. Review or performance of functional studies at the cell, tissue, or animal level.
4. Examination of family members for segregation of the variant and associated phenotype (typically starting with the individual and biologic parents, known as trio analysis).

HOW IS WHOLE EXOME SEQUENCING USED CLINICALLY?

Although the exome consists of 20–25,000 genes, in clinical practice, typically fewer genes are studied by WES. WES can be very useful in testing a large number of genes at the same time, and in cases in which a genetic disorder is suspected, but a specific diagnosis is not evident. However, pretest counseling for WES is important to assure individuals understand the range of results and limitations. First, the degree of certainty of disease associated with an identified variant is important. Anxiety around "uncertain" or "likely" designations is common. Second, discovery of variants in genes unrelated to the reason for testing is possible. Such secondary findings may include detection of carrier states for autosomal recessive and X-linked disorders, increased risks of cancer, and increased risks of adult onset disorders. These incidental findings may be clinically relevant to all the individuals being tested—the parents, the child or fetus, and possibly the extended family. The ACMG endorses a specific list of pathogenic variants that should be assessed and disclosed, as they are considered potentially actionable (e.g., cancer predisposition genes that may indicate a need for surveillance). Many of the genes are related to cardiac health as well as cancer risk. Some laboratories have chosen to expand this list with additional genes (Table 6.4).[15]

Guidelines for use of WES in prenatal diagnosis have been published and represent the opinions of experts across a wide range of disciplines including genetics, maternal fetal medicine, and imaging.[16] Key points include the need for further research and data sharing, restriction of WES to cases in which fetal anomalies are present, use of a trio approach (testing of the fetus and both parents), and the need for extensive pretest and posttest counseling from experts with an understanding of the challenges of interpretation and the limitations of testing.

Although WES can detect numerous gene changes, several limitations exist. Because these techniques are new, many novel variants are identified for which the significance is uncertain. Identification of such novel variants can require considerable evaluation to ascertain whether they are likely disease causing or benign, and the turnaround time for results is often lengthy. Not all types of genetic variants that cause single gene disorders are detected by WES. In particular, small insertions and deletions of DNA (indels) are typically not identified although in some cases these can be disease causing. In addition, it is recognized that some genetic diseases are caused by disorders of gene regulation due to variants in the introns and such variants are not detected by WES, which only studies the exons.

WHAT IS WHOLE GENOME SEQUENCING?

Whereas exome sequencing looks at the 2% of the genome that encodes proteins, WGS sequences the entire genome of an individual, including both the exons and introns. Although this has advantages in more rapid sequencing, the additional data obtained means that the analysis is more complex. It has been suggested that WGS may increase detection of exome containing disease variants as well as capture those variants outside of the exome that have clinical significance. However, there is less clinical experience with WGS, and in one series, the combined increase in disease detection was estimated to be <1% (0.8%).[17]

WHAT OTHER TOOLS ARE USED FOR MOLECULAR GENETIC ANALYSIS?

PCR is an extremely common technique that is used to amplify a single copy or a few copies of a segment of DNA in a short amount of time (Fig. 6.3). PCR is used in a number of testing scenarios, including to identify methylation-specific alterations that may lead to disease (such as Beckwith–Weidemann syndrome [BWS][18]). In BWS, more than half of the causative genetic changes would be undetected by sequencing as they are methylation changes that suppress gene action rather than changes in the gene sequence (Fig. 6.4).[19] For BWS, specialized testing is required to assess methylation.

Another specialized PCR technique is multiplex ligation-dependent probe amplification (MLPA). MLPA can discriminate sequences that differ in only a single nucleotide. One clinical use of MLPA is for spinal muscular atrophy (SMA), a neuromuscular

TABLE 6.4
American College of Medical Genetics and Genomics version 2.0 genes and associated phenotypes recommended for return of secondary findings in clinical sequencing.

Disease name and Molecular Interaction Map (MIM) number	Gene
Adenomatous polyposis coli (MIM 175100)	APC (MIM 611731)
Aortic aneurysm, familial thoracic 4 (MIM 132900)	MYH11 (MIM 160745)
Aortic aneurysm, familial thoracic 6 (MIM 611788)	ACTA2 (MIM 102620)
Arrhythmogenic right ventricular cardiomyopathy, type 5 (MIM 604400)	TMEM43 (MIM 612048)
Arrhythmogenic right ventricular cardiomyopathy, type 8 (MIM 607450)	DSP (MIM 125647)
Arrhythmogenic right ventricular cardiomyopathy, type 9 (MIM 609040)	PKP2 (MIM 602861)
Arrhythmogenic right ventricular cardiomyopathy, type 10 (MIM 610193)	DSG2 (MIM 125671)
Arrhythmogenic right ventricular cardiomyopathy, type 11 (MIM 610476)	DSC2 (MIM 125645)
Breast-ovarian cancer, familial 1 (MIM 604370)	BRCA1 (MIM 113705)
Breast-ovarian cancer, familial 2 (MIM 612555)	BRCA2 (MIM 600185)
Brugada syndrome 1 (MIM 601144)	SCN5A (MIM 600163)
Catecholaminergic polymorphic ventricular tachycardia (MIM 604772)	RYR2 (MIM 180902)
Dilated cardiomyopathy 1A (MIM 115200)	LMNA (MIM 150330)
Dilated cardiomyopathy 1A (MIM 115200)	MYBPC3 (MIM 600958)
Ehlers-Danlos syndrome, type 4 (MIM 130050)	COL3A1 (MIM 120180)
Fabry's disease (MIM 301500)	GLA (MIM 300644)
Familial hypercholesterolemia (MIM 143890)	APOB (MIM 107730)
	LDLR (MIM 606945)
Familial hypertrophic cardiomyopathy 1 (MIM 192600)	MYH7 (MIM 160760)
Familial hypertrophic cardiomyopathy 3 (MIM 115196)	TPM1 (MIM 191010)
Familial hypertrophic cardiomyopathy 4 (MIM 115197)	MYBPC3 (MIM 600958)
Familial hypertrophic cardiomyopathy 6 (MIM 600858)	PRKAG2 (MIM 602743)
Familial hypertrophic cardiomyopathy 7 (MIM 613690)	TNNI3 (MIM 191044)
Familial hypertrophic cardiomyopathy 8 (MIM 608751)	MYL3 (MIM 160790)
Familial hypertrophic cardiomyopathy 10 (MIM 608758)	MYL2 (MIM 160781)
Familial hypertrophic cardiomyopathy 11 (MIM 612098)	ACTC1 (MIM 102540)
Familial medullary thyroid carcinoma (MIM 155240)	RET (MIM 164761)
Hypercholesterolemia, autosomal dominant, 3 (MIM 603776)	PCSK9 (MIM 607786)
Juvenile polyposis syndrome, (MIM 174900)	BMPR1A (MIM 601299)
Juvenile polyposis syndrome, (MIM 174900)	SMAD4 (MIM 600993)
Left ventricular noncompaction 6 (MIM 601494)	TNNT2 (MIM 191045)
Li-Fraumeni syndrome 1 (MIM 151623)	TP53 (MIM 191170)
Loeys-Dietz syndrome type 1A (MIM 609192)	TGFBR1 (MIM 190181)
Loeys-Dietz syndrome type 1B (MIM 610168)	TGFBR2 (MIM 190182)
Loeys-Dietz syndrome type 2A (MIM 608967)	TGFBR1 (MIM 190181)
Loeys-Dietz syndrome type 2B (MIM 610380)	TGFBR2 (MIM 190182)

Continued

TABLE 6.4

American College of Medical Genetics and Genomics version 2.0 genes and associated phenotypes recommended for return of secondary findings in clinical sequencing.—cont'd

Disease name and Molecular Interaction Map (MIM) number	Gene
Loeys-Dietz syndrome type 3 (MIM 613795)	SMAD3 (MIM 603109)
Long QT syndrome 1 (MIM 192500)	KCNQ1 (MIM 607542)
Long QT syndrome 2 (MIM 613688)	KCNH2 (MIM 152427)
Long QT syndrome 3 (MIM 603830)	SCN5A (MIM 600163)
Lynch syndrome (MIM 120435)	MLH1 (MIM 120436)
	MSH2 (MIM 609309)
	MSH6 (MIM 600678)
	PMS2 (MIM 600259)
Malignant hyperthermia (MIM 145600)	RYR1 (MIM 180901)
	CACNA1S (MIM 114208)
Marfan's syndrome (MIM 154700)	FBN1 (MIM 134797)
Marfan's syndrome (MIM 154700)	TGFBR1 (MIM 190181)
Multiple endocrine neoplasia, type 1 (MIM 131100)	MEN1 (MIM 613733)
Multiple endocrine neoplasia, type 2a (MIM 171400)	RET (MIM 164761)
Multiple endocrine neoplasia, type 2b (MIM 162300)	RET (MIM 164761)
MYH-associated polyposis (MIM 608456)	MUTYH (MIM 604933)
Neurofibromatosis, type 2 (MIM 101000)	NF2 (MIM 607379)
Ornithine carbamoyltransferase deficiency (MIM 311250)	OTC (MIM 300461)
Paragangliomas 1 (MIM 168000)	SDHD (MIM 602690)
Paragangliomas 2 (MIM 601650)	SDHAF2 (MIM 613019)
Paragangliomas 3 (MIM 605373)	SDHC (MIM 602413)
Paragangliomas 4 (MIM 115310)	SDHB (MIM 185470)
Peutz-Jeghers syndrome (MIM 175200)	STK11 (MIM 602216)
Pilomatrixoma (MIM 132600)	MUTYH (MIM 604933)
PTEN hamartoma tumor syndrome (MIM 153480)	PTEN (MIM 601728)
Retinoblastoma (MIM 180200)	RB1 (MIM 614041)
Tuberous sclerosis 1 (MIM 191100)	TSC1 (MIM 605284)
Tuberous sclerosis 2 (MIM 613254)	TSC2 (MIM 191092)
Von Hippel-Lindau syndrome (MIM 193300)	VHL (MIM 608537)
Wilms' tumor (MIM 194070)	WT1 (MIM 607102)
Wilson disease (MIM 277900)	ATP7B (MIM 606882)

(From Kalia et al. 2017.)

disorder with progressive muscle weakness. Although SMA is generally due to a homozygous deletion in the *SMN1* gene, the disease severity can be modified by the number of copies of *SMN2*. Because *SMN1* and *SMN2* differ only by one nucleotide, the MLPA amplification is useful for copy number detection.

Other molecular testing strategies include gel electrophoresis, restriction enzyme digestion, and hybridization.

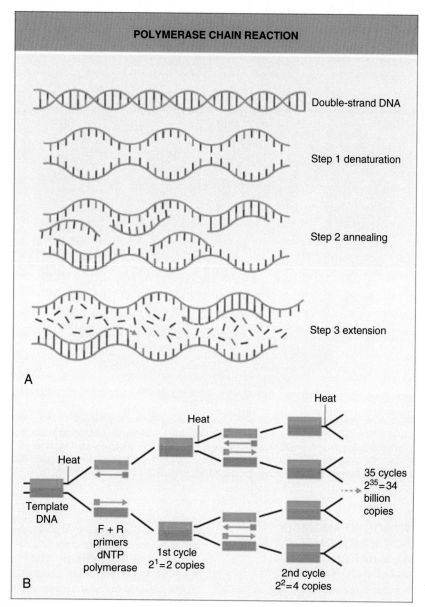

POLYMERASE CHAIN REACTION

Double-strand DNA

Step 1 denaturation

Step 2 annealing

Step 3 extension

A

Heat

Heat

Heat

Template
DNA

F + R
primers
dNTP
polymerase

1st cycle
2^1=2 copies

2nd cycle
2^2=4 copies

35 cycles
2^{35}=34
billion
copies

B

FIG. 6.3 PCR involves application of primers, nucleotides, and polymerase and cycles of heating and cooling where the polymerase extends the nucleotide chain doubling the content of DNA with each cycle. From Jean L. Bolognia, Joseph L. Jorizzo, Julie V. Schaffer, Dermatology. 2012. Elsevier.

These processes separate mixtures of DNA, RNA, or proteins according to their molecular size and charge,[20] often following specialized preparation with restriction enzyme digestion. These approaches are commonly used for "DNA fingerprinting," determining paternity, and for locating the presence or absence of genetic sequences of known size. The Southern blot method combines many of the above techniques to test for disorders of DNA expansion such as myotonic dystrophy, Huntington disease, and fragile X syndrome.

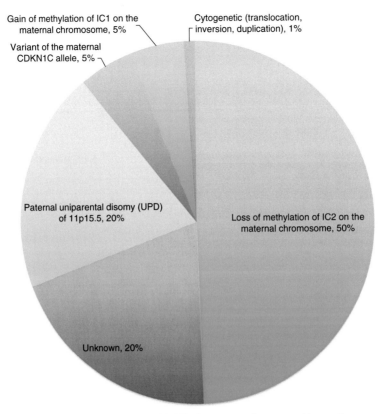

FIG. 6.4 Multiple genetic etiologies of Beckwith-Wiedemann syndrome requiring a diverse array of testing. *IC1* and *IC2*, Imprinting centers. Image from GeneReviews. (Shuman C, Beckwith JB, Weksberg R. Beckwith-Wiedemann Syndrome. 2000 Mar 3 [Updated 2016 Aug 11]. In: Adam MP, Ardinger HH, Pagon RA, et al., editors. GeneReviews® [Internet]. Seattle (WA): University of Washington, Seattle; 1993–2018. Available from: https://www.ncbi.nlm.nih.gov/books/NBK1394/)

WHEN AN ULTRASOUND ANOMALY IS PRESENT AND CHROMOSOMAL CAUSES ARE EXCLUDED, WHAT ADDITIONAL TESTING SHOULD BE CONSIDERED?

With increased ultrasound resolution as well as rapid advances in molecular testing, more robust genetic assessment of the fetus is possible. However, although such analyses are possible, the selection of the appropriate test, pretest and posttest counseling, and integration of the result with the fetal and neonatal phenotype is challenging. The approach to assessment of fetal anomalies ideally incorporates individuals from various disciplines including genetics, maternal fetal medicine, radiology, neonatology, and other pediatric subspecialists. The approach to molecular testing may include a specific gene test if a disorder is suspected (e.g., Noonan syndrome with a cystic hygroma), a gene panel if a category of disorders including a limited number of genetic disorders or genes is suspected (e.g., skeletal dysplasia), or WES if a genetic disorder is highly suspected. When compared head with head, targeted panels fail to detect an additional 5%–10% of alterations eventually found by WES.[12,21,22] Although targeted panels can be cost saving and directed to the prenatal phenotype, care should be individualized as many limitations remain. For most fetal ultrasound anomalies, the phenotypic presentation of a syndrome may not be clear, or may in fact differ from the newborn/pediatric characteristics. In addition, sequential testing can increase the time to find an answer and, occasionally, the amount of DNA available for testing may be limited. A multidisciplinary team can assess the range of possible genetic conditions, select the appropriate testing and prioritize diagnostics. This team also

TABLE 6.5
Review of perinatal Genomic Tests. (From Bodurtha et al, 2012)

Type of Test	Chorionic Villi	Amniocytes	Nucleated Fetal Cells	Cell-free DNA/RNA	Polar Bodies	Biopsy of Blastomere or Blastocyst	Potential for Genomewide Analysis
Karyotype	Yes	Yes	No	No	No	No	Yes
FISH	Yes	Yes	Yes	No	Yes	Yes	No
Quantitative PCR	Yes	Yes	Yes	Yes	Yes	Yes	No
SNP or comparative genomic hybridization array (CMA)	Yes	Yes	Yes	Yes	Yes	Yes	Yes
Shotgun sequencing or massively parallel sequencing	Yes	Yes	Yes	Yes	Yes	Yes	Yes
Whole exome sequencing (WES)	Yes	Yes	Yes	Yes	Yes	Yes	Yes
Variant detection	Yes	Yes	Yes	Yes	Yes	Yes	No

plays a fundamental role in conveying the limitations and uncertainties of the genetic testing to the individual (see Chapter 11).

WHAT TYPES OF TISSUES ARE USED FOR MOLECULAR GENETIC TESTING IN PRENATAL GENETICS?

Molecular genetic testing is performed on DNA, which can be retrieved from a variety of sources. Fetal DNA is abundant in amniotic fluid, chorionic villi, and fetal blood (obtained from a percutaneous umbilical blood sampling). Although less plentiful in the maternal circulation, cell-free DNA, which includes some fragments of placental DNA, can be retrieved and is increasingly being studied for testing for single gene disorders (see Chapter 9). Intact fetal cells from the maternal circulation continue to be of interest for prenatal genetic testing, as well (Table 6.5).[23]

WHEN ARE PARENTAL SAMPLES NEEDED?

Parental samples can be helpful when a genetic variant of unknown significance is detected in a sequencing prenatal test. Parental DNA from a blood or sputum sample can be used to determine if one of the parents have the same genetic variant identified in the fetus or newborn. Although parental information can help refine counseling based on the parental phenotype, many genes have variable penetrance and

expressivity and the parental phenotype may not be the same as their offspring.

WHAT PREIMPLANTATION TESTS CAN BE PERFORMED ON AN EMBRYO?

Many genetic tests can be performed on a small sample of DNA and therefore can be applied to an embryo created through in vitro fertilization. For families at risk of inherited genetic disorders, this is often a desirable approach to avoid detection of a serious genetic disorder during the pregnancy or at birth. Genetic material is generally obtained now from a day 5 trophoblast biopsy or less often a day 3 blastomere. The genetic material can be amplified with PCR and then analyzed with array comparative genomic hybridization, a single nucleotide (SNP) array, quantitative PCR, or multiplex PCR. Additionally, new techniques such as NGS and karyomapping have been successfully applied and are areas of continued investigation[24] (see Chapter 15).

WHAT IS GENE EDITING AND HOW IS IT BEING USED (CRISPR-CAS9)?

As the ability to read DNA sequences became readily available, investigators turned to whether altering DNA (gene editing) could be accomplished. Much as sequencing has been automated and made simpler and faster, gene editing has undergone tremendous advances in recent years. In 2012, investigators at University of

California, Berkley and soon thereafter at the Broad Institute reported on both approaches to capitalize on an existing molecular system to locate and "cut out" precise segments of DNA.[25,26] A technique referred to as CRISPR-cas9 (Clustered Regularly Interspaced Short Palindromic Repeats) targets the desired DNA using a site-specific RNA and removes it with the attached Cas9 enzyme. Either insertion of a normal sequence, or repair using the normal allele, completes the edit (Fig. 6.5).[25] Gene editing differs from the prior methods of genetic engineering, which relied on permanent, random incorporation of target DNA along with a viral vector.[27]

Potential gene editing in humans using CRISPR-cas9 includes somatic cell editing in individuals with an inherited disease such as Duchenne muscular dystrophy or sickle cell anemia.[28] In addition, germline editing has been proposed and performed in pilot studies in embryos to prevent transmission of genetic diseases.[29,30] Such techniques have raised ethical and other concerns (see Chapter 16).

WHAT IS GENE WRITING?

A progression from gene reading to gene editing may be gene writing, or building a complete genome from scratch. A Human Genome Project—Write (HG-W), initiative launched in 2016 to construct an entire genome including wrapping of the DNA around histones and reproducing the control by the epigenome and other forces driving gene transcription.[31] Current abilities to write genomes are confined to short segments and smaller genomes from bacteria. The project's 10-year plan moves to writing human genomes by 2021 and completing expansions to medicine, the environment, and population sustainability by 2026.[31] Currently, in humans, gene writing and editing remain largely investigational.

Cas9 programmed by crRNA:tracrRNA duplex

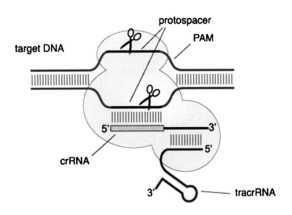

Cas9 programmed by single chimeric RNA

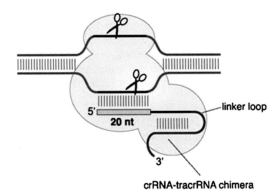

FIG. 6.5 Schematic of use of CRISP-cas9 to identify a specific gene target, remove the identified segment and replace with new DNA sequence (Jinek et al. 2012).

REFERENCES

1. Boycott KM, Rath A, Chong JX, et al. International cooperation to enable the diagnosis of all rare genetic diseases. *Am J Hum Genet.* 2017;100(5):695–705. https://doi.org/10.1016/j.ajhg.2017.04.003.
2. Hershfield M. *Adenosine Deaminase Deficiency.* Seattle: University of Washington; 1993. http://www.ncbi.nlm.nih.gov/pubmed/20301656.
3. Alberts B, Johnson A, Lewis J, et al. *Molecular Biology of the Cell.* 4th ed. New York: Garland Science; 2002. https://www.ncbi.nlm.nih.gov/books/NBK26834/.
4. Lu JT, Campeau PM, Lee BH. Genotype-phenotype correlation–promiscuity in the era of next-generation sequencing. *N Engl J Med.* 2014;371(7):593–596. https://doi.org/10.1056/NEJMp1400788.
5. Antonarakis SE, Cooper DN. Human gene variant in inherited disease: molecular mechanisms and clinical consequences. In: Rimoin D, Pyeritz R, Korf B, eds. *Emery and Rimoin's Principles and Practice of Medical Genetics.* 6th ed. Elsevier; 2013:1–48. (Chapter 7).
6. Origa R. *Beta-thalassemia. GeneReviews(R).* Seattle: University of Washington; 1993. http://www.ncbi.nlm.nih.gov/pubmed/20301599.
7. Kedar-Barnes I, Paul R. The Jewish people: their ethnic history, genetic disorders and specific cancer susceptibility. *Fam Cancer.* 2004;3(3–4):193–199. https://doi.org/10.1007/s10689-004-9544-0.
8. Gross SJ, Pletcher BA, Monaghan KG. Carrier screening in individuals of Ashkenazi Jewish descent. *Genet Med.* 2008;10(1):54–56. https://doi.org/10.1097/GIM.0b013e31815f247c.

9. Mehta N, Lazarin GA, Spiegel E, et al. Tay-sachs Carrier screening by enzyme and molecular analyses in the New York city minority population. *Genet Test Mol Biomarkers*. 2016;20(9):504–509. https://doi.org/10.1089/gtmb.2015.0302.

10. Strom CM, Redman JB, Peng M. The dangers of including nonclassical cystic fibrosis variants in population-based screening panels: P.L997F, further genotype/phenotype correlation data. *Genet Med*. 2011;13(12):1042–1044. https://doi.org/10.1097/GIM.0b013e318228efb2.

11. Macek M, Mackova A, Hamosh A, et al. Identification of common cystic fibrosis variants in African-Americans with cystic fibrosis increases the detection rate to 75%. *Am J Hum Genet*. 1997;60(5):1122–1127. http://www.ncbi.nlm.nih.gov/pubmed/9150159.

12. LaDuca H, Farwell KD, Vuong H, et al. Exome sequencing covers >98% of variants identified on targeted next generation sequencing panels. *PLoS One*. 2017;12(2):1–11. https://doi.org/10.1371/journal.pone.0170843.

13. Richards S, Aziz N, Sherri B, Bick D, Das S, Gastier-Foster J. Standards and guidelines for the interpretation of sequence variants: a joint consensus recommendation of the American College of Medical Genetics and Genomics and the Association for Molecular Pathology. *Genet Med*. 2015;17(5):405–424. https://doi.org/10.1038/gim.2015.30.Standards.

14. Cantarel BL, Lei Y, Weaver D, et al. Analysis of archived residual newborn screening blood spots after whole genome amplification. *BMC Genomics*. 2015;16(1):602. https://doi.org/10.1186/s12864-015-1747-2.

15. Kalia SS, Adelman K, Bale SJ, et al. Recommendations for reporting of secondary findings in clinical exome and genome sequencing, 2016 update (ACMG SF v2.0): a policy statement of the American College of Medical Genetics and Genomics. *Genet Med*. 2017;19(2):249–255. https://doi.org/10.1038/gim.2016.190.

16. Joint Position Statement from the International Society for Prenatal Diagnosis (ISPD), the Society for Maternal Fetal Medicine (SMFM), and the Perinatal Quality Foundation (PQF) on the use of genome-wide sequencing for fetal diagnosis. *Prenat Diagn*. 2018;38(1):6–9. https://doi.org/10.1002/pd.5195.

17. Meienberg J, Bruggmann R, Oexle K, Matyas G. Clinical sequencing: is WGS the better WES? *Hum Genet*. 2016;135(3):359–362. https://doi.org/10.1007/s00439-015-1631-9.

18. Kurdyukov S, Bullock M. DNA methylation analysis: choosing the right method. *Biology*. 2016;5(1):3. https://doi.org/10.3390/biology5010003.

19. Shuman C, Beckwith JB, Weksberg R. *Beckwith-Wiedemann Syndrome*; 1993. http://www.ncbi.nlm.nih.gov/pubmed/20301568.

20. Kim SY, Park G, Han K-H, et al. Prevalence of p.V37I variant of GJB2 in Mild or Moderate Hearing Loss in a Pediatric Population and the Interpretation of its Pathogenicity. Khudyakov YE, ed. *PLoS One*. 2013;8(4):e61592. https://doi.org/10.1371/journal.pone.0061592.

21. Saudi Mendeliome Group. Comprehensive gene panels provide advantages over clinical exome sequencing for Mendelian diseases. *Genome Biol*. 2015;16(1):134. https://doi.org/10.1186/s13059-015-0693-2.

22. Meienberg J, Zerjavic K, Keller I, et al. New insights into the performance of human whole-exome capture platforms. *Nucleic Acids Res*. 2015;43(11):e76. https://doi.org/10.1093/nar/gkv216.

23. Bodurtha J, Strauss JF. Genomics and perinatal care. Feero WG, Guttmacher AE, eds. *N Engl J Med*. 2012;366(1):64–73. https://doi.org/10.1056/NEJMra1105043.

24. Dahdouh EM, Qc M, Balayla J, et al. Technical update: preimplantation genetic diagnosis and screening. *J Obs Gynaecol Can*. 2015;37(232):451–463.

25. Jinek M, Chylinski K, Fonfara I, Hauer M, Doudna JA, Charpentier E. A programmable dual-RNA-guided DNA endonuclease in adaptive bacterial immunity. *Science*. 2012;337(6096):816–821. https://doi.org/10.1126/science.1225829.

26. Ran FA, Hsu PD, Wright J, Agarwala V, Scott DA, Zhang F. Genome engineering using the CRISPR-Cas9 system. *Nat Protoc*. 2013;8(11):2281–2308. https://doi.org/10.1038/nprot.2013.143.

27. Abdallah NA, Prakash CS, McHughen AG. Genome editing for crop improvement: challenges and opportunities. *GM Crops Food*. 2015;6(4):183–205. https://doi.org/10.1080/21645698.2015.1129937.

28. Long C, Li H, Tiburcy M, et al. Correction of diverse muscular dystrophy variants in human engineered heart muscle by single-site genome editing. *Sci Adv*. 2018;4(1):eaap9004. https://doi.org/10.1126/sciadv.aap9004.

29. Ma H, Marti-Gutierrez N, Park S-W, et al. Correction of a pathogenic gene variant in human embryos. *Nature*. 2017;548(7668):413–419. https://doi.org/10.1038/nature23305.

30. Liang P, Xu Y, Zhang X, et al. CRISPR/Cas9-mediated gene editing in human tripronuclear zygotes. *Protein Cell*. 2015;6(5):363–372. https://doi.org/10.1007/s13238-015-0153-5.

31. Boeke JD, Church G, Hessel A, et al. The genome project-write we need technology and an ethical framework for genome-scale engineering. *Science*. 2016;353(6295):126–127. https://doi.org/10.1126/science.aaf6850.

CHAPTER 7

Carrier Screening for Genetic Conditions

MICHAEL H. GUO, MD, PHD • ANTHONY R. GREGG, MD, MBA

INTRODUCTION

Prenatal genetic carrier screening has evolved over a period of about 25 years. Advances in technology and health policy have ushered this evolution. With these changes, new terminology has appeared, whereas old terms and their definitions have evolved. It is helpful for the reader to understand the current core terminology around the topic of carrier screening.

Definitions

Condition: There has been a general trend to replace the term "disease" with "condition." Genetic testing and screening, when applied to populations of healthy people, will commonly uncover health risk to either themselves or their offspring. This can provoke unnecessary anxiety. Furthermore, there is less stigmatization associated with "condition" compared with "disease."

Primary prevention: A public health strategy aimed at preventing or minimizing the impact on health, such as vaccination in preventing infectious diseases. Prenatal genetic carrier screening can play a role in primary prevention when at risk couples use assisted reproductive technologies (ARTs) in their reproductive planning.

Secondary prevention: A public health strategy aimed at identifying and limiting early disease. Papanicolaou screening for cervical cancer is an example. Carrier genetic screening can play a role in secondary prevention. Postconception decision-making falls into this category of secondary prevention.

Mutation: When referring to changes in the sequence of a gene, this term has generally been replaced by "variant." Variant has less stigmatization and is less definitive, allowing for classification according to its relationship with a condition of interest (e.g., benign, pathogenic).

Pathogenic variant (i.e., PV): A category assigned to variants in a gene that are associated with a condition. The caution here is that penetrance may not be 100%, and there may be variable expressivity (see below).

Likely pathogenic variant: A category assigned to pathogenic variants in a gene where the association with a condition is less certain.

Benign variant: A category assigned to variants in a gene that are clearly not associated with a condition.

Likely benign variant: A category assigned to variants in a gene that are most likely not associated with a condition, but where the benign nature is less certain.

Variant of uncertain significance (i.e., VUS): A category of variants in a gene where the variant cannot be placed into either of the above four categories. These variants are numerous and are often the most challenging for clinicians, as they bring uncertainty into management and treatment decisions.

Residual risk: The risk that remains after a negative screening test result. Applied to genetic carrier screening, residual risk is conceptualized by the following formula:

$$\text{Carrier frequency of a condition} \times (1 - \text{detection rate})$$

Next-generation sequencing (NGS): Generally applied to sequencing technologies that allow simultaneous sequence multiple distinct regions of the genome. It is considerably faster and cheaper than traditional Sanger sequencing.

Whole-genome sequencing (WGS): (Now referred to as genome-sequencing by the American College of Medical Genetics and Genomics (ACMG)) Sequencing the entire genome of an individual. This requires NGS.

Whole-exome sequencing (WES): (Now referred to as exome-sequencing by ACMG) Sequencing that selectively targets the protein-coding regions of the genome. Most known pathogenic variants are in these protein-coding regions; therefore, selectively sequencing these regions can reduce cost relative to WGS.

Genotyping: A technological method of assaying genetic variants that targets known pathogenic variants. This approach is faster and less expensive compared with NGS. It allows for simultaneous assay of up

Perinatal Genetics. https://doi.org/10.1016/B978-0-323-53094-1.00007-2

to hundreds of thousands of variants. Variants that are not part of the prespecified genotyping platform will not be assayed.

Pan-ethnic screening: This is an approach to carrier screening where all ethnic groups are screened the same way. For example, if pan-ethnic screening for sickle cell disease is the goal, then it is not only performed among individuals of African descent but also applied to all ethnic groups in the same fashion.

Expressivity: Expressivity reflects how a genetic variant can manifest phenotypically. It recognizes that a pathogenic variant can be associated with a range of phenotypes (i.e., variable expressivity). For example, a variant causing Alagille syndrome may present with hepatic dysfunction in some individuals, but not in others.

Penetrance: The percentage of people with a pathogenic variant who develop the associated phenotype. Population-based genotyping has uncovered that many pathogenic alleles are not highly penetrant. Incomplete penetrance makes selecting variants for testing on a carrier screening panel challenging. Incomplete penetrance also challenges interpretation of screening results and downstream clinical decision-making.

WHAT ARE THE PRINCIPLES OF GENETIC SCREENING?

Traditionally, carrier screening, as recognized by Wilson and Jungner,[1] was a form of secondary prevention. Its application was largely in public health in the same realm as infectious diseases (e.g., tuberculosis [TB], syphilis). In public health, screening tests are applied to populations broadly (e.g., testing children before enrollment into school) or in a more targeted fashion based on known risk factors (e.g., prisoners). Historically, screening tests were inexpensive and noninvasive. They are generally low technology or amenable to automation, which allows high throughput. Examples include the rapid plasma reagin blood test (RPR) for syphilis or the Mantoux skin test for TB. Because screening tests have an associated false-positive rate, they are often followed with confirmatory diagnostic testing before treatments begin. Diagnostic tests generally have lower false-positive and false-negative rates but can be more expensive and/or more invasive.

Prenatal genetic carrier screening is distinct from primary or secondary prevention screening in several ways that contrast with those described by Wilson and Jungner for traditional screening tests[1] and are important for the clinician to appreciate (Table 7.1):
1. Targets a broad population (like primary prevention screening).
2. It is noninvasive (like primary prevention screening).

TABLE 7.1 Wilson and Yunger Characteristics of Screening Tests	
Conditions Screened	Condition with a personal/societal burden
	Well known natural history
	Detectable at an early stage
	Early stage treatment beneficial
Test Characteristics	Suitable for early stage detection
	Acceptable by patients
	Repeat testing intervals determined
Social	Health care supervision is adequate for increased work burden
	Physical and psychologic benefits are greater than risks of screening
	Costs and benefits are balanced

3. The same test/method can be used for screening and diagnosis in that there may be no follow-up diagnostic test available or required.
4. It is generally expensive (like a diagnostic test).
5. Excluding VUS, the false-positive rate is low (like a diagnostic test).
6. There is almost always a false-negative rate (e.g., residual risk).
7. Screening generally has health implications for the offspring and not the person being screened (some exceptions apply).

Unlike most screening examinations and laboratory tests in which there is a high detection rate and low specificity, prenatal genetic carrier screening generally has high detection rate (DR) for the variants being examined. However, because all variants may not be tested or reported, the false-negative rate can be quite high. This has the potential to yield a low negative predictive value (NPV) compared with what is seen with traditional primary screening, but the low prevalence of specific conditions screened tempers this potential. Residual risk is a surrogate for NPV in clinical genetics practice where carrier screening is the focus. The key components of residual risk are carrier frequency within the population of interest and the screening test DR. There is a residual risk for nearly every condition screened.

These characteristics that distinguish prenatal genetic carrier screening from traditional screening modalities make it a unique entity in public health. These distinguishing features equate to unique challenges around

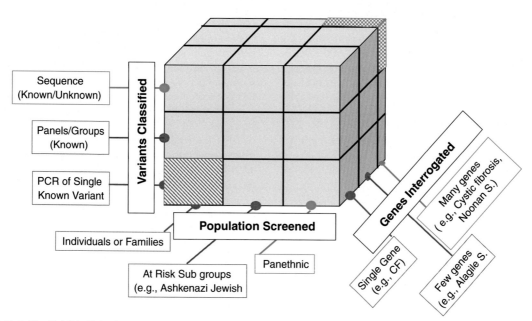

FIG. 7.1 The Rubik's Cube has three axes. The horizontal axis represents population screened. The vertical axis represents variants classified, and the diagonal axis represents the genes interrogated. Each of the 18 cubes corresponds to a combination of points along each axis. Screening has its origin in the red striped cube (foreground bottom left) and is progressing rapidly to the green checkered cube (background top right). (Modified from Gregg AR. Expanded carrier screening. *Obstet Gynecol Clin N Am*. 2018;45:103–112.)

policy, education of patients and providers, as well as implementation.

WHAT IS EXPANDED CARRIER SCREENING?

Unlike screening for one condition at a time (i.e., *a la carte* testing), expanded carrier screening (ECS) adds breadth (more conditions) and depth (interrogation of or reporting on more variants within a gene). It has a reduced false-negative rate for specific genes (because of the increased number of variants examined) and higher sensitivity for detecting carriers across a broad spectrum of conditions.

Carrier screening has three dimensions: (1) population(s) screened, (2) gene(s) interrogated, and (3) variant(s) classified. A Rubik cube model illustrates the three axes involved[2] (Fig. 7.1). When prenatal genetic screening first began, small groups of people were the focus (the bottom left cube with red stripes). These small groups included families with an affected proband for a condition or an ethnic group at risk for certain genetic conditions such as individuals of Ashkenazi Jewish descent.[3] Specific conditions were the focus, and a limited number of genetic variants were probed for.[4] With enhanced sequencing technology that included higher

throughput, there was an expansion to targeting subpopulations and the number of variants categorized grew. There was no longer an ethnic-based focus on conditions, and screening became less restricted to conditions observed in the family.[5] Over time, screening has allowed for a pan-ethnic paradigm for some conditions.[6,7]

HOW DOES PRENATAL SCREENING UTILIZE THE STRUCTURE OF THE HUMAN GENOME?

The human genome comprises approximately 3 billion nucleotides (or letters; A's, C's, G's, and T's) that serve as the blueprint for all of life. The DNA sequence comprised of these nucleotides, which can be thought of as a string of combinations of the above-mentioned letters/nucleotides, encode for all of the proteins that become part of cells, tissues, and organs. These 3 billion nucleotides are separated into 23 different chromosomes, which are densely packaged segments of DNA. The DNA sequence codes for approximately 20,000 different genes, which are the functional unit of the genome; in general, each gene encodes for a single protein. For example, the *CFTR* gene encodes for the cystic fibrosis transmembrane conductance regulator protein, a transporter protein that helps transport chloride in and out of cells. However, the fraction of DNA that codes for genes only comprises a small proportion (approximately 1.5%) of the whole genome.[8] Interspersed between the gene "coding" sequences are long stretches of DNA that are "noncoding." These noncoding regions of the genome have critical regulatory roles in that they determine which genes are turned on in a given cell type or condition.[9] By turning on different genes in different cell types, each cell type can have a specific form and function.

The sequence of everyone's genome is largely the same. However, the DNA sequence differs at approximately 1 in 1000 nucleotides between any two individuals.[10] These differences in the DNA sequence are called genetic variants. All genetic variants originally arise in a single individual as a mutational event, where the sequence of the genome is copied incorrectly when DNA is passed from one generation to the next. These variants can have a wide range of downstream effects. If the variant occurs in a noncoding region of the genome, it may affect the gene regulatory potential of that DNA sequence, or it may have no effect at all. Similarly, if the variant occurs in a region of the genome that codes for a gene, it may have no effect at all on the resultant protein product, or it may have tremendous deleterious effects on its function, or in some cases even improve the function of that encoded protein.

Genetic variation comes in many forms. The simplest and most common form of variation is single nucleotide polymorphisms, or SNPs, which are single nucleotide changes in the genome. Next are indels, which are short insertions or deletions of several nucleotides in the genome. Lastly, copy number variants (CNVs) and structural variants (SVs) are large structural changes of much greater size (hundreds of nucleotides or more).

The fundamental challenge of diagnostic and prenatal screening is identifying which variants in a gene can cause genetic conditions. Most of the genetic variants in the population are common and thus shared by many individuals in the population. Furthermore, most variants are benign, with no apparent effect on downstream protein function or known condition. Each gene contains many different variants, which have a wide range of effects. There have been considerable coordinated efforts such as ClinGen to distinguish which variants are benign versus pathogenic for disease.[11] It should be noted that the clear majority of variants in a given gene are not pathogenic.

WHAT TECHNOLOGIES ARE USED TO SCREEN FOR GENETIC CONDITIONS?

To screen for genetic variants capable of causing disease, we need to be able to read the DNA sequence of an individual and compare it with a reference sequence.

Over the years, the technology used to sequence DNA has changed rapidly and with it has changed how we perform gene screening.

The oldest method of DNA sequencing is Sanger sequencing.[12] Despite still being the most accurate form of sequencing, this method has very low throughput and is expensive and generally manually intensive. In a given sequencing reaction, only a short segment of DNA (generally less than 1000 nucleotides) can be interrogated. However, given its accuracy, it is still used as confirmation for findings from other sequencing technologies as described below.

Over the past decade, the advent of next-generation sequencing (NGS) has transformed our ability to screen and diagnose genetic conditions.[13] NGS refers to high-throughput sequencing methods, which allow for simultaneous sequencing of multiple distinct regions of the genome (i.e., parallelization), which contrasts with traditional Sanger sequencing. NGS technologies generate sequencing "reads," which are simply readouts (As, Ts, Cs, and Gs) of the sequence of a segment of an individual's DNA. Once the sequence of each read is determined, the reads can be mapped to a reference genome sequence, and computational methods can be applied to identify differences from the reference genome (i.e., genetic variants). NGS can allow for sequencing of the entire genome (i.e., WGS) or a select panel of regions of the genome such as the set of all protein-coding genes (i.e., WES).

A separate technology that is commonly used is genotyping. In contrast to NGS or Sanger sequencing where entire stretches of DNA are read, genotyping assays just one nucleotide at a time. A genotyping reaction thus allows us to determine the genotype at prespecified variant sites but does not allow us to uncover variants that are not part of the designed genotyping assay. However, genotyping is much cheaper, and with higher throughput than NGS or Sanger sequencing—in one genotyping reaction, hundreds of thousands of variants can be assayed. It is particularly applicable when there are known genetic variants that have a large disease burden, such as the sickle cell mutation, allowing for rapid and high-throughput screening of that variant in many individuals.

It should be noted that prenatal genetic carrier screening panels can use any of the three above technologies. Furthermore, a single panel may use multiple different modalities, with different technologies used for different genes/variants because of technical considerations.

WHAT IS THE GOAL OF PRENATAL GENETIC CARRIER SCREENING?

Prenatal genetic carrier screening identifies individuals and couples at risk of transmitting genetic variants to their offspring at the time of fertilization. The genetic variants that are of interest in the context of prenatal genetic screening are those that can result in undesired developmental abnormalities and/or function. Birth defects and developmental delay are examples of conditions for which it may be desirable to screen.

The major goal of prenatal genetic screening is to provide desired information to individuals or couples. The information gained from carrier screening can be used in reproductive decision-making. The clinical utility of screening is related to the time it takes to make screening results available to couples.

Identification of at-risk couples ideally takes place during the preconception period, but the reality is that screening most often occurs once a pregnancy is established. In some ethnic communities, knowledge of carrier status can even impact whether a couple decides to marry (such as Ashkenazi Jewish communities). Knowledge of carrier status before conception may impact the reproductive choices a couple makes. For example, a couple where each partner carries a pathogenic variant in *CFTR* may decide not to conceive because of concern of having a child with cystic fibrosis. Knowledge of a couple's carrier status may also impact the decision to use donor games (i.e., sperm or egg) or to opt for preimplantation genetic diagnosis. However, as described below, knowledge of carrier status before conception can also impact the other benefits of carrier screening.

When prenatal genetic carrier screening occurs after conception, it can impact decision-making. This includes whether to proceed with diagnostic testing (e.g., chorionic villous sampling or amniocentesis), perinatal management, and/or discontinuing a pregnancy. Knowledge that both parents are carriers of recessive pathogenic variants for a given condition greatly increases the likelihood of having a child who is affected. In this scenario, diagnostic testing would provide the opportunity to ascertain whether a fetus did in fact receive both pathogenic variants from the parents. For some conditions, it may also influence the management provided in the perinatal period. For example, the diagnosis of a genetic condition associated with congenital cardiac defects may spur additional screening for cardiac anomalies and preparation at delivery with the appropriate medical personnel (e.g., delivering at a medical center with extensive expertise in high-risk obstetrics, cardiac surgery, and neonatology). Furthermore, when results are delivered after conception but early in pregnancy, couples can learn about the care of a child/adult with conditions for which they are at risk, and with this information determine whether they will continue to carry a pregnancy. *In summary*, carrier screening aims to provide couples information about their risk of conceiving or carrying a child with a genetic condition characterized by Mendelian inheritance.

WHAT FACTORS DETERMINE THE APPROPRIATENESS OF SCREENING FOR A GENE OR CONDITION?

For the most part, prenatal genetic carrier screening applies to recessive conditions, where a pathogenic variant within a gene transmitted from each parent would result in a defined genetic condition. In this scenario, the parents are unaffected. Carrier screening is less applicable in dominant conditions because the parent transmitting the pathogenic variant would also be affected with the condition, assuming full penetrance. Genes that are more suitable for screening also tend to have genetic variants that are highly penetrant, as interpretation of low-penetrant variants can be very challenging. Most genes suitable for screening are reliably sequenced. However, there are exceptions. Genes responsible for fragile X mental retardation syndrome (FMR), spinal muscular atrophy (SMA), and congenital adrenal hyperplasia (CAH) offer special challenges. They require special methods to determine carrier status because of the repetitive nature of the variant (trinucleotide repeats in FMR) or the presence of pseudogenes in the same region (CAH and SMA). The added complexity in screening these genes does not disqualify them for screening, although these genes require special attention during the screening process.[14]

Following the tenets of Wilson and Jungner,[1] the genes screened should be associated with severe conditions. However, determining which conditions are "severe" is a challenging task. One study surveyed a large group of healthcare professionals and found that consensus can be reached when stratifying severity of specific conditions.[15] The study found that conditions associated with intellectual disability and reduction in life span during infancy, childhood, or adolescence were found to be the characteristics that led to high severity ratings. Defining the severity of conditions is further complicated by the wide phenotypic spectrum of some conditions and the different values that patients place on the clinical features of some conditions. Furthermore, our ability to treat some conditions is changing rapidly such that some conditions viewed as "severe" in the past may now be treated and lead to a new perception of severity for that condition. Counseling after the return of results in prenatal carrier screening should remain sensitive to varied perceptions of severity.

TABLE 7.2
Ashkenazi Jewish Conditions ACOG Perspective

SCREEN		CONSIDER SCREENING	
Condition	Carrier frequency	Condition	Carrier frequency
Canavan disease	1:40	Bloom syndrome	1:102
Cystic fibrosis	1:26	Familial hyperinsulinism	1:100
Familial dysautonomia	1:32	Fanconi anemia	1:89
Tay-Sachs disease	1:30	Gaucher disease	1:15
		Glycogen storage disease type I	1:91
		Joubert syndrome	1:150
		Maple syrup urine disease	1:81
ACOG Committee Opinion		Mucolipidosis type IV	1:22
Number 691, March 2017		Niemann-Pick disease	1:90
Carrier screening for genetic conditions		Usher syndrome	1:95

In summary, there is general agreement that the conditions appropriate for screening are actionable. This term has broad connotation and encompasses medical interventions and patient values.

WHAT ARE THE RECOMMENDATIONS BY PROFESSIONAL ORGANIZATIONS FOR CARRIER SCREENING?

In 2015 the status of carrier screening guidelines was reviewed by five professional organizations.[16] Hemoglobinopathies, conditions prevalent in Ashkenazi Jewish individuals (e.g., Tay-Sachs disease), and spinal muscular atrophy were the only conditions listed in that set of guidelines. At the time, cystic fibrosis was the only condition agreed upon for pan-ethnic screening.

In March 2017, in the wake of wide spread adoption of NGS technology, the American College of Obstetricians and Gynecologists (ACOG) revised its recommendations.[17] In addition to recommending pan-ethnic screening for cystic fibrosis, spinal muscular atrophy was added. A complete blood count (CBC) was proposed as first-line screening in all patients not only for anemia but also for hemoglobinopathies in general. Fragile X carrier screening was recommended in those with a family history of fragile X or intellectual disabilities. Some conditions such as Tay Sachs disease were recommended for individuals of high-risk ethnic backgrounds (Ashkenazi Jewish, French Canadian or Cajun). Providers were also instructed to "consider" 10 conditions in the Ashkenazi population as optional

for screening (Table 7.2). In a separate 2017 Committee Opinion,[7] ACOG recommended ECS be limited to conditions with carrier frequency greater than 1 in 100, which includes the optional ethnic-specific conditions described.

In summary, there is consensus that cystic fibrosis and spinal muscular atrophy are appropriate for pan-ethnic screening. NGS allows for high-throughput screening for more conditions with a carrier frequency threshold lower than recommended by ACOG.

IS THERE AN "IDEAL" PAN-ETHNIC GENE/ CONDITION SCREENING PANEL?

This is a challenging question and one for which existing evidence is insufficient to provide clear guidance. To frame this question, there are two factors that influence which gene(s) would be part of an ideal pan-ethnic panel. First is how much residual risk one is willing to tolerate. This issue was discussed above and is similarly applicable to the design of an ideal pan-ethnic panel. The second factor is which ethnicities are being screened for in an ideal pan-ethnic panel. This is important because each ethnicity has different conditions that are more prevalent. For example, sickle cell anemia is more prevalent among individuals of African descent, whereas cystic fibrosis is more prevalent among individuals of European descent. If a pan-ethnic panel was designed for just individuals of European or African descent, then the panel might just include the union of genes that are desirable to be screened for in the component populations. However, in an ethnically diverse population such as the United States, there are many ethnic populations that constitute the component population. Therefore, a pan-ethnic panel will be more complex to design. Some of these ethnic populations (e.g., Amish or Hutterites) only comprise a small proportion of the population but may add many genes for which screening would be needed. Thus, the decision regarding which population(s) the pan-ethnic panel is designed for would influence the genes that comprise an ideal panel.

There is little empiric evidence to guide the design and benefits of a pan-ethnic expanded carrier screening panel. However, an industry database provided evidence in favor of a pan-ethnic panel.[6] A custom panel that screens for 94 conditions that meet some criteria described by Wilson and Yunger[1] was applied to 350,000 individuals across 15 ethnic populations. They found that this ECS panel greatly improved yields when compared with the yield that would be obtained from the recommended ethnicity-based screening.[17] For example, for couples of Ashkenazi Jewish descent, ACMG recommended Ashkenazi screening genes would identify approximately 131 fetuses that would be expected to be affected per 100,000 pregnancies. However, the pan-ethnic ECS panel would identify an additional 115 affected fetuses per 100,000. The enhanced carrier detection derives from adding conditions not recommended for screening by ACOG and expanding the number of variants reported. Additional data regarding the yields of all genes and conditions will be needed to guide the benefits and composition of pan-ethnic screening panels.

In summary, the most appropriate pan-ethnic carrier screening panel remains elusive. This is due in part to the many variables that define clinical utility, patient desires, and public perception.

WHAT ARE THE PITFALLS TO RELYING ON SEQUENCING TO DETERMINE CARRIER STATUS?

Although carrier screening is now largely performed by sequencing, the technology is by no means perfect. This imperfection is related to the inability of sequencing to detect some forms of genetic variation.

Most carrier screening approaches, either based on Sanger sequencing or NGS, only cover gene-coding regions. However, there are many known pathogenic variants that occur in noncoding regions of the genome and would thus be missed by sequencing. Additionally, some forms of genetic variation, including longer insertions/deletions (indels) and CNV/SVs, are poorly captured by sequencing approaches due to inherit technological limitations. For example, many known pathogenic variants in *CYP21A2*, which cause congenital adrenal hyperplasia, are caused by deletions of all or portions of the gene.[18] As another example of variants that are poorly captured, sequencing is currently largely incapable of resolving the length of repeats in trinucleotide repeat disorders such as some forms of spinocerebellar ataxia.[19] These problems are particularly salient for screening approaches based on genotyping, because genotyping selects a priori the variants to be detected and usually focuses on single nucleotide substitutions that are known to cause a condition.

For some conditions, sequencing alone is inadequate and relying on an alternate method of screening is preferred (e.g., hemoglobin electrophoresis). For Tay-Sachs screening, pairing with another method enhances detection, as relying solely on sequencing leads to an unacceptable residual risk. In one study of Tay-Sachs carriers, gene sequencing had a sensitivity of 52% as compared with 91% for a hexosaminidase A enzymatic assay.[20] When both methods were combined, the highest detection of carriers was seen (100%). Enzymatic screening is preferred in the non-Ashkenazi population as the common genetic mutations seen in the Ashkenazi population are not typically found. As another example, hemoglobin electrophoresis is recommended as a means of rapidly and accurately screening for hemoglobinopathies.[17] In cases of high suspicion and normal electrophoresis, NGS can be used, but not as a first-line screening approach.[21] In at-risk families, NGS has proven value in identifying carriers of rare thalassemias that have the potential to impact the fetus.[22] These examples highlight the pitfall of relying solely on sequencing for screening.

In summary, sequencing methods do not identify all genetic variations. In one study, applying a more complex screening process was required to identify nearly 30% of variation.[23] Some conditions are more accurately screened by evaluating the function of the gene product (e.g., hexosaminidase A in Tay-Sachs disease) or structure (hemoglobin electrophoresis in hemoglobinopathies).

HOW MANY ADDITIONAL CARRIERS ARE IDENTIFIED WITH ECS COMPARED WITH CONVENTIONAL APPROACHES?

One study that addressed this question evaluated the yield of a commercial NGS panel and compared it with yields obtained after conventional genotyping targeting known pathogenic variants. The study was performed in 11,691 individuals and identified 447 variant carriers across 14 genes.[24] The study found that approximately one quarter of the variants detected by NGS would not have been detected using conventional targeted genotyping of known pathogenic variants.

A large study of 474,644 individuals in a commercial dataset examined the yield of ECS using NGS.[25] Sequencing was performed for genes responsible for 110 conditions, including several technically challenging conditions such as congenital adrenal hyperplasia (*CAH*), spinal muscular atrophy (*SMN1*), alpha thalassemia (*HBA1*), and fragile X (*FMR1*). They found that these technically challenging genes comprised 28.9% of the yield of ECS. They also modeled the yield from a hypothetical conventional genotyping panel targeting 500 of the most common pathogenic variants in these 110 conditions. The genotyping panel would miss 7.6% of the sequence variants detected by NGS-based ECS.

Another study evaluated 506 individuals of Ashkenazi Jewish descent.[26] A commercially available NGS-based panel was used to interrogate 84 genes associated with autosomal recessive conditions plus *FMR1* (for Fragile X). The study found that 288 individuals (57%) were carriers. There were 434 pathogenic variants detected in the study. However, only 312 of these variants would have been detected by genotyping. Thus, 28% of the variants detected by ECS using NGS would have been missed using genotyping methods.

In summary, the number of carriers identified when NGS is used for carrier screening is increased over that seen with conventional genotyping. There are limited data addressing the clinical utility of this increase in yield.

DOES COST ANALYSIS FAVOR CARRIER SCREENING WITH NGS OVER CONVENTIONAL SCREENING?

Although NGS offers an opportunity to enhance screening efficiency, sequencing costs are increased relative to other technologies such as genotyping. One study modeled 1 million US couples and compared conventional genotyping with NGS for 14 conditions.[27] NGS-based screening would avert an additional 21 affected births and reduce costs by $13 million dollars (based on a 2014-dollar value) when compared with genotyping-based screening. Compared with no screening, NGS-based screening would avert 223 additional affected births. One problem with using cost-benefit analyses is that the entity bearing the cost is not always the entity acquiring the benefit—lifetime savings in healthcare

costs may not be accumulated to the same health plan that bore the cost of the testing.

The dollar value of screening may be disparate from a couple's willingness to pay for screening. After receiving carrier screening results by NGS for 728 conditions and 121 secondary findings, about 40% of participants were willing to pay $20–$100 and nearly 15% were willing to pay $300 to $1000 for this information.[28] Interestingly, two factors seem to be most related to willingness to pay: annual household income and whether the individuals considered themselves spiritual.

Increasingly, the cost of performing ECS is shifting away from the cost of sequencing to test interpretation and counseling. Currently, the interpretation of variants is not fully automated, requiring some manual curation. Additionally, the cost in time spent by genetic counselors in follow-up of carrier screening results has been raised as a barrier to population-wide screening using NGS. One study examined counseling time spent to discuss results to 107 participants across 101 different genes.[29] Participants had a mean of 1.9 positive results per person (range of 1–4). The median time for results disclosure was 64 min, with a range from 5 to 229 min. As carrier screening panels become more comprehensive in terms of genes and variants interrogated, this will likely increase the number of positive results returned and the amount of time spent on downstream counseling.

In summary, there are currently insufficient data to answer the question of cost-effectiveness of NGS. The lack of pricing transparency across commercial entities and healthcare systems adds to the lack of information. Limited evidence suggests that society may experience a cost savings if an NGS-based approach to carrier screening is adopted. Furthermore, patients seem willing to pay. However, the burden on the genetics community in the form of hours (often not compensated) spent discussing results will be large.

HOW ARE VARIANTS SELECTED FOR REPORTING?

The selection of variants for reporting is a challenging task, even when they are within genes that are deemed worthy of inclusion on a screening panel. The fundamental challenge is that we currently are unable to perfectly distinguish between variants that are pathogenic and those that are not. There are several characteristics of variants that make them more likely to be pathogenic.[30] First, variants that are rare in the general population are more likely to be pathogenic because natural selection operates to suppress the frequency of deleterious variants. Second, variants that are predicted to perturb an encoded protein's function are more likely to be pathogenic, although our ability to predict these effects is quite inaccurate. Third, variants that have been observed in other individuals with the same condition are more likely to be pathogenic, but this can also be misleading. Many variants that meet these characteristics turn out to not be pathogenic. On the other hand, many pathogenic variants do not meet all of these characteristics. There are many large-scale collaborative efforts, such as ClinGen, aimed at teasing out which variants are pathogenic.[11]

The challenge of selecting which variants are reported is compounded by variable expressivity and incomplete penetrance. Many pathogenic variants display variable expressivity in the range of phenotypic characteristics it is associated with. Thus, a pathogenic variant can in some individuals cause a severe condition that is worthy of reporting but in other individuals cause a mild condition that would not be acted upon in a clinical setting. With incomplete penetrance, a pathogenic variant may only cause the condition some of the time. Often, a pathogenic variant may cause the condition only in 1% (or even less) of individuals who carry that variant. Both factors make selection of variants more challenging.

Opinions vary over which variants should be reported, particularly in variants where the pathogenicity is not clear (e.g., variants of uncertain significance), or those that are incompletely penetrant. When variants are overreported, uncertainty and concern resulting in unnecessary follow-up testing can result. When variants are underreported, increased residual risk is the result. Regardless, it is the job of the clinician ordering the test to frame the results for the patients and help guide clinical care.

In summary, the selection process for variants has been evolving. Rules have been established that categorize variants according to pathogenicity. One confounder to variant classification emanates from reduced penetrance and variable expressivity.

HOW DOES PRETEST COUNSELING FOR ECS COMPARED WITH CONVENTIONAL SCREENING?

It has been a long dictum in genetics that counseling should be informative, while remaining "nondirective," thus allowing patients to make decisions that are most suitable for them.[31] Professional organizations have identified several steps that providers can take to prepare for patients who decide to pursue ECS using NGS. Distinct concepts should be shared with patients during pretest counseling, and the return of results will be different, as reflected by a greater number of positive results.[16] These pre- and posttest counseling concepts are outlined in Table 7.3.

TABLE 7.3
Counseling for ECS

Provider Homework	Pre-test Counseling Concepts	Post – test counseling session
Be aware of the conditions being screened	Screening is voluntary.	Prepare in advance
Understand the difference between penetrance and variable expressivity	Results are confidential.	When serial screening is under-taken and results are positive, offer to screen the biologic father.
Consider other approaches to screening when variants have low penetrance.	Conditions screened have variable severity.	When a Tay-Sachs disease carrier is identified and the partner is a non-carrier by molecular testing, screening with enzyme analysis is recommended.
Establish a genetics professional consultant.	Many conditions screened are rare.	Provide reliable information directed at positive results.
Develop a plan for communicating results.	Paternity must be accurate to determine pregnancy risk.	Consider referral to a genetics professional when positive results are returned for both partners.
It is impractical and unnecessary to explain each condition. Consider a few examples.	It is common to be a carrier for at least one condition.	Offer fetal testing when both partners test positive.

TABLE 7.3
Counseling for ECS—cont'd

Provider Homework	Pre-test Counseling Concepts	Post – test counseling session
Disease prevalence, mutation frequencies, and detection rates may be imprecise.	It is possible that carrier screening identifies health risk or explains signs/symptoms in the person screened.	Offer to provide reliable information to other family members.
After NGS carrier screening, re-screening is not recommended in subsequent pregnancies.	Some conditions screened are X-linked and semi- dominant.	
Screening paradigms for hemoglobinopathies rely on mean corpuscular volume and hemoglobin electrophoresis.	A negative screen reduces risk but does not eliminate risk. There is always a residual risk.	
Hexosaminidase A enzyme analysis using blood (leukocytes during pregnancy) add to detection rates seen after ECS using NGS.	Residual risk is impractical to calculate for the many conditions screened.	

There have been concerns that patients are generally afraid of genetic screening using NGS, but these concerns have not been backed by available information.[32] Rather than portraying ECS in a tone that incites fear around screening, some authors prefer to use the term "uncertain." One study defined and evaluated domains of uncertainty expressed by patients during pre and posttest counseling. These domains were organized into a construct called the "perception of uncertainties around genomic screening" (PUGS).[33] This construct for counseling was merged with specific points articulated by professional organizations and grouped into "PUGS domains" (Tables 7.4 and 7.5).[2] It remains to be established whether this construct is useful to patients in the prenatal setting and whether providers find this construct helpful and facile to implement.

In summary, ECS that incorporates NGS places specific demands on obstetric care providers in the pre- and posttest period. A novel construct around counseling offers promise to simplify counseling while addressing patient perceptions of uncertainty.

HOW CAN ECS USING NGS BE IMPLEMENTED?

The terms "offer" and "make available" have historic importance. The clinical distinction was first made in 2001 when the American Academy of Pediatrics (AAP), ACOG, and ACMG concluded that screening for cystic fibrosis should extend beyond those with a positive family history.[34] In this set of recommendations,

TABLE 7.4
10 Point PUGS Pretest Counseling Domains

Domain	Consideration by those screened
Clinical	Conditions reported have varied severity
	Conditions screened are often rare
	Conditions screened are severe
Affective	Screening is voluntary
	Results are confidential and protected
	Plan for returning results
Effective	Requires accurate paternity information
	Residual risk remains after a negative screen
	May identify a recessive condition in an asymptomatic person.
	Asymptomatic carriers of semi-dominant, dominant and X-linked disorders may be identified.

Modified from Gregg AR Obstet and Gynecol Clinics of NA

different levels of clinical responsibility were assigned according to patient classification into a high- or low-risk group. Those in a high-risk ethnic group received a higher level of responsibility by providers. In contrast, those in a low-risk ethnic group were provided written materials in accordance with the terms "make available." However, as ECS has become more widely and

TABLE 7.5
7 Point PUGS Post-test Counseling Domains

Domain	Consideration by those screened
Clinical	Access to reliable information regarding conditions for which both members of couple screen positive should be provided.
Affective	A copy of carrier screening results should be provided.
	Provide written information that can be used for sharing positive screening results with other family members if desired.
	Plan for returning results
Effective	Pregnancies are considered low risk when couples have discordant results (one screens negative and the other positive).
	When one partner screens positive and the other negative for Tay-Sachs, the negative partner should be screened with enzyme analysis.
	Offer fetal testing when both partners test positive.

Modified from Gregg AR Obstet and Gynecol Clinics of NA

easily available, this hierarchical paradigm of "offer" and "make available" seems less applicable.

ACOG's recommendations are sufficiently nondirective that practitioners have flexibility to offer carrier screening *a la carte*, only offering carrier screening for the pan-ethnic conditions already discussed (e.g., SMA and cystic fibrosis), or expanded testing.[7] ACOG emphasized consistency within one's practice. However, this view was challenged in a recent round table discussion around specific aspects of carrier screening that included maternal fetal medicine physicians, geneticists, and genetic counselors; the group was unanimous in its view that patients should understand all options (including no screening at all). They were also in agreement that the specific approach to screening should be a patient's choice and not driven solely by provider preference.[35]

In summary, offering ECS is recognized as a major leap in prenatal carrier screening. Education and a general sentiment that ECS is not ready for prime time are the primary obstacles to pan-ethnic ECS.

CONCLUSION

Prenatal carrier screening has taken on a level of complexity that requires providers of prenatal care to become better educated. Terminology is new, and in some cases,

the definitions have changed. As ethnic groups become intermixed, pan-ethnic approaches to prenatal carrier screening become more relevant. ECS using NGS while addressing the specific complexity of genes will undoubtedly replace conventional genotyping.

REFERENCES

1. Wilson JMG, Jungner G. Principles and practice of screening for disease. *Publ Health Pap.* 1968;34:7–151.
2. Gregg AR. Expanded carrier screening. *Obstet Gynecol Clin N Am.* 2018;45:103–112.
3. Workshop on Population Screening for the Cystic Fibrosis Gene. Statement from the national institutes of health workshop on population screening for the cystic fibrosis gene. *N Engl J Med.* 1990;323:70–71.
4. Abeliovich D, Lavon IP, Lerer I, et al. Screening for five mutations detects 97% of cystic fibrosis (CF) chromosomes and predicts a carrier frequency of 1:29 in the Jewish Ashkenazi population. *Am J Hum Genet.* 1992;51:951–956.
5. Rohlfs EM, Zhou Z, Heim RA, et al. Cystic fibrosis carrier testing in an ethnically diverse US population. *Clin Chem.* 2011;57:841–848.
6. Prior TW, Professional Practice and Guidelines Committee. Carrier screening for spinal muscular atrophy. *Genet Med.* 2008;10:840–842.
7. Committee opinion No. 690 summary: carrier screening in the age of genomic medicine. *Obstet Gynecol.* 2017;129:595–596.
8. International Human Genome Sequencing Consortium, Human I, and Sequencing G. Initial sequencing and analysis of the human genome. *Nature.* 2001;409:860–921.
9. Bernstein BE, Birney E, Dunham I, Green ED, Gunter C, Snyder M. An integrated encyclopedia of DNA elements in the human genome. *Nature.* 2012;489:57–74.
10. Auton A, Abecasis GR, Altshuler DM, et al. A global reference for human genetic variation. *Nature.* 2015;526:68–74.
11. Rehm HL, Berg JS, Brooks LD, et al. ClinGen — the clinical genome resource. *N Engl J Med.* 2015;372:2235–2242.
12. Sanger F, Coulson AR. A rapid method for determining sequences in DNA by primed synthesis with DNA polymerase. *J Mol Biol.* 1975;94.
13. Mardis ER. Next-generation sequencing platforms. *Annu Rev Anal Chem.* 2013;6:287–303.
14. Greene CN, Cordovado SK, Turner DP, Keong LM, Shulman D, Mueller PW. Novel method to characterize CYP21A2 in Florida patients with congenital adrenal hyperplasia and commercially available cell lines. *Mol Genet Metab Rep.* 2014;1:312–323.
15. Lazarin GA, Hawthorne F, Collins NS, Platt EA, Evans EA, Haque IS. Systematic classification of disease severity for evaluation of expanded Carrier screening panels. *PLoS One.* 2014;9:e114391.
16. Edwards JG, Feldman G, Goldberg J, et al. Expanded Carrier screening in reproductive medicine—points to consider. *Obstet Gynecol.* 2015;125:653–662.

17. Romero S, Biggio Jr JR, Saller DN, Giardine R. Committee opinion No. 691: carrier screening for genetic conditions. *Obstet Gynecol.* 2017;129:e41–e55.

18. New MI, Abraham M, Gonzalez B, et al. Genotype-phenotype Correlation in 1,507 Families with Congenital Adrenal Hyperplasia Owing to 21-hydroxylase Deficiency.

19. Jayadev S, Bird TD. Hereditary ataxias: overview. *Genet Med.* 2013;15:673–683.

20. Park NJ, Morgan C, Sharma R, et al. Improving accuracy of Tay Sachs Carrier screening of the non-jewish population: analysis of 34 carriers and six late-onset patients with HEXA enzyme and DNA sequence analysis. *Pediatr Res.* 2010;67:217–220.

21. Hooven TA, Hooper EM, Wontakal SN, Francis RO, Sahni R, Lee MT. Diagnosis of a rare fetal haemoglobinopathy in the age of next-generation sequencing. *BMJ Case Rep.* 2016;2016. https://doi.org/10.1136/bcr-2016-215193.

22. Sabath DE. Molecular diagnosis of thalassemias and hemoglobinopathies. *Am J Clin Pathol.* 2017;148:6–15.

23. Haque IS, Lazarin GA, Kang HP, Evans EA, Goldberg JD, Wapner RJ. Modeled fetal risk of genetic diseases identified by expanded Carrier screening. *J Am Med Assoc.* 2016;316:734.

24. Hallam S, Nelson H, Greger V, et al. Validation for clinical use of, and initial clinical experience with, a novel approach to population-based Carrier screening using high-throughput, next-generation DNA sequencing. *J Mol Diagn.* 2014;16:180–189.

25. Beauchamp KA, Muzzey D, Wong KK, et al. Systematic design and comparison of expanded carrier screening panels. *Genet Med.* 2018;20:55–63.

26. Arjunan A, Litwack K, Collins N, Charrow J. Carrier screening in the era of expanding genetic technology. *Genet Med.* 2016;18:1214–1217.

27. Azimi M, Schmaus K, Greger V, Neitzel D, Rochelle R, Dinh T. Carrier screening by next-generation sequencing: health benefits and cost effectiveness. *Mol Genet Genomic Med.* 2016;4:292–302.

28. Clarke EV, Schneider JL, Lynch F, et al. Assessment of willingness to pay for expanded Carrier screening among women and couples undergoing preconception Carrier screening. *PLoS One.* 2018;13:e0200139.

29. Lynch FL, Himes P, Gilmore MJ, et al. Time costs for genetic counseling in preconception Carrier screening with genome sequencing. *J Genet Counsel.* 2018;27:823–833.

30. Richards S, Aziz N, Bale S, et al. Standards and guidelines for the interpretation of sequence variants: a joint consensus recommendation of the American College of medical genetics and genomics and the association for molecular pathology. *Genet Med.* 2015;17:405–424.

31. Rogers CR. *Counseling and Psychotherapy.* Cambridge, MA: Houghton Mifflin Co; 1942.

32. Gonzalez-Garay ML, McGuire AL, Pereira S, Caskey CT. Personalized genomic disease risk of volunteers. *Proc Natl Acad Sci USA.* 2013;110:16957–16962.

33. Biesecker BB, Woolford SW, Klein WMP, et al. PUGS: a novel scale to assess perceptions of uncertainties in genome sequencing. *Clin Genet.* 2017;92:172–179.

34. American College of Obstetricians and Gynecologists and American College of Medical Genetics. *Preconception and Prenatal Carrier Screening for Cystic Fibrosis: Clinical and Laboratory Guidelines.* Bethesda, MD: American College of Obstetricians and Gynecologists; 2001.

35. Gregg AR, Edwards JG. Prenatal genetic carrier screening in the genomic age. *Semin Perinatol.* 2018;42:303–306.

CHAPTER 8

Serum and Ultrasound Based Screening Tests for Aneuploidy

BARBARA M. O'BRIEN, MD • LAUREN LICHTEN, MS, CGC

WHAT IS THE HISTORY OF SERUM SCREENING?

Prenatal screening for aneuploidy has evolved dramatically over a short period of time. The purpose of prenatal screening for aneuploidy is to identify women who are at an increased risk for the most common aneuploidies. Down syndrome is the most common aneuploidy seen in live births.[1] Chromosomal abnormalities occur in approximately 1 in 150 live births with Down syndrome being the most common with a prevalence of 1 in 800.[2]

Screening tests for open neural tube defects started in the 1970s after the discovery that elevated levels of maternal serum alpha-fetoprotein (MSAFP) in the second trimester were associated with open spina bifida and anencephaly.[3] The combination of reduced serum levels of second trimester AFP and maternal age was used to screen for Down syndrome beginning in 1984.[4] Test performance improved with the introduction of other second trimester analytes namely unconjugated estriol (uE3), human chorionic gonadotropin (hCG), free beta hCG, and dimeric inhibin A,[5-9]. Decreased maternal serum levels of uE3 and increased levels of hCG and inhibin A are associated with Down syndrome. Second trimester screening using maternal age and the quadruple serum markers alpha fetoprotein, total hCG, uE3, and inhibin A has been validated as an effective tool for Down syndrome.[10-13]

First trimester maternal serum analytes were introduced in the mid-1980s, including pregnancy-associated plasma protein A (PAPP-A) and free beta hCG.[14,15] Decreased levels of PAPP-A and increased levels of free beta hCG are associated with Down syndrome. The nuchal translucency (NT) is the most effective first trimester ultrasound marker for fetal aneuploidy and was first used in 1990.[16] First trimester screening, using NT, combined with maternal age and serum analytes (the combined test) was found to be equivalent in performance to the second trimester quadruple test.[17]

The integrated test was introduced in 1993 and includes first trimester NT and PAPP-A and the second trimester quad screen markers with the final interpretation provided only after analysis of the second trimester analyte levels.[18] Integrated screening can also be performed using first and second trimester analytes without an NT. This may prove to be beneficial in cases in which women do not have access to first trimester NT assessment or in cases in which the NT is not obtainable.

Both the stepwise sequential and the contingent sequential screen are a type of integrated test. The results are available in the first trimester for both tests. In the stepwise sequential screen, the first trimester and the quadruple screen are performed with the results available after the first trimester screen. If a patient returns with a high risk for aneuploidy, this allows for earlier options. In the contingent screen, all women undergo the first trimester screen. They then get stratified into high-, medium-, and low-risk groups. The low-risk group does not require any further testing. The intermediate group is offered quadruple screening and the high-risk group is offered diagnostic testing.

Cell-free DNA (cfDNA) screening became commercially available in 2011 after Palomaki et al. conducted a blinded nested case–control study designed within a cohort of more than 4600 pregnancies at high risk for Down syndrome.[19] The Down syndrome detection rate was 98.6% with a 0.8% false-positive rate. cfDNA screening is reviewed in Chapter 9.

WHO SHOULD BE OFFERED SERUM SCREENING FOR ANEUPLOIDY?

All women should be offered the option of screening or diagnostic testing for aneuploidy regardless of age.[20] There are identifiable risk factors that increase a woman's risk of having a child affected with aneuploidy including advancing age (Table 8.1). Other risk factors

Perinatal Genetics. https://doi.org/10.1016/B978-0-323-53094-1.00008-4

TABLE 8.1
Risk of Chromosomal Abnormalities Based on Maternal Age at Term

Age at Term	Risk of Trisomy 21	Risk of Any Chromosome Abnormality
15	1:1578	1:454
16	1:1572	1:475
17	1:1565	1:499
18	1:1556	1:525
19	1:1544	1:555
20	1:1480	1:525
21	1:1460	1:525
22	1:1440	1:499
23	1:1420	1:499
24	1:1380	1:475
25	1:1340	1:475
26	1:1290	1:475
27	1:1220	1:454
28	1:1140	1:434
29	1:1050	1:416
30	1:940	1:384
31	1:820	1:384
32	1:700	1:322
33	1:570	1:285
34	1:456	1:243
35	1:353	1:178
36	1:267	1:148
37	1:199	1:122
38	1:148	1:104
39	1:111	1:80
40	1:85	1:62
41	1:67	1:48
42	1:54	1:38
43	1:45	1:30
44	1:39	1:23
45	1:35	1:18
46	1:31	1:14
47	1:29	1:10
48	1:27	1:8
49	1:26	1:6
50	1:25	§

From ACOG Bulletin 163.

for aneuploidy are as follows: a history of a prior fetus with aneuploidy, a fetal anomaly or structural malformation, or a parental translocation.[20] The decision to perform screening and/or diagnostic testing depends on the woman's goals and desires for her pregnancy. Some women choose screening for knowledge, whereas others want to obtain information to make decisions regarding pregnancy continuation versus termination. Patients considering aneuploidy screening should have pretest counseling regarding the benefits, risks, and limitations of the test.

WHAT ARE THE DIFFERENT SERUM SCREENING TESTS? WHAT ARE THE BENEFITS AND LIMITATIONS OF EACH ONE?

Screening tests for aneuploidy include serum screening, ultrasound, and cfDNA. Fetal aneuploidy risk can be evaluated on the basis of maternal age, maternal serum results and ultrasound markers. No one screening test is superior for all testing characteristics, and not all tests are available in all centers. Factors to be considered in the choice of screening tests are the availably of NT assessment, gestational age at the time of presentation, cost, screening test sensitivity, and limitations. An overview of serum screening tests is described below and summarized in Table 8.2. Detection rates and false-positive rates for common screening tests for aneuploidy are displayed. Each test has advantages and disadvantages that should be discussed with the patient before screening.

First-Trimester Screening

Screening based on the NT alone is insufficient for aneuploidy risk evaluation because of a lower detection rate of approximately 70%, although NT alone may be used to screen women with high-order multiple gestations (triplets or quadruplets), as there are currently no effective serum screening options for these pregnancies. The first trimester screen includes NT measurement by ultrasound along with serum testing for free beta hCG or total hCG, and PAPP-A levels. First trimester screening can be performed between 10 0/7 and 13 6/7 weeks' gestation. The NT is dependent on the crown-rump length (CRL) of the fetus being within the appropriate range (36–84 mm) at the time of ultrasound. The NT and serum marker data are combined with gestational age and information regarding maternal factors such as maternal age, prior history of aneuploidy, weight, race and number of fetuses, to calculate a risk estimate for the risk of aneuploidy.[21] The first trimester screen

TABLE 8.2
Detection Rates and False Positives for Common Screening Tests for Aneuploidy

Test	Gestational Age	Detection Rate T21, %	Detection Rate of All Aneuploidies, %	Screen-Positive Rate, %[b]
First trimester screen[a] (PAPP-A, hCG and NT)	10 0/7 to 13/67	80	69	5
Sequential screen[a] 1st trimester PAPP-A, hCG, NT and 2nd trimester MSAFP, hCG, uE3, and inhibin A)	10 0/7 to 13/67, then 15 0/7 to 22 6/7	93	82	5
Cell-free DNA	10 0/7 to term	99	72	1–9
Chorionic villus sampling	10 0/7–13/67	>99	>99	1
Amniocentesis	15 0/7 to term	>99	>99	0.2

[a]Based on the NT performed at 12 weeks' gestational age.
[b]Includes all results requiring follow-up (i.e., failed result, false-positive result, and mosaicism). Adapted from Am J Obstet Gynecol 2015; 212:711–6.

detects approximately 85% of cases of trisomy 21 at a 5% false-positive rate.[22]

Trisomy 18 is characterized by increased NT and decreased free beta hCG and PAPP-A.[14,23] Screening using the combination of all three markers can detect 86%–89% of trisomy 18 at a 0.5–1.0% false-positive rate.[24] The benefits of first trimester screening include the early gestational age at which results are provided. cfDNA or diagnostic testing can then be offered and pursued at an earlier gestational age. A limitation of first trimester screening is the accuracy required for the NT scan.

Quadruple Screen

The quadruple screen can be performed between 15 0/7 and 22 6/7 weeks of gestation, but for optimal screening of neural tube defects the ideal timing is between 16 and 18 weeks.[12,13,20] The test is comprised of hCG, AFP, dimeric inhibin A, and uE3. Similar to the first trimester screen, these results, along with maternal factors including maternal age, weight, race, the presence of diabetes, and number of fetuses, are used to calculate an estimate for the specific risk of aneuploidy or neural tube defect. First trimester and quad screening have similar detection rates for Down syndrome with comparable false-positive rates.[12,20] There is an 80% detection rate with a 5% false-positive rate[20] for Down syndrome.

The benefits of the quadruple screen are that it screens for open neural tube defects in addition to aneuploidy. A skilled sonographer is not needed as there is no ultrasound component to the exam. The limitation is the late gestational age at which it is performed.

Sequential Screening

Sequential screening combines the first trimester screen and the quadruple screen for increased aneuploidy detection rates over either test in isolation. In the sequential screen, results from the first trimester screen are shared with the patient. This offers women the opportunity for early diagnostic testing if the early risk for aneuploidy is increased. Women without an increased risk of aneuploidy after the early screen then undergo quadruple screening in the second trimester, which is incorporated with their first trimester screen results for a final estimate of the risk of aneuploidy.

Integrated Screening

An integrated screen offers both first and second trimester testing but without disclosing the results of the first trimester screen. The detection rate for Down syndrome is approximately 96% with a false-positive rate of 5%.[12] The benefit of integrated screening is the high detection rate. The limitation is the unavailability of a result until the second trimester.

Stepwise Sequential and Contingent Screening

The stepwise sequential screen is a combination of the first trimester portion of the integrated screen with an NT scan and serum analytes. Patients at very high risk for aneuploidy with greater or equal to 1 in 50 or at the highest 0.5% of having an affected fetus are offered counseling and diagnostic testing. Women who do not have an increased risk (less than 1 in 50) proceed to the second trimester portion of the test. These women at lower risk for not receiving the first trimester results do not receive their results until the second trimester. The limitations of this approach are the withholding of first trimester results to some women until the second trimester and the potential for nonadherence of the second blood draw.[20]

Both the stepwise sequential screen and the contingent sequential make the first trimester screening results available to patients. In the stepwise sequential screen, both the first trimester screen and the quad screen are performed. The results are available after their first trimester screen. This allows for earlier counseling for patients at high risk for aneuploidy. In the contingent screen, all women undergo the first trimester screen and then get stratified into high-, medium-, and low-risk groups. The high-risk group is then offered cfDNA screening or diagnostic testing.[20] The low-risk group requires no further testing. The intermediate-risk group is offered quad screening. The detection rate for the contingent screen is between 80%–94% with a false-positive rate of 5%.

WHAT IS THE ROLE OF FIRST TRIMESTER ULTRASOUND MARKERS IN THE DETECTION OF ANEUPLOIDY?

First trimester ultrasound can be used to assess the risk for fetal aneuploidy. Markers of interest are summarized below.

Increased Nuchal Translucency and Cystic Hygroma

NT is the subcutaneous fluid-filled space between the back of the fetal neck and overlying skin.[25] The fetal NT should be measured between 10 and 14 weeks' gestation, when the CRL is between 36 and 84 mm, by a clinician with expertise in this technique.[26] A cystic hygroma is an enlarged hypoechoic space at the back of the fetal neck, extending along the length of the fetal back, and in which septations are clearly visible.[27]

Increased NT is associated with an increased risk for chromosomal abnormalities, including trisomy 21, 13, 18, and monosomy X.[13,28,29] The detection rate for Down syndrome using NT ranges between 63% and 77% with a 5% false-positive rate.[12,17,30] The risk for fetal aneuploidy increases with NT measurement.[31,32] One study examined 11,315 pregnancies, which included 19% (2168) with an abnormal karyotype.[31] In that study, an NT measurement less than 3 mm was associated with a 7% risk for a chromosome abnormality, whereas the risk increased to 75% when the NT measured 8.5 mm or greater. Furthermore, the NT measurement varied

depending on the fetal karyotype with the majority of fetuses affected with trisomy 21 having an NT measurement less than 4.5 mm, fetuses affected with trisomy 13 or 18 between 4.5 and 8.4 mm, and fetuses affected with Turner syndrome above 8.5 mm. A cystic hygroma is associated with approximately 50% risk for chromosome abnormalities, particularly trisomy 21, trisomy 18, and Turner syndrome.[27,33] Some studies have shown that septated cystic hygromas have a higher risk of aneuploidy than simple cystic hygromas,[34] but other studies have not found this association.[35]

NT measurement is currently used as a component of first trimester screening, integrated screening, and sequential screening.[20] Comstock and colleagues evaluated data from 36, 120 subjects enrolled in the FASTER Trial to determine the utility of serum analytes in the setting of an increased NT.[36] In this study, 32 patients had an NT measurement greater than 4 mm, and 128 patients had an NT measurement between 3 and 4 mm. There was minimal benefit of measuring serum analytes in cases with an NT measurement between 3 and 4 mm, and no benefit to measuring serum analytes when the NT measurement is above 4 mm. The authors concluded that chorionic villus sampling (CVS) should be offered to patients with an NT of 3 mm or greater.

NT measurement may not be useful in identifying aneuploidy for woman already undergoing cfDNA screening. The DNA*First* study examined 2691 women in Rhode Island who had cfDNA testing as the primary mode of aneuploidy screening between September 2014 and July 2015. Ten women had an NT above 3 mm or a cystic hygroma as well as cfDNA testing, and the cfDNA testing was able to correctly identify both euploid and aneuploid fetuses.[37] In 2017, the Society for Maternal Fetal Medicine issued a statement recommending that NT measurement is not useful for women already undergoing cfDNA testing.[38]

In contrast, first trimester ultrasound can still be useful for women who are deciding between aneuploidy screening and diagnostic testing via CVS. In one retrospective study of more than 2400 women of advanced maternal age, 2337 were eligible for cfDNA testing, and 237 of those women had an ultrasound abnormality at the time of testing that could have changed the testing strategy such as an anomaly, incorrect dating, multiple gestation, or nonviable pregnancy.[39] Similarly, a retrospective cohort study examined 1739 women at increased risk for aneuploidy based on age or medical history who had negative cfDNA testing.[40] Sixty women had an unexpected fetal finding: 33 had an NT measurement above 3 mm (4 of these cases had a cystic hygroma, and 3 had a structural abnormality); 13 had unrecognized twins; and 10 had a fetal demise. A normal karyotype was confirmed in 98.7% of these cases. Another retrospective cohort study examined 1906 women undergoing first trimester ultrasound between 2013 and 2014.[41] Negative cfDNA testing results were available for half of the women (956), and 37% of these women had a clinically significant first trimester ultrasound finding (42 fetal, 286 gynecological, and 317 placental). Fetal findings included NT abnormalities (8, 19%), fetal abnormality with NT abnormality (8, 19%), and fetal abnormality without NT abnormality (26, 61%). Gynecological abnormalities included ovarian (148, 52%) and uterine findings (138, 48%). Placental abnormalities included location (258, 81%), placentation (1, 0.3%), bleeding (56, 18%), and cord insertion (2, 0.6%).

Fetuses with increased NT and cystic hygroma that have normal karyotypes are at increased risk for structural abnormalities, particularly cardiac defects.[42-44] The risk of cardiac defects increases with increasing NT measurement,[45] with approximately one-third risk for cardiac defects when a cystic hygroma is detected.[27] A metaanalysis that included 20 studies involving 205,232 fetuses, including 537 diagnosed with a congenital heart defect,[46] reported a pooled positive likelihood ratio of 30.5 (95% CI, 24.3–38.6) for NT > 99th percentile. Other fetal anomalies that have been seen in association with increased NT have involved the neurologic, gastrointestinal, urogenital, and skeletal systems.[27] Therefore, a detailed fetal survey and fetal echocardiogram are recommended for all fetuses with an increased NT or cystic hygroma.

Several genetic syndromes have been associated with an increased NT and cystic hygroma,[27] with Noonan syndrome being the most frequent syndrome diagnosed. Lee et al.[47] performed a retrospective review of 134 fetuses tested for mutations in PTPN11, which is the most common gene associated with Noonan syndrome and 12/134 fetuses had a PTPN11 mutation. Cystic hygroma had a higher likelihood of a positive result (16%) than increased NT (2%). Another study performed by Croonen et al.[48] found a mutation in genes associated with Noonan syndrome in 13/75 fetuses with a normal karyotype and abnormal ultrasound (PTPN11, KRAS, RAF1) and 10/60 fetuses with an abnormal ultrasound only (PTPN11, RAF1, BRAF, MAP2K1). The authors recommended prenatal testing for Noonan syndrome (PTPN11, RAF1, KRAS) in fetuses with an increased NT and at least one additional ultrasound finding such as polyhydramnios, hydrops, renal abnormalities, distended jugular lymphatic sac, hydrothorax, cardiac abnormalities, cystic hygroma, and ascites. They also recommended considering mutation analysis of BRAF and MAP2K1. A recent study calculated a 10% risk for Noonan syndrome in fetuses with an NT over 3 mm based on findings of a Noonan syndrome–related mutation in 4/39 fetuses with an NT over 3 mm and a normal karyotype.[49] Testing for other genetic syndromes should be determined based on additional ultrasound findings at the time of the fetal survey ultrasound.

Chromosome microarray should be considered for all fetuses with an increased NT or cystic hygroma. A metaanalysis showed that an NT measurement above 3.5 mm was associated with a 5% pooled rate of copy number variants on chromosome microarray.[50] The most common findings were 22q11.2 deletion, 22q11.2 duplication, 10q26.12q26.3 deletion, and 12q21q22 deletion. Variants of uncertain significance occurred 1% of the time. Fetuses with additional abnormalities were more likely to have a copy number variant. Similarly, Yang et al.[51] identified a submicroscopic chromosomal abnormality in 20 of 220 fetuses with an increased NT and normal karyotype (9.1%). Fetuses with additional ultrasound abnormalities on a second-trimester ultrasound were more likely to have a submicroscopic abnormality (26.9%) than those with otherwise normal ultrasounds (6.7%). Maya et al.[52] assessed NT cut-off levels as an indication for CMA by examining 462 fetuses with a normal NT (less than 3 mm), 170 with NT between 3–3.4 mm, and 138 with an NT greater than 3.5 mm. Pathogenic copy number variants were detected more often when NT was larger (1.7% NT less than 3 mm, 6.5% NT 3–3.4 mm 13.8% NT greater than 3.5 mm).

Some studies have examined long-term neurodevelopmental outcomes in fetuses with increased NT. There does not appear to be an increased risk for neurodevelopmental problems in early childhood for children with normal karyotypes, no structural abnormalities, and a history of an increased NT measurement or cystic hygroma.[53,54] Iculano et al.[55] reported that the risk for adverse outcome in school age children with a history of an increased NT is comparable with the general population.

Nasal Bone

Multiple studies have identified an association between absent fetal nasal bone in the first trimester and trisomy 21.[56-58] Nasal bone sonography has been shown to improve the detection rate and lower the false-positive rate for trisomy 21 on first trimester screening.[59] However, nasal bone measurement is not uniformly included in all first trimester screening protocols because there are multiple factors besides fetal aneuploidy that can impact the nasal bone and measurement requires an experienced sonographer.[60] Cicero et al.[61] noted that the incidence of absent nasal bone was related to the ethnic origin of the mother (less common in Caucasians than African Americans or Asians), fetal CRL (less common as CRL increases), and NT thickness (more common with increasing NT thickness). Another concern about nasal bone sonography is its lack of sensitivity. Malone et al.[62] studied 6324 patients who had an NT ultrasound and nasal bone sonography. Of the 4801 patients who had an acceptable nasal bone measurement, 0.5% had an absent nasal bone (22). The majority of fetuses with trisomy 21 had a nasal bone (9/11), whereas 50% of the fetuses with trisomy 18 had a nasal bone (1/2). Overall, the authors found the absence of a nasal bone to have a sensitivity of 7.7% for fetal aneuploidy, positive predictive value of 4.5%, and false-positive rate of 0.3%. Chanprapaph et al.[63] also found nasal bone sonography to be specific, but lacking sensitivity.

Ductus Venosus Blood Flow

There are differences in ductus venosus blood flow between aneuploid and euploid fetuses.[64,65] Reversed flow at the time of atrial contraction has been associated with aneuploidy and fetal cardiac defects, while forward triphasic pulsatile ductus venosus flow is normal. Abnormal ductus venosus blood flow has been observed in 59%–93% of aneuploid fetuses and 3%–21% of euploid fetuses.[66] Measurement of ductus venosus blood flow and NT increases the sensitivity of first trimester ultrasound in the detection of Down syndrome to 94%.[67,68] Measurement of ductus venosus flow can be helpful in identifying increased risks for adverse fetal outcomes. One study showed adverse outcomes in 11/42 (26.2%) fetuses with a normal NT and reversed or absent ductus venosus blood flow.[69] Adverse outcomes included heart defects, fetal growth restriction, and multiple fetal anomalies.

Tricuspid Regurgitation

Tricuspid regurgitation (TR) diagnosed by pulse wave Doppler studies between 11 and 13 weeks 6 days gestation has been shown to be a marker for fetal aneuploidy, particularly trisomy 21.[70,71,72] A metaanalysis of 15 studies showed that TR detected at 11–14 weeks of gestation has a likelihood ratio of 25 for the fetus to have Down syndrome (95% CI 14.9–41.9).[73] Additionally, many studies have suggested that TR is a marker for heart defects in euploid fetuses. A metaanalysis showed that the strength of association between TR and heart defects persisted when there was another factor associated with heart defects, such as an increased NT, but no association between TR and CHD when screening a low-risk population for heart defects.[74] Overall, the sensitivity of TR was 35.2%, and the specificity was 98.6%.

WHAT IS THE ROLE OF SECOND TRIMESTER ULTRASOUND IN THE DETECTION OF FETAL ANEUPLOIDY?

There are several second trimester markers that are useful in estimating the risk of fetal aneuploidy. These markers are summarized in Chapter 10.

HOW SHOULD A SCREEN-POSITIVE SERUM SCREEN FOR FETAL ANEUPLOIDY BE INTERPRETED? WHAT OTHER TESTS SHOULD BE OFFERED IN THE CASE OF SCREEN-POSITIVE SERUM SCREENING?

A positive screen should not be interpreted as diagnostic for aneuploidy. The age-related risk for aneuploidy should be discussed in the light of the serum screening result cutoff[20] and the patients' understanding documented. Patients with a positive screen should be offered genetic counseling. Repeat serum screening is not recommended. Diagnostic testing should be discussed and offered (see Chapter 14). Patients should be counseled regarding the small risk of loss associated with the procedure including a 1/450 risk of loss with CVS and a 1/900 risk of loss with amniocentesis.[75] cfDNA may be offered, especially to women who do not opt for diagnostic testing by CVS or amniocentesis. Counseling on the benefits and limitations of cfDNA in this setting must be discussed. The gestational age of the patient should be considered as cfDNA test results can take up to 10 days to return, therefore, she may desire to opt for diagnostic testing to avoid a delay in definitive diagnosis and management. The patient should be informed that there is a 2% residual risk of chromosomal abnormalities after a normal cfDNA in the setting of a positive serum screen.[76]

Diagnostic testing should include discussions of the small risk of loss with the procedure including 1/450 risk of loss with CVS and 1/900 risk of loss with amniocentesis.[75]

WHAT OPTIONS ARE AVAILABLE FOR SCREENING FOR FETAL ANEUPLOIDY IN MULTIPLE GESTATIONS?

NT is the only available method for screening in higher-order multiples (greater than twins) at this time. At this time, the American College of Obstetrics and Gynecology and the Society for Maternal-Fetal Medicine (SMFM) do not recommend the use of cfDNA in multiple gestations because of the limited evidence regarding its efficacy.[20] Diagnostic testing can be performed in women with multiple gestations who desire definitive testing for genetic abnormalities. Diagnostic testing should include discussion of the small risk of loss associated with the procedure.[75] The procedure-associated pregnancy loss rate is slightly higher compared with the loss rate in singletons, reported to be 1%–1.8%.[77]

WHAT IS THE ROLE OF SERUM SCREENING IN THE PREDICTION OF ADVERSE PREGNANCY OUTCOMES?

Hypersensitive disorders of pregnancy have been shown to affect up to 5%–10% of pregnancies[78] and are associated with adverse pregnancy outcomes such as preterm birth, maternal morbidity and mortality, and long-term cardiovascular disease.[79] Prevention and early identification and management could potentially identify women who could benefit from intensive monitoring in pregnancy. Abnormal screening results in the first and second trimester have been associated with adverse pregnancy outcomes in the absence of aneuploidy or neural tube defects. Low PAPP-A and uE3 levels and elevated hCG, inhibin A, and MSAFP levels have been associated with a number of adverse obstetric outcomes including preeclampsia, stillbirth, preterm birth, and birth weight less than the 10th percentile. The likelihood of an adverse pregnancy outcome increases as the values of the markers become more extreme and as the number of abnormal markers increase.[80,81] Although many of the associations between maternal serum markers for aneuploidy are statistically significant, the sensitivity and positive predictive values are too low to be clinically useful for screening tests. Furthermore, there are currently no proven management strategies to manage patients with abnormal aneuploidy markers. Future research to determine optimal management strategies for women with abnormal markers as well as identification of additional markers to improve the sensitivity and specificity of a prediction model for adverse obstetric outcomes is needed.[80,81]

REFERENCES

1. Morris JK, Alberman E. Trends in down's syndrome live births and antenatal diagnoses in England and Wales from 1989 to 2008: analysis of data from the national down syndrome cytogenetic register. *BMJ.* 2009;339:b3794.
2. Nussbaum RL, McInnes RR, Willard HF. Principles of clinical cytogenetics and genome analysis. In: *Thompson and Thomson Genetics in Medicine.* Philadelphia (PA): Elsevier; 2016:57–74.
3. Wald NJ, et al. Maternal serum-alpha-fetoprotein measurement in antenatal screening for anencephaly and spina bifida in early pregnancy. Report of UK collaborative study on alpha-fetoprotein in relation to neural-tube defects. *Lancet.* 1977;1(8026):1323–1332.
4. Merkatz IR, et al. An association between low maternal serum α-fetoprotein and fetal chromosomal abnormalities. *Am J Obstet Gynecol.* 1984;148(7):886–894.
5. Bogart MH, Pandian MR, Jones OW. Abnormal maternal serum chorionic gonadotropin levels in pregnancies with fetal chromosome abnormalities. *Prenat Diagn.* 1987;7(9):623–630.
6. Canick JA, et al. Low second trimester maternal serum unconjugated oestriol in pregnancies with Down's syndrome. *BJOG An Int J Obstet Gynaecol.* 1988;95(4):330–333.
7. Cuckle HS, et al. Maternal serum dimeric inhibin A in second-trimester Down's syndrome pregnancies. *Prenat Diagn.* 1995;15(4):385–386.
8. Knight GJ, et al. hCG and the free β-subunit as screening tests for Down syndrome. *Prenat Diagn.* 1998;18(3):235–245.
9. Ozturk M, et al. Abnormal maternal serum levels of human chorionic gonadotropin free subunits in trisomy 18. *Am J Med Genet.* 1990;36(4):480–483.
10. Benn PA, et al. Incorporation of inhibin-A in second-trimester screening for Down syndrome. *Obstet Gynecol.* 2003;101(3):451–454.
11. Jaques AM, et al. Using record linkage and manual follow-up to evaluate the Victorian maternal serum screening quadruple test for Down's syndrome, trisomy 18 and neural tube defects. *J Med Screen.* 2006;13(1):8–13.
12. Malone FD, et al. First-trimester or second-trimester screening, or both, for Down's syndrome. *N Engl J Med.* 2005b;353(19):2001–2011.
13. Wald NJ, Huttly WJ, Hackshaw AK. Antenatal screening for Down's syndrome with the quadruple test. *Lancet.* 2003;361(9360):835–836.
14. Spencer K, et al. Free β-hCG as first-trimester marker for fetal trisomy. *Lancet.* 1992;339(8807):1480.
15. Wald N, et al. First trimester concentrations of pregnancy associated plasma protein A and placental protein 14 in Down's syndrome. *BMJ Br Med J (Clin Res Ed).* 1992;305(6844):28.
16. Szabo J, Gellen J. Nuchal fluid accumulation in trisomy-21 detected by vaginosonography in first trimester. *Lancet.* 1990;336(8723):1133.
17. Wald NJ, et al. First and second trimester antenatal screening for Down's syndrome: the results of the Serum, Urine and Ultrasound Screening Study (SURUSS). *J Med Screen.* 2003;10(2):56–104.
18. Wald NJ, Watt HC, Hackshaw AK. "Integrated screening for Down's syndrome based on tests performed during the first and second trimesters. *N Engl J Med.* 1999;341(7):461–467.
19. Palomaki GE, et al. DNA sequencing of maternal plasma to detect Down syndrome: an international clinical validation study. *Genet Med.* 2011;13(11):913.

20. American College of Obstetricians and Gynecologists Committee on Practice Bulletins—Obstetrics, Committee on Genetics, and the Society for Maternal-Fetal Medicine. Practice Bulletin No. 163: Screening for Fetal Aneuploidy. *Obstet Gynecol.* 2016;127(5):e123–e137.

21. Kagan KO, et al. Screening for trisomy 21 by maternal age, fetal nuchal translucency thickness, free beta-human chorionic gonadotropin and pregnancy-associated plasma protein-A. *Ultrasound Obstet Gynecol.* 2008;31(6):618–624.

22. Canick JA, Lambert-Messerlian GM, Palomaki GE, et al. Comparison of serum markers in first-trimester down syndrome screening. *Obstet Gynecol.* 2006;108:1992.

23. Sherod C, Sebire NJ, Soares W, Snijiders RJM, Nicolaides KH. Prenatal diagnosis of trisomy 18 at the 10–14 week ultrasound scan. *Ultrasound Obstet Gynecol.* 1997;10:387–390.

24. Tul N, Spencer K, Nobie P, Chan C, Nicolaides KH. Screening for trisomy 18 by fetal nuchal translucency and maternal serum screening free beta hCG and PAPP-A at 10–14 weeks of gestation. *Prenat Diagn.* 1999;19. 10350 1042.

25. Nicolaides KH, Brizot ML, Snijders RJM. Fetal nuchal translucency: ultrasound screening for fetal trisomy in the first trimester of pregnancy. *BJOG An Int J Obstet Gynaecol.* 1994;101(9):782–786.

26. Abuhamad A. Technical aspects of nuchal translucency measurement. *Semin Perinatol.* 2005;29(6). Elsevier.

27. Malone FD, et al. First-trimester septated cystic hygroma: prevalence, natural history, and pediatric outcome. *Obstet Gynecol.* 2005;106(2):288–294.

28. Malone FD, et al. First-trimester screening for aneuploidy: research or standard of care? *Am J Obstet Gynecol.* 2000;182(3):490–496.

29. Nicolaides KH, Heath V, Cicero S. Increased fetal nuchal translucency at 11–14 weeks. *Prenat Diagn.* 2002;22(4):308–315.

30. Snijders RJM, et al. UK multicentre project on assessment of risk of trisomy 21 by maternal age and fetal nuchal-translucency thickness at 10–14 weeks of gestation. *Lancet.* 1998;352(9125):343–346.

31. Kagan, Oliver K, et al. Relation between increased fetal nuchal translucency thickness and chromosomal defects. *Obstet Gynecol.* 2006;107(1):6–10.

32. Scholl J, et al. First-trimester cystic hygroma: relationship of nuchal translucency thickness and outcomes. *Obstet Gynecol.* 2012;120(3):551–559.

33. Graesslin O, et al. Characteristics and outcome of fetal cystic hygroma diagnosed in the first trimester. *Acta Obstet Gynecol Scand.* 2007;86(12):1442–1446.

34. Rosati P, Guariglia L. Prognostic value of ultrasound findings of fetal cystic hygroma detected in early pregnancy by transvaginal sonography. *Ultrasound Obstet Gynecol.* 2000;16(3):245–250.

35. Johnson, Paul M, et al. First-trimester simple hygroma: cause and outcome. *Am J Obstet Gynecol.* 1993;168(1):156–161.

36. Comstock CH, et al. Is there a nuchal translucency millimeter measurement above which there is no added benefit from first trimester serum screening? *Am J Obstet Gynecol.* 2006;195(3):843–847.

37. O'brien BM, et al. Nuchal translucency measurement in the era of prenatal screening for aneuploidy using cell free (cf) DNA. *Prenat Diagn.* 2017;37(3):303–305.

38. Society for Maternal-Fetal Medicine (SMFM), Electronic address: pubs@smfm.org, Norton ME, Biggio JR, et al. The role of ultrasound in women who undergo cell-free DNA screening. *Am J Obstet Gynecol.* 2017;216:B2.

39. Vora NL, et al. The utility of a prerequisite ultrasound at 10–14 weeks in cell free DNA fetal aneuploidy screening. *Ultrasound Obstet Gynecol.* 2016.

40. Reiff ES, et al. What is the role of the 11-to 14-week ultrasound in women with negative cell-free DNA screening for aneuploidy? *Prenat Diagn.* 2016;36(3):260–265.

41. Rao RR, et al. The value of the first trimester ultrasound in the era of cell free DNA screening. *Prenat Diagn.* 2016;36(13):1192–1198.

42. Souka AP, et al. Defects and syndromes in chromosomally normal fetuses with increased nuchal translucency thickness at 10–14 weeks of gestation. *Ultrasound Obstet Gynecol.* 1998;11(6):391–400.

43. Souka AP, et al. Outcome of pregnancy in chromosomally normal fetuses with increased nuchal translucency in the first trimester. *Ultrasound Obstet Gynecol.* 2001;18(1):9–17.

44. Souka AP, et al. Increased nuchal translucency with normal karyotype. *Am J Obstet Gynecol.* 2005;192(4):1005–1021.

45. Shamshirsaz AA, et al. Nuchal translucency and cardiac abnormalities in euploid singleton pregnancies. *J Matern Fetal Neonatal Med.* 2014;27(5):495–499.

46. Sotiriadis A, et al. Nuchal translucency and major congenital heart defects in fetuses with normal karyotype: a meta-analysis. *Ultrasound Obstet Gynecol.* 2013;42(4):383–389.

47. Lee KA, et al. PTPN11 analysis for the prenatal diagnosis of Noonan syndrome in fetuses with abnormal ultrasound findings. *Clin Genet.* 2009;75(2):190–194.

48. Croonen EA, et al. Prenatal diagnostic testing of the Noonan syndrome genes in fetuses with abnormal ultrasound findings. *Eur J Hum Genet.* 2013;21(9):936.

49. Ali MM, Chasen ST, Norton ME. Testing for Noonan syndrome after increased nuchal translucency. *Prenat Diagn.* 2017.

50. Grande M, et al. Genomic microarray in fetuses with increased nuchal translucency and normal karyotype: a systematic review and meta-analysis. *Ultrasound Obstet Gynecol.* 2015;46(6):650–658.

51. Yang X, et al. Submicroscopic chromosomal abnormalities in fetuses with increased nuchal translucency and normal karyotype. *J Matern Fetal Neonatal Med.* 2017;30(2):194–198.

52. Maya I, et al. Cut-off value of nuchal translucency as indication for chromosomal microarray analysis. *Ultrasound Obstet Gynecol.* 2017;50(3):332–335.

53. Hellmuth SG, et al. Increased nuchal translucency thickness and risk of neurodevelopmental disorders. *Ultrasound Obstet Gynecol.* 2017;49(5):592–598.

54. Sotiriadis A, Papatheodorou S, Makrydimas G. Neurodevelopmental outcome of fetuses with increased nuchal translucency and apparently normal prenatal and/or

postnatal assessment: a systematic review. *Ultrasound Obstet Gynecol.* 2012;39(1):10–19.

55. Iuculano A, et al. Pregnancy outcome and long-term follow-up of fetuses with isolated increased NT: a retrospective cohort study. *J Perinat Med.* 2016;44(2):237–242.

56. Cicero S, et al. Absence of nasal bone in fetuses with trisomy 21 at 11–14 weeks of gestation: an observational study. *Lancet.* 2001;358(9294):1665–1667.

57. Otano L, et al. Association between first trimester absence of fetal nasal bone on ultrasound and Down syndrome. *Prenat Diagn.* 2002;22(10):930–932.

58. Zoppi MA, et al. Absence of fetal nasal bone and aneuploidies at first-trimester nuchal translucency screening in unselected pregnancies. *Prenat Diagn.* 2003;23(6):496–500.

59. Kagan KO, et al. Fetal nasal bone in screening for trisomies 21, 18 and 13 and Turner syndrome at 11–13 weeks of gestation. *Ultrasound Obstet Gynecol.* 2009;33(3):259–264.

60. Cicero S, et al. Learning curve for sonographic examination of the fetal nasal bone at 11–14 weeks. *Ultrasound Obstet Gynecol.* 2003;22(2):135–137.

61. Cicero S, et al. Absent nasal bone at 11–14 weeks of gestation and chromosomal defects. *Ultrasound Obstet Gynecol.* 2003b;22(1):31–35.

62. Malone FD, et al. First-trimester nasal bone evaluation for aneuploidy in the general population. *Obstet Gynecol.* 2004;104(6):1222–1228.

63. Chanprapaph P, Dulyakasem C, Phattanchindakun B. Sensitivity of multiple first trimester sonomarkers in fetal aneuploidy detection. *J Perinat Med.* 2015;43(3):359–365.

64. Borrell A, et al. Abnormal ductus venosus blood flow in trisomy 21 fetuses during early pregnancy. *Am J Obstet Gynecol.* 1998;179(6):1612–1617.

65. Matias A, et al. Screening for chromosomal abnormalities at 10–14 weeks: the role of ductus venosus blood flow. *Ultrasound Obstet Gynecol.* 1998;12(6):380–384.

66. Malone FD, D'alton ME. First-trimester sonographic screening for Down syndrome. *Obstet Gynecol.* 2003;102(5):1066–1079.

67. Mavrides E, et al. Screening for aneuploidy in the first trimester by assessment of blood flow in the ductus venosus. *BJOG An Int J Obstet Gynaecol.* 2002;9:1015–1019.

68. Timmerman E, et al. Ductus venosus pulsatility index measurement reduces the false-positive rate in first-trimester screening. *Ultrasound Obstet Gynecol.* 2010;36(6):661–667.

69. Oh C, Harman C, Baschat AA. Abnormal first-trimester ductus venosus blood flow: a risk factor for adverse outcome in fetuses with normal nuchal translucency. *Ultrasound Obstet Gynecol.* 2007;30(2):192–196.

70. Huggon IC, DeFigueiredo DB, Allan LD. Tricuspid regurgitation in the diagnosis of chromosomal anomalies in the fetus at 11–14 weeks of gestation. *Heart.* 2003;89(9):1071–1073.

71. Faiola S, Tsoi E, Huggon IC, Allan LD, Nicolaides KH. Likelihood ratio for trisomy 21 in fetuses with tricuspid regurgitation at the 11 to 13 + 6-week scan. *Ultrasound Obstet Gynecol.* 2005;26(1):22–27.

72. Falcon O, Faiola S, Huggon I, Allan L, Nicolaides KH. Fetal tricuspid regurgitation at the 11 + 0 to 13 + 6-week scan: association with chromosomal defects and reproducibility of the method. *Ultrasound Obstet Gynecol.* 2006; 27(6):609–612.

73. Scala C, et al. P11. 08: tricuspid regurgitation as a screening marker for Trisomy 21: systematic review and meta-analysis. *Ultrasound Obstet Gynecol.* 2016;48(S1):200.

74. Scala C, et al. Fetal tricuspid regurgitation in the first trimester as a screening marker for congenital heart defects: systematic review and meta-analysis. *Fetal Diagn Ther.* 2017;42.1:1–8.

75. American College of Obstetricians and Gynecologists. Practice Bulletin No. 162: prenatal diagnostic testing for genetic disorders. *Obstet Gynecol.* 2016b;127(5):e108.

76. Norton ME, Jelliffe-Pawlowski LL, Currier RJ. Chromosome abnormalities detected by current prenatal screening and noninvasive prenatal testing. *Obstet Gynecol.* 2014;124(5):979–986.

77. Agarwal K, Alfirevic Z. Pregnancy loss after chorionic villus sampling and genetic amniocentesis in twin pregnancies: a systematic review. *Ultrasound Obstet Gynecol.* 2012;40:128–134.

78. Wallis AB, et al. Secular trends in the rates of preeclampsia, eclampsia, and gestational hypertension, United States, 1987–2004. *Am J Hypertens.* 2008;21(5):521–526.

79. American College of Obstetricians and Gynecologists. Hypertension in pregnancy. Report of the American College of Obstetricians and Gynecologists' task force on hypertension in pregnancy. *Obstet Gynecol.* 2013;122(5):1122.

80. Dugoff L, et al. First-trimester maternal serum PAPP-A and free-beta subunit human chorionic gonadotropin concentrations and nuchal translucency are associated with obstetric complications: a population-based screening study (the FASTER Trial). *Am J Obstet Gynecol.* 2004;191(4):1446–1451.

81. Dugoff L. First-and second-trimester maternal serum markers for aneuploidy and adverse obstetric outcomes. *Obstet Gynecol.* 2010;115(5):1052–1061.

FURTHER READING

1. American College of Obstetricians and Gynecologists. ACOG Committee Opinion no. 638. First Trimester risk assessment for early-onset preeclampsia. *Obstet Gynecol.* 2015;126:e25–e27.

2. American College of Obstetrics and Gynecologists. Cell–free DNA screening for Aneuploidy" no. 640. *Obstet Gynecol.* 2015;126:e31–e37.

3. Baer RJ, et al. Detection rates for aneuploidy by first-trimester and sequential screening. *Obstet Gynecol.* 2015; 126(4):753–759.

4. Santorum M, et al. Accuracy of first-trimester combined test in screening for trisomies 21, 18 and 13. *Ultrasound Obstet Gynecol.* 2017;49(6):714–720.

5. Syngelaki A, et al. Challenges in the diagnosis of fetal non-chromosomal abnormalities at 11–13 weeks. *Prenat Diagn.* 2011;31(1):90–102.

6. Wapner R, et al. First-trimester screening for trisomies 21 and 18. *N Engl J Med.* 2003;349(15):1405–1413.

CHAPTER 9

Cell-Free DNA Screening

SOHA S. PATEL, MD, MS, MSPH • LORRAINE DUGOFF, MD[a]

OVERVIEW

Cell-free DNA (cfDNA) screening has been rapidly introduced into prenatal care since it became clinically available in 2011. cfDNA screening can detect more than 99% of cases of trisomy 21 and also has high sensitivity and specificity for the detection of trisomy 13 and 18 and the common sex chromosome aneuploidies. cfDNA screens for aneuploidy by sequencing cfDNA from the maternal serum, which includes fetal cfDNA, largely derived from the placenta from apoptotic trophoblasts.

Pretest counseling should be performed for all women considering cfDNA screening, and all women with positive tests or test failures should receive posttest counseling. Confirmatory testing with chorionic villus sampling (CVS) or amniocentesis should be recommended to women with positive results as false-positive results occur and may be due to confined placental mosaicism (CPM) as well as other rare biologic causes including an underlying maternal chromosomal abnormality, a vanishing twin and in very rare cases, a maternal tumor or malignancy.

The entire fetal genome is represented in short cell-free fragments in the maternal plasma. Additional potential applications using cfDNA technology include screening for microdeletions, fetal Rh-determination, and detection of single gene disorders.

WHAT IS CELL-FREE DNA AND HOW IS IT USED FOR SCREENING FOR FETAL ANEUPLOIDY?

cfDNA is increasingly being used to screen for the common fetal aneuploidies because of the higher sensitivity and specificities compared with conventional serum screening.[1] Prenatal cfDNA screening was initially described in 1997 and became clinically available in 2011.[2] The cfDNA in the maternal plasma consists of free-floating small fragments of maternal DNA and placental DNA. Placental cfDNA is primarily derived from apoptotic trophoblasts. It can be detected in maternal blood as early as 4 weeks' gestation. The fetal fraction, which is the proportion of cfDNA of fetal (placental) origin to maternal cfDNA, exceeds 4% in the majority of pregnant women beginning at about 10 weeks' gestation. It continues to increase by 0.1% per week through 21 weeks' gestation and approximately 1% per week after 21 weeks' gestation.[3] Data suggest that a fetal fraction of at least 4% is needed to obtain a reliable result with cfDNA screening.[4,5]

cfDNA screening is currently used to detect trisomies 21, 18, and 13; 45 X; and 47 XXX, XXY, and XYY. The American College of Medical Genetics and Genomics (ACMG) has endorsed the acronym NIPS (noninvasive prenatal screening) to emphasize the fact that cfDNA is a screening test and not a diagnostic test.[6] In this chapter, we use the terminology "cell-free DNA" instead of "noninvasive prenatal screening," as all current screening tests are considered noninvasive.

Placental cfDNA has a very short half-life; therefore, a cfDNA screening result will not be affected by a previous pregnancy.[7] Screening is available after approximately 9–10 weeks of gestation when the fetal fraction is generally above 4%. cfDNA screening may be used either as a primary screening test or as a secondary screening test. Traditional serum screening (first trimester screening or second trimester maternal serum screening) is not recommended after cfDNA screening, and concurrent testing with cfDNA and traditional serum screening is also not recommended.[1]

WHAT TECHNIQUES ARE USED IN CELL-FREE DNA SCREENING?

Several different methods of assaying cfDNA are currently in use for aneuploidy screening using next-generation sequencing technology: whole-genome sequencing (massively parallel sequencing), chromosome-selective (or targeted) sequencing, and single-nucleotide polymorphism (SNP) analysis. Although all the three methods appear to have similar sensitivities

[a]**Financial Disclosures:** Lorraine Dugoff, MD has received research support from Progenity, Inc.

Perinatal Genetics. https://doi.org/10.1016/B978-0-323-53094-1.00009-6

and specificities,[8] there are advantages and limitations associated with each method.

Massively parallel sequencing randomly analyzes DNA from the entire genome. It sequences the entire DNA that is extracted from the maternal sample, counts cfDNA fragments, and assigns them to their specific chromosomal origin.[9]

Targeted sequencing, also known as chromosome-specific sequencing, specifically amplifies chromosomal areas that are of interest and subsequently evaluates if there is an excess of one specific chromosome over another.[10] An advantage of this technique is increased efficiency and overall lower cost (because only specific chromosomal areas are sequenced).[10] A microarray-based technology that does not require next-generation sequencing has been used to quantify the relative contributions from specific chromosomes. This approach yielded high sensitivities and specificities that were comparable with next-generation sequencing approaches.[11] This approach may result in additional decreased cost and turnaround time and testing of samples with a lower fetal fraction because of individual hybridization instead of sample multiplexing.[11,12]

The third method uses a single-nucleotide polymorphism-based approach with analysis of the quantitative contributions of maternal and fetal DNA.[7] The SNP-based approach cannot be used in pregnancies involving egg donors because this approach uses maternal genotypic information. This approach may identify consanguinity or uniparental disomy, in which both copies of a chromosome are inherited from the same parent.

Although the sensitivities and specificities for the detection of aneuploidy are similar for all three approaches, the whole genome sequencing approach is reported to have the lowest failure rate at 1.58%, followed by targeted sequencing at 3.56%, and SNP-based approach at 6.39%. The etiology of these failure rates is multifactorial and varies depending on quality control metrics, measurement of fetal fraction, and patient factors.[13]

HOW EFFECTIVE IS CELL-FREE DNA IN SCREENING FOR FETAL ANEUPLOIDY?

cfDNA screening has a higher sensitivity and lower false-positive rate than conventional screening modalities (see Chapter 8) in detecting fetal aneuploidy. Clinical studies have demonstrated that the detection rates and false-positive rates for fetal aneuploidy do not differ with maternal age.[14] The performance characteristics of cfDNA screening for fetal aneuploidy are summarized in Table 9.1. A metaanalysis that included data from 35 studies reported cfDNA screening detection rates of 99.7% for trisomy 21, 97.9% for trisomy 18, and 99.0% for trisomy 13. The detection rates for sex chromosome aneuploidies were greater than 95% (Table 9.1).[8] Of note, it is important to recognize that the cases of fetal aneuploidy in women who did not receive a cfDNA test result were not included in the calculation of the detection rates. As expected, the positive predictive values (PPVs) for trisomy 21, 18, and 13 are higher in older women as the prevalence of these conditions increases with advancing maternal age.[15]

WHAT IS THE ACCURACY OF SCREENING FOR SEX CHROMOSOME ANEUPLOIDIES?

The performance characteristics are presented in Table 9.1. Although the overall false-positive and false-negative rates for the detection of sex chromosome

---

TABLE 9.1
Cell-Free DNA Screening Performance Characteristics

Chromosomal Abnormality	Number of Affected Cases[8]	Detection Rate (%); 95% CI[8]	False-Positive Rate (%); 95% CI[8]	POSITIVE PREDICTIVE VALUE[a]	
				25-Year Old	40-Year Old
Trisomy 21	1963	99.7 (99.1–99.9)	0.04 (0.02–0.07)	51%	93%
Trisomy 18	563	97.9 (94.9–99.1)	0.04 (0.03–0.07)	15%	69%
Trisomy 13	119	99.0 (65.8–100.0)	0.04 (0.02–0.07)	7%	50%
Monosomy X	36	95.8 (70.3–99.5)	0.14 (0.05–0.38)	41%	41%
47 XXY	17[b]	100.00 (83.6–97.8)[b]	0.004 (0.0–0.08)[b]	29%	52%
47 XYY				25%	25%
47 XXX				27%	45%

[a]Positive predictive values obtained using PPV calculator from https://www.perinatalquality.org/Vendors/NSGC/NIPT/.
[b]Pooled for 47 XXY, 47 XYY, and 47 XXX.

aneuploidies are very low, the PPV appears to be limited. Bianchi et al. reported a low frequency (0.26%–1.05%) of false-positive results for sex chromosome aneuploidy in a cohort of approximately 18,000 women who had cfDNA testing.[16] Although clinical follow-up was only obtained for 44 of the 148 cases predicted to have monosomy X, 35 (79.5%) of the cases were false positives. Among 38 screen positive cases of XXX, 12 of 13 (92.3%) with clinical follow-up were false positive. Of the 12 false-positive cases, 2 were due to a maternal XXX cell line. Among six XYY cases, two had follow-up. One was confirmed as XYY and the other as XXY. Of the 12 XXY cases, 2 had follow-up and were confirmed to be true positives. These findings raise concerns about the limitations of cfDNA in screening for sex chromosome aneuploidy and highlight the importance of pretest counseling and confirmatory diagnostic testing following a screen-positive cfDNA test result.[16] False-negative cases are likely to remain largely undetected because of the absence of fetal and neonatal findings in the most common sex chromosome aneuploidies. More information about performance characteristics of cfDNA for detection of sex chromosome aneuploidies will likely be forthcoming from future large prospective studies.[17]

WHAT ARE THE POTENTIAL ADVANTAGES AND DISADVANTAGES ASSOCIATED WITH CELL-FREE DNA SCREENING FOR FETAL ANEUPLOIDY COMPARED WITH CONVENTIONAL SCREENING TESTS?

cfDNA is the most sensitive screening option for trisomy 13, 18, and 21. The false-positive rates associated with cfDNA screening are lower compared with conventional screening. Conventional screening tests (first trimester screening, second trimester screening, or stepwise sequential screening) have detection rates of 80%–95% with false-positive rates of 5%.[1] This could potentially lead to an increased number of diagnostic procedures in women who have conventional screening compared with cfDNA screening.

In addition, the PPV (the likelihood that a woman with a positive test has an affected fetus) is considerably higher with cfDNA screening compared with conventional screening. In a study of approximately 1900 women with a mean age of 29.6 years, the PPVs for the detection of trisomy 21 were 45.5% with cfDNA screening and 4.2% with conventional screening.[15]

An additional potential benefit of cfDNA is the option for earlier genetic screening results compared with some traditional screening methods. This allows for definitive diagnostic testing at an earlier gestational age.

cfDNA screening does not include screening for open neural tube defects. Patients should be offered MSAFP level at approximately 16–18 weeks' gestation unless the fetal anatomy is adequately evaluated with a second trimester ultrasound by a provider with experience in the detection of neural tube defects, ventral wall defects, and other fetal disorders.

A study of a cohort of 1.3 million women who had traditional aneuploidy screening through the California State screening program showed that 506 (17%) of the 2993 women with a positive aneuploidy screen and an abnormal result on invasive diagnostic testing had chromosomal abnormalities that would not be detectable with cfDNA screening.[18] The abnormalities characterized as undetectable by cfDNA screening included mosaic cases of trisomy 21, trisomy 18 and trisomy 13, mosaic sex chromosome aneuploidies, other trisomies (nonmosaic and mosaic), balanced rearrangements, unbalanced rearrangements, insertions and deletions, triploidy, tetraploidy, and cases with extra structurally abnormal chromosomes. There were 45 cases with CPM. Of note, the clinical outcomes associated with these abnormalities ranged from mild to having a significant disability. Some of the undetected abnormalities including the triploidy cases and the tetraploidy case would likely have resulted in spontaneous pregnancy loss, and the fetuses with balanced translocations would likely have been phenotypically normal. Of note, although cfDNA screening currently does not report on the detection of rare autosomal trisomies, it is possible to detect these abnormalities using this technology. However, with present methods, traditional multiple marker screening is a broader screen for the detection of fetal anomalies compared with the high precision of cfDNA screening. Large-scale prospective studies are needed to evaluate the clinical validity and utility of reporting information on the rare autosomal trisomies.[19]

A decision analytic model comparing clinical outcomes, quality-adjusted life-years and costs associated with different strategies for Down syndrome testing using cost estimates from 2015 determined that cfDNA is the optimal and most cost-effective screen for women of 40 years and older.[20] The authors assessed the outcomes of six testing strategies incorporating diagnostic testing with chromosomal microarray, multiple marker screening, cfDNA screening, and nuchal translucency screening alone, in combination, or in sequence. Multiple marker screening with optional follow-up diagnostic testing was the most effective (highest quality-adjusted life-years) and least expensive strategy at ages of 20–38 years.

WHAT ARE OTHER POTENTIAL USES FOR CELL-FREE DNA IN PRENATAL TESTING?

Determination of Fetal Sex

A metaanalysis involving 60 studies (11,179 cfDNA tests) reported a sensitivity of 98.9% (95% CI 0.980–0.994) and a specificity of 99.6% (95% CI 0.989–0.998) for the detection of fetal sex.[14] Determination of fetal sex allows for refinement of risk for couples at increased risk of having a child with an X-linked recessive condition. Female carriers of X-linked recessive disorders have a 50% risk of transmitting the mutant allele to their male offspring, and thus, having an affected son. Females, themselves, generally are not significantly affected with X-linked recessive disorders because of the protection from a normal X chromosome and lyonization (see Chapter 1). Common X-linked recessive disorders include Duchenne muscular dystrophy, hemophilia, and fragile X Syndrome.

Detection of Microdeletions

cfDNA screening panels have been extended by some laboratories to include microdeletion syndromes including 22q11 deletion syndrome (DiGeorge syndrome), Wolf–Hirschhorn syndrome (4p deletion), Cri-du-chat (5p minus syndrome), 1p36 deletion syndrome, and Prader Willi and Angelman syndromes, which both may result from a 15q deletion. Because of the low prevalence of these conditions and the low number of plasma samples available from affected pregnancies to help validate the testing, there is a paucity of data on the performance characteristics (sensitivity and specificity, positive predictive value, and false-positive and false-negative results) associated with screening for microdeletion syndromes.

22q11.2 deletion syndrome is the most frequent microdeletion syndrome, occurring in 1/3000–6000 live births.[21,22] Approximately, 5%–10% of cases of prenatally diagnosed congenital heart defects have 22q11.2 deletions, depending on the specific defect. Conotruncal defects including Tetralogy of Fallot, truncus arteriosus, and interrupted aortic arch are associated with 22q11.2 deletion syndrome.[23,24] Prenatal diagnosis of 22q11.2 deletion syndrome may reduce the associated early mortality and morbidity and potentially reduce medical, emotional, and financial costs. Although diagnostic testing with chromosomal microarray analysis is recommended when a fetal heart defect or other structural abnormality is identified on early prenatal ultrasound,[25] cell-free DNA screening for microdeletions including 22q11.2 deletion syndrome may be an option for patients who would not consider invasive prenatal diagnostic testing. Patients with fetal structural abnormalities detected at an advanced gestational age may opt for cfDNA screening including microdeletions as a means of avoiding the risk associated with amniocentesis but potentially influencing decisions including delivery location to optimize neonatal care. In these situations, it should be made clear that cfDNA screening is not diagnostic, that the false-positive and false-negative rates are not known, and that diagnostic testing will likely be performed after delivery.[26]

Based on the low prevalence of the microdeletion syndromes, the PPVs are anticipated to be low. Furthermore, it is possible that screening for microdeletion syndromes may increase the overall false-positive rate and potentially lead to an increased rate of invasive diagnostic testing.[27] The American College of Obstetricians and Gynecologists (ACOG) and Society for Maternal-Fetal Medicine (SMFM) do not endorse routine cfDNA screening for microdeletion syndromes due to a lack of clinical validation.[1]

Wapner and colleagues reported a 1.7% (1 in 60) incidence of clinically relevant microdeletions and microduplications in a cohort of 3118 pregnancies sampled for indications other than fetal structural abnormalities.[28] Women who desire testing for microdeletions (copy number variants) should be offered diagnostic testing with chromosomal microarray. This may be performed by CVS or amniocentesis (see Chapter 14).

Single Gene Disorders (see Chapter 1)

cfDNA to screen for single gene disorders has been reported and is available clinically in some laboratories.[29] Initial cfDNA testing for single gene disorders focused on conditions in which the mother did not carry the mutant allele. This included screening for some autosomal dominant disorders in which the variant is carried on the paternal allele, de novo autosomal dominant disorders in which a new variant occurs in the offspring, and autosomal recessive conditions in cases where the parents carry different variants in the affected gene. The diagnosis in these cases was based on detection or exclusion of the paternally inherited allele.[29,30] Examples of single gene disorders potentially amenable to cfDNA screening include achondroplasia, Noonan syndrome, osteogenesis imperfecta, craniosynostosis syndromes, Rett syndrome, myotonic dystrophy, neurofibromatosis type 1, cystic fibrosis, and congenital adrenal hyperplasia. De novo autosomal dominant disorders are associated with advanced paternal age. The risk for de novo autosomal dominant mutations is 0.3%–0.5%

among the offspring of fathers aged greater than 40 years, which is comparable with the risk of Down syndrome among the offspring of 35- to 40-year-old mothers.[31] Panels to screen for such de novo autosomal dominant disorders are available, but the clinical utility has not been proven and use of such panels is not routinely recommended.

Advances in digital polymerase chain reaction (PCR) and next-generation DNA sequencing technology have made it possible to discriminate affected from unaffected fetuses by determining the relative contribution of the normal and abnormal allele in cases including those involving inheritance of a maternal mutant allele. This has made it possible to detect X-linked recessive and additional autosomal recessive conditions using cfDNA.[30]

Concerns regarding the use of cfDNA in the diagnosis of single gene disorders include the costs of testing, as well as the potential for disparities in access among women of lower socioeconomic groups. Many of these genetic diseases are rare and require individualized testing approaches developed on a family-specific basis.[32] Use of cfDNA for the diagnosis of single gene disorders has not been endorsed by ACOG, SMFM, or ACMG to date.

RhD Determination

cfDNA testing can be used to screen for fetal RhD status in RhD-negative women. Fetal RhD genotyping can be performed as early as 10 weeks of gestation. RhD detection is based on real-time PCR of cfDNA that distinguishes fetal RhD sequences from the maternal plasma. Mackie etal. conducted a bivariate metaanalysis that showed that fetal RhD genotyping with cfDNA is highly sensitive (99.3%) and specific (98.4%) with low false-negative results.[8] In general, earlier testing with cfDNA is preferred because 40% of Rh-negative women will carry an Rh-negative fetus.[33,34] Identification of RhD-negative fetuses could potentially save unnecessary administration of Rh immune globulin in unsensitized women and avoid screening for fetal anemia (i.e., serial middle cerebral artery Doppler assessments) and unnecessary invasive procedures (i.e., amniocentesis and intrauterine transfusion) in sensitized women.[33,34] cfDNA determination of fetal RhD status is used in the first trimester in several European countries, where Rh immune globulin is less readily available, as well as in Canada, and may prove to be a cost-effective approach in the management of RhD-negative women in the United States.[33,34] Future cost-effective studies are indicated.

WHAT ARE THE POTENTIAL CAUSES OF A FALSE-POSITIVE CELL-FREE DNA RESULT?

When screening for trisomies 21, 18, and 13, approximately 0.5% of cases will have a false-positive result.[1] CPM, a vanishing twin, incidental maternal findings, organ transplantation, or human and/or laboratory errors may result in false-positive cfDNA results.[35]

Confined Placental Mosaicism

CPM refers to a phenomenon in which a chromosomal abnormality is present only in the placenta and not in the fetus (see Chapter 5). CPM is detected in approximately 1%–2% of viable pregnancies studied by CVS. False-positive cfDNA results can occur when there is CPM.[36]

Vanishing Twin

The placental tissue can remain after an early twin demise; thus contribution of a vanishing twin to the cfDNA in the maternal plasma can result in a false-positive or false-negative cfDNA result. False-positive results are expected more commonly as many fetal deaths are due to aneuploidy.[7] For this reason, it is not advisable to use cfDNA screening in pregnancies with a diagnosed vanishing twin. An ultrasound examination is useful before cfDNA screening to rule out a vanishing twin.

Incidental Maternal Findings: Maternal Aneuploidy

False-positive cfDNA results have been associated with maternal chromosomal abnormalities, including a 47, XXX karyotype, mosaicism for Turner syndrome, and 22q11.2 deletion syndrome.[37,38]

Incidental Maternal Findings: Maternal Malignancy

Apoptotic malignant cells release cfDNA into the maternal circulation. A variety of underlying maternal malignancies have been associated with false-positive cfDNA results. In these cases, typically multiple nonspecific copy number gains and losses are observed across multiple chromosomes. Bianchi etal. reported 10 cases of women with cfDNA results that were positive for one or more aneuploidies involving chromosome 13, 18, 21, X, or Y who were diagnosed with malignancies.[39] The 10 cancer cases were clinically diverse and included three cases of B-cell lymphoma and one case each of T-cell leukemia, leiomyosarcoma, unspecified adenocarcinoma, and neuroendocrine, colorectal, and anal carcinomas, ovarian carcinoma, a follicular lymphoma, and a Hodgkin lymphoma.[39] Further studies are needed to assess the clinical relevance of these results and determine the appropriate protocol for follow-up clinical evaluation.[39]

Organ Transplantation

Incorrect fetal sex determination with cfDNA screening can result in cases in which women carrying female fetuses received a bone marrow or solid organ transplantation from a male donor.[16] The ACMG recommends offering aneuploidy screening other than cfDNA screening to patients with a history of bone marrow or organ transplantation from a male donor or donor of uncertain biologic sex.[6] In addition, a blood transfusion less than 4 weeks before blood draw for cfDNA has also been reported to result in discordant biologic sex.[6]

Sample Mix-Up/Human Error

As with any test, human error can lead to an incorrect result if the incorrect specimen was taken, if it was sent to the wrong laboratory, or if the incorrect analyses were conducted on a sample.

WHAT IS THE SIGNIFICANCE OF FAILED OR "NO CALL" SCREENING FOR FETAL ANEUPLOIDY? WHAT ARE SOME POTENTIAL CAUSES OF A LOW FETAL FRACTION LEADING TO A FAILED CFDNA SCREEN?

Inability of the laboratory to provide results may occur because of problems associated with sample collection and transportation of samples to the lab, assay failure, and low fetal fraction (usually below 4%). A recent metaanalysis reported no-call rates ranging from 0.03% to 12.2%. The incidence of no-call rates due to a low fetal fraction ranged from 0.1% to 6.1% depending on the cfDNA testing approach and the laboratory. An analysis of the three studies that reported no-call rates separately for sex chromosome aneuploidies and trisomies showed that the incidence of no-call rates was higher for the sex chromosome aneuploidies (11.7%) compared with the trisomies (5.9%).[8]

A no-call result due to a low fetal fraction has been associated with fetal aneuploidy,[40] obesity,[41] early gestational age,[42] and treatment with low-molecular-weight heparin.[2]

Fetal Aneuploidy

Trisomies 13, 18, 21 and triploidy have all been associated with a no-call result because of a low fetal fraction. In the NEXT trial, 488 (3.0%) of the 16,329 women who underwent cfDNA screening did not have a reported result; 192 (1.2%) had a fetal fraction less than 4%; 83 (0.5%) had a fetal fraction that could not be measured; and 213 (1.3%) had a high assay variance (sequencing results that were difficult to interpret) or an assay failure.[40] There was a 2.7% incidence of aneuploidy in the group with no result reported, compared with a 0.4% incidence of aneuploidy in the overall cohort. The incidence of aneuploidy was highest (4.7%) in women with a fetal fraction of less than 4%.[40] Pergament et al. reported an OR of 9.2 (CI 4.4–19.0) for fetal aneuploidy in cases with no result due to a low fetal fraction.[43] In this study, the no-call cases due to a low fetal fraction included three trisomy 21, four trisomy 18, two trisomy 13, one monosomy X, and six cases of triploidy.[43] Trisomy 18 and 13 and triploidy are more frequent when the fetal fraction is very low, which has been attributed to a small placental volume.[44]

Obesity

Fetal fraction decreases with increasing maternal weight.[41,42] This may result from a dilutional effect or accelerated turnover of adipocytes with increased amounts of cfDNA of maternal origin released into the circulation, and a lower proportion of fetal cfDNA.[42] Ashoor and colleagues observed that the mean fetal fraction decreased from 11.7% at 60 kg to 3.9% at 160 kg at 12 weeks of gestation. The estimated proportion of women with fetal fraction below 4% increased with maternal weight from <1% at 60 kg to >50% at 160 kg. Thus, cfDNA testing may not be the optimal approach for obese women.[42]

Treatment With Low–Molecular-Weight Heparin

Burns and colleagues reported that enoxaparin therapy is associated with an increased incidence of a failed cfDNA test because of a low fetal fraction (adjusted OR 37.53; 95% CI 11.19–125.87).[2] Additional smaller studies and case reports have reported a similar association.[44] The mechanism by which this alters the cfDNA test functionality is unknown. It is possible that the low fetal fraction may be associated with the underlying maternal medical condition associated with the indication for anticoagulation and not the anticoagulant itself.

HOW SHOULD PATIENTS WITH NO RESULT DUE TO A LOW FETAL FRACTION BE COUNSELED AND MANAGED?

Patients with failed cfDNA screening because of a low fetal fraction should be offered diagnostic testing because of the increased risk of fetal aneuploidy. The current ACOG guidelines recommend a genetics consultation, follow-up ultrasound, and diagnostic testing in cases with a low fetal fraction.[1] ACOG does not preclude a repeat blood draw as an option.[1] Conversely, the ACMG recommends offering diagnostic testing for a no-call result because of low fetal fraction if maternal blood was drawn at an appropriate age, which is defined at 9 or 10 weeks and beyond depending on the laboratory used. The ACMG states that "a repeat blood draw is NOT appropriate."[6] The choice to reattempt cfDNA screening may depend on a number of factors including gestational age and the presence of ultrasound findings as well as other serum screening results suggestive of fetal aneuploidy. It is important to consider that an obese patient or a patient receiving treatment with low-molecular-weight heparin with no result due to a low fetal fraction may have a lower risk for fetal aneuploidy compared with a woman with a normal BMI not receiving treatment with low-molecular-weight heparin. If a patient desires to repeat a cfDNA test, there is a 46%–87% chance of obtaining a reportable result.[45–48]

WHAT INFORMATION SHOULD BE PROVIDED ABOUT CELL-FREE DNA IN PRETEST COUNSELING?

All pregnant women have three options: screening, diagnostic testing, and no screening or testing. All pregnant women should be counseled regarding the risks, benefits, and limitations of each screening and diagnostic testing option. This information should include the difference between a screening test and a diagnostic test as well as the detection rate and false-positive rate for each test offered, the implications of a false-positive screen, and, if applicable, the cost to the patient. Women should be counseled regarding their specific risk for fetal aneuploidy based on their age and history.

Pretest counseling points regarding cfDNA screening should include the following:

- cfDNA screening appears to be the most accurate screening test for trisomy 21.
- cfDNA also screens for trisomy 13 and 18 and the most common sex chromosome abnormalities. It does not screen for all chromosomal conditions and birth defects.
- Women who desire definitive information about chromosome conditions and microdeletions in their pregnancy should be offered the option of amniocentesis or CVS.
- False-positive and false-negative results occur with cfDNA.
- Diagnostic confirmation with CVS or amniocentesis is recommended for women with abnormal cfDNA results.

- A negative cfDNA result indicates a decreased risk and does not definitively rule out trisomy 21 or other chromosome conditions.
- cfDNA does not screen for neural tube defects. Screening with MSAFP at approximately 16 weeks' gestation, and/or detailed ultrasound is recommended.
- There is a chance that a cfDNA test may lead to the detection of an underlying chromosomal abnormality or malignant condition in the pregnant woman.
- cfDNA screening may be used as a follow-up test for patients with a positive traditional screen who do not choose to have a diagnostic test. In this case, patients should be counseled that the residual risk of a chromosome abnormality with a normal cfDNA test after an abnormal traditional screening test has been reported to be 2%.[1,18]

WHAT INFORMATION SHOULD BE PROVIDED IN POSTTEST COUNSELING FOR A POSITIVE RESULT?

It is critical that patients understand that cfDNA is a screening test and that positive results require confirmation with a diagnostic test before changes in management of the pregnancy. A study of approximately 30,000 women undergoing cfDNA screening reported that 6.2% of women with positive results chose to terminate the pregnancy without invasive test confirmation.[45] This underscores the importance of posttest counseling in women with positive results.

The PPV should be discussed with women with positive cfDNA test results. PPVs for trisomy 21, 13, and 18 are higher in older women because of the increased prevalence of these conditions as a result of an increase in meiotic nondisjunction. Patient-specific PPVs based on age can be obtained using an online PPV calculator (https://www.perinatalquality.org/Vendors/NSGC/NIPT/).

OTHER CONSIDERATIONS
SHOULD CELL-FREE DNA BE USED IN MULTIPLE GESTATIONS?

There are limited studies describing the performance of cfDNA screening for aneuploidy in twins and scant data are available regarding higher-order multiples. Although preliminary data have demonstrated that cfDNA screening may prove to be the most effective aneuploidy screening strategy in twins,[5,49–55] additional studies are required. The median fetal fraction in twins is lower compared with that of singletons, and the failure rates appear to be higher. For dizygotic twins and higher multiples, cfDNA screening is limited because only a single result for the entire pregnancy is provided with no potential to distinguish if one fetus is euploid and the other is aneuploid. This limitation also applies to conventional serum screening in multiple gestations. Nuchal translucency screening can be used to assign an individual risk of aneuploidy to each fetus. A combination of maternal age and nuchal translucency assessment is currently the optimal strategy to determine risk assessment in higher-order multiples. The ACOG and the SMFM do not currently recommend the use of cfDNA screening in multiple pregnancies due to the lack of adequate validation.[1]

WHAT IS THE ROLE OF FIRST TRIMESTER ULTRASOUND IN PATIENTS CONSIDERING CELL-FREE DNA SCREENING?

A recent retrospective study of 2337 advanced maternal age women who had 10–14 week ultrasound at a tertiary care center reported that 16.1% of the women had a first trimester ultrasound finding (fetal anomaly, incorrect dating, multiple gestation, and nonviable pregnancy) that would have altered the counseling for a screening or diagnostic testing strategy for fetal aneuploidy.[56]

The following potential benefits may be associated with performing an ultrasound before cfDNA screening:

- Accurate gestational age assessment
- Identification of anembryonic gestations, vanishing twins, and fetal demises
- Detection of multiple gestations
- Identification of major structural fetal abnormalities
- Identification of aneuploidy markers (including increased nuchal translucency, cystic hygroma)

WHAT IS THE ROLE OF CELL-FREE DNA AS A FOLLOW-UP SCREEN FOR WOMEN WITH POSITIVE TRADITIONAL SERUM SCREENING RESULTS?

For women found to be at increased risk for aneuploidy based on traditional serum screening, cell-free DNA is an option that is often discussed. Although cfDNA can detect the common aneuploidies in such patients, traditional screening is relatively nonspecific and such women are at risk for other, rare aneuploidies as well. It has been reported that in women with positive serum screening, 17% of the chromosome abnormalities detected by follow-up diagnostic testing would not be detected by most cfDNA screening tests. Overall, women with abnormal traditional screening results have a 2%, or 1 in 50, chance of having a fetus with one of these rarer chromosomal abnormalities, and this limitation should be discussed.[18]

REFERENCES

1. American College of Obstricians and Gynecologists. Practice bulletin No. 163: screening for fetal aneuploidy. *Obstet Gynecol.* 2016;127(5):e123–e137.
2. Burns W, Koelper N, Barberio A, et al. The association between anticoagulation therapy, maternal characteristics, and a failed cfDNA test due to low fetal fraction. *Prenat Diagn.* 2017;37:1125–1129.
3. Wang E, Batey A, Struble C, Musci T, Song K, Oliphant A. Gestational age and maternal weight effects on fetal cell-free DNA in maternal plasma. *Prenat Diagn.* 2013;33:662–666.
4. Norton ME, Brar H, Weiss J, et al. Non-Invasive Chromosomal Evaluation (NICE) Study: results of a multicenter prospective cohort study for detection of fetal trisomy 21 and trisomy 18. *Am J Obstet Gynecol.* 2012;207(2):137.e1–e8.
5. Canick JA, Kloza EM, Lambert-Messerlian GM, et al. DNA sequencing of maternal plasma to identify Down syndrome and other trisomies in multiple gestations. *Prenat Diagn.* 2012;32(8):730–734.
6. Gregg AR, Skotko BG, Benkendorf JL, et al. Noninvasive prenatal screening for fetal aneuploidy, 2016 update: a position statement of the American College of Medical Genetics and Genomics. *Genet Med.* 2016;18(10):1056–1065.
7. Benn P. Non-invasive prenatal testing using cell-free DNA in maternal plasma: recent developments and future prospects. *J Clin Med.* 2014;3:537–565.
8. Gil MM, Accurti V, Santacruz B, et al. Analysis of cell-free DNA in maternal blood in screening for aneuploidies: updated meta-analysis. *Ultrasound Obstet Gynecol.* 2017;50(3):302–314.
9. Chiu RW, Chan KC, Gao Y, et al. Noninvasive prenatal diagnosis of fetal chromosomal aneuploidy by massively parallel genomic sequencing of DNA in maternal plasma. *Proc Natl Acad Sci U S A.* 2008;105:20458–20463.
10. Sparks AB, Wang ET, Struble CA, et al. Selective analysis of cell-free DNA in maternal blood for evaluation of fetal trisomy. *Prenat Diagn.* 2012;32:3–9.
11. Juneau K, Bogard PE, Huang S, et al. Microarray-based cell-free DNA analysis improves noninvasive prenatal testing. *Fetal Diagn Ther.* 2014;36(4):282–286. .
12. Stokowski R, Wang E, White K, et al. Clinical performance of non-invasive prenatal testing (NIPT) using targeted cell-free DNA analysis in maternal plasma with microarrays or next generation sequencing (NGS) is consistent across multiple controlled clinical studies. *Prenat Diagn.* 2015;35(12):1243–1246.
13. Yaron T. The implications of non-invasive prenatal testing failures: a review of an under-discussed phenomenon. *Prenat Diagn.* 2016;36:391–396.
14. Mackie FL, Hemming K, Allen S, et al. The accuracy of cell-free fetal DNA-based non-invasive prenatal testing in singleton pregnancies: a systematic review and bivariate meta-analysis. *BJOG.* 2016;124(1):32–46.

15. Bianchi DW, Parker RL, Wentworth J, et al. DNA sequencing versus standard prenatal aneuploidy screening. *N Engl J Med.* 2014;370(9):799–808.

16. Bianchi DW, Parsa S, Bhatt S, et al. Fetal sex chromosome testing by maternal plasma DNA sequencing: clinical laboratory experience and biology. *Obstet Gynecol.* 2015;125(2):375–382.

17. Mennuti MT, Chandrasekaran S, Khalek N, Dugoff L. Cell-free DNA screening and sex chromosome aneuploidies. *Prenat Diagn.* 2015;35(10):980–985.

18. Norton ME, Jelliffe-Pawlowski LL, Currier RJ. Chromosome abnormalities detected by current prenatal screening and noninvasive prenatal testing. *Obstet Gynecol.* 2014;124:979–986.

19. Bianchi DW. Should we 'open the kimono' to release the results of rare autosomal aneuploidies following noninvasive prenatal whole genome sequencing? *Prenat Diagn.* 2017;37:123–125.

20. Kaimal AJ, Norton ME, Kuppermann M. Prenatal testing in the genomic age: clinical outcomes, quality of life, and costs. *Obstet Gynecol.* 2015;126:737–746.

21. Devriendt K, Fryns JP, Mortier G, et al. The annual incidence of DiGeorge/velocardiofacial syndrome. *J Med Genet.* 1998;35:789–790.

22. Tezenas Du Montcel S, Mendizabai H, Ayme S, et al. Prevalence of 22q11 microdeletion. *J Med Genet.* 1996;33:719.

23. Manji S, Roberson JR, Wiktor A, et al. Prenatal diagnosis of 22q11.2 deletion when ultrasound examination reveals a heart defect. *Genet Med.* 2001;3(1):65–66.

24. Lee MY, Won HS, Baek JW, et al. Variety of prenatally diagnosed congenital heart disease in 22q11.2 deletion syndrome. *Obstet Gynecol Sci.* 2014;57(1):11–16.

25. American College of Obstetricians and Gynecologists (ACOG). Committee Opinion No. 581. The use of chromosomal microarray analysis in prenatal diagnosis. *Obstet Gynecol.* 2013;122(6):1374–1377.

26. Dugoff L, Mennuti MT, McGinn-McDonald D. The benefits and limitations of cell-free DNA screening for 22q11 deletion syndrome. *Prenat Diagn.* 2017;37(1):53–60.

27. Dondorp W, de Wert G, Bombard Y, et al. Non-invasive prenatal testing for aneuploidy and beyond: challenges of responsible innovation in prenatal screening. *Eur J Hum Genet.* 2015;23:1438–1450.

28. Wapner RJ, Martin CL, Levy B, et al. Chromosomal microarray versus karyotyping for prenatal diagnosis. *N Engl J Med.* 2012;367(23):2175–2184.

29. Drury S, Mason S, McKay F, et al. Implementing noninvasive prenatal diagnosis (NIPD) in a National Health Service laboratory; from dominant to recessive disorders. *Adv Exp Med Biol.* 2016;924:71–75.

30. Lench N, Barrett A, Fielding S, et al. The clinical implementation of non-invasive pre- natal diagnosis for single-gene disorders: challenges and progress made. *Prenat Diagn.* 2013;33(6):555–562.

31. Friedman JM. Genetic disease in the offspring of older fathers. *Obstet Gynecol.* 1981;57:745–749.

32. Korpi-Steiner N, Chiu RWK, Chandrasekharan S, et al. Emerging considerations for noninvasive prenatal testing. *Clin Chem.* 2017;63(5):946–953. https://doi.org/10.1373/clinchem.2016.266544.

33. Moise Jr KJ, Gandhi M, Boring NH, et al. Circulating cell-free DNA to determine the fetal RHD status in all three trimesters of pregnancy. *Obstet Gynecol.* 2016;128(6):1340–1346.

34. Moise Jr KJ, Argoti PS. Management and prevention of red cell alloimmunization in pregnancy: a systematic review. *Obstet Gynecol.* 2012;120(5):1132–1139.

35. Mennuti MT, Cherry AM, Morrissette JJ, Dugoff L. Is it time to sound an alarm about false-positive cell-free DNA testing for fetal aneuploidy? *Am J Obstet Gynecol.* 2013;209(5):415–419.

36. Mardy A, Wapner RJ. Confined placental mosaicism and its impact on confirmation of NIPT results. *Am J Med Genet.* 2016;172:118–122.

37. Wang Y, Chen Y, Tian F, et al. Maternal mosaicism is a significant contributor to discordant sex chromosomal aneuploidies associated with noninvasive prenatal testing. *Clin Chem.* 2014;60(1):251–259.

38. Yao H, Zhang L, Zhang H, et al. Noninvasive prenatal genetic testing for fetal aneuploidy detects maternal trisomy X. *Prenat Diagn.* 2012;32(11):1114–1116.

39. Bianchi DW, Chudova D, Sehnert AM, et al. Noninvasive prenatal testing and incidental detection of occult maternal malignancies. *J Am Med Assoc.* 2015;314(2):162–169.

40. Norton ME, Jacobsson B, Swamy GK, et al. Cell-free DNA analysis for noninvasive examination of trisomy. *N Engl J Med.* 2015;372(17):1589–1597.

41. Livergood M, LeChien KA, Trudell AS. Obesity and cell-free DNA "no calls": is there an optimal gestational age at time of sampling?. *Am J Obstet Gynecol.* 2017;216: 413e1–413e9.

42. Ashoor G, Syngelaki A, Poon LC, Rezende JC, Nicolaides KH. Fetal fraction in maternal plasma cell-free DNA at 11-13 weeks' gestation: relation to maternal and fetal characteristics. *Ultrasound Obstet Gynecol.* 2013;41:26–32.

43. Pergament E, Cuckle H, Zimmermann B, et al. Single-nucleotide polymorphism-based noninvasive prenatal screening in a high-risk and low-risk cohort. *Obstet Gynecol.* 2014;124:210–218.

44. Ma GC, Wu WJ, Lee MH, et al. Low molecular weight heparin associated with reduced fetal fraction and subsequent false-negative cell-free DNA test result for trisomy 21. *Ultrasound Obstet Gynecol.* 2018;51(2):276–277.

45. Dar P, Curnow KJ, Gross SJ, et al. Clinical experience and follow-up with large scale single-nucleotide polymorphism-based noninvasive prenatal aneuploidy testing. *Am J Obstet Gynecol.* 2014;211:527.e1–e17.

46. Willems PJ, Dierickx H, Vandenakker ES, et al. The first 3,000 non-invasive prenatal tests (NIPT) with the Harmony test in Belgium and The Netherlands. *Facts Views Vis Obgyn.* 2014;6:7–12.

47. Sago H, Sekizawa A. Japan NIPT consortium. Nationwide demonstration project of next-generation sequencing of cell-free DNA in maternal plasma in Japan: one-year experience. *Prenat Diagn.* 2015;35:331–336.

48. Benn P, Valenti E, Shah S, et al. Factors associated with informative redraw after an initial no result in noninvasive prenatal testing. *Obstet Gynecol.* 2018/07/10. Ahead of print. PMID: 29995728.

49. Huang X, Zheng J, Chen M, et al. Noninvasive prenatal testing of trisomies 21 and 18 by massively parallel sequencing of maternal plasma DNA in twin pregnancies. *Prenat Diagn.* 2014;34:335–340.

50. Del Mar Gil M, Quezada MS, Breant B, et al. Cell-free DNA analysis for trisomy risk assessment in first trimester twin pregnancies. *Fetal Diagn Ther.* 2014;35:204–211.

51. Bevilacqua E, Bil MM, Nicolaides KH, et al. Performance of screening for aneuploidies by cell-free DNA analysis of maternal blood in twin pregnancies. *Ultrasound Obstet Gynecol.* 2015;45(1):61–66.

52. Zhang H, Gao Y, Jiang F, et al. Non-invasive prenatal testing for trisomies 21, 18, and 13: clinical experience from 146, 958 pregnancies. *Ultrasound Obstet Gynecol.* 2015;45(5):530–538.

53. Benachi A, Letourneau A, Kleinfinger P, et al. Cell-free DNA analysis in maternal plasma in cases of fetal abnormalities detected on ultrasound examination. *Obstet Gynecol.* 2015;125(6):1330–1337.

54. Tan Y, Gao Y, Ge L, et al. Noninvasive prenatal testing (NIPT) in twin pregnancies with treatment of assisted reproductive techniques (ART) in a single center. *Prenat Diagn.* 2016;36(7):672–679.

55. Le Conte G, Letourneau A, Jani J, et al. Cell-free DNA analysis in maternal plasma as a screening test for trisomy 21, 18 and 13 in twin pregnancies. *Ultrasound Obstet Gynecol.* 2017. https://doi.org/10.1002/uog.18838.

56. Vora NL, Robinson S, Hardisty EE, Stamilio DM. Utility of ultrasound examination at 10-14 weeks prior to cell-free DNA screening for fetal aneuploidy. *Ultrasound Obstet Gynecol.* 2017;49:465–469.

CHAPTER 10

Ultrasound Markers for Aneuploidy in the Second Trimester

MALAVIKA PRABHU, MD • JEFFREY A. KULLER, MD • JOSEPH R. BIGGIO JR., MD, MS

INTRODUCTION

Soft ultrasound markers were initially described as a screening method for trisomy 21 to improve the detection rate over that based on age-related risk alone. Soft markers are not structural abnormalities; rather, they are minor ultrasound findings identified in the midtrimester that may be a variant of normal but are noteworthy because they have been associated with an increased risk of fetal aneuploidy. Commonly identified soft markers addressed in this chapter include echogenic intracardiac focus (EIF), choroid plexus cyst (CPC), single umbilical artery (SUA), echogenic bowel, urinary tract dilation (UTD) (previously known as pyelectasis or pelviectasis), short humerus and/or femur, and thickened nuchal fold.[1–4]

Contemporaneous with the advancement in aneuploidy detection using soft markers was the development of improved screening methods to predict aneuploidy risk, including first-trimester screening with maternal serum analytes and nuchal translucency measurement.[5] In 2011, the introduction of cell-free DNA (cfDNA) techniques greatly improved the ability to screen for common aneuploidies. The American College of Obstetricians and Gynecologists (ACOG) and the Society for Maternal-Fetal Medicine (SMFM) recommend that cfDNA screening be offered to patients with a higher risk for common aneuploidies, although any patient who desires aneuploidy screening may elect to pursue cfDNA screening.[6]

Given the high sensitivity of maternal serum screening algorithms and cfDNA for trisomy 21, 18, and 13, the role of ultrasound-based screening for aneuploidy is in evolution. The purpose of this chapter is to focus on the evaluation and management of isolated ultrasound soft markers diagnosed in the second trimester.

WHAT IS THE INITIAL APPROACH AFTER A SOFT MARKER IS IDENTIFIED?

Once a soft marker is identified, a detailed ultrasound examination is recommended to ensure the finding is isolated (i.e., there is only a single soft marker that does not co-occur with any structural abnormality or other soft marker), as the presence of multiple soft markers increases the risk of aneuploidy.[7] In the case of multiple soft markers or a structural abnormality, the approach to evaluation should be individualized. If an isolated soft marker is confirmed, subsequent evaluation and counseling depends on the nature of the soft marker and associations with nonaneuploid conditions.

The presence or absence of specific soft markers has been used to modify the probability of trisomy 21, and secondarily that of trisomy 18, using positive and negative likelihood ratios (LRs).[8] This approach requires an accurate assessment of (1) the a priori, or pretest, risk (age-related risk at the time of delivery or age-related risk in the midtrimester) of the aneuploidy of interest; (2) the posttest risk based on a screening test, if performed; (3) validated and reproducible sonographic definitions for the identification of each soft marker; and (4) accurate estimates of sensitivity and specificity to generate the positive and negative LRs of an isolated soft marker for a particular aneuploidy.[7,9] Once the risk estimates and LRs are determined, then a final risk estimate incorporating the presence or absence of an ultrasound soft marker for the aneuploidy of interest can be calculated.

In general, positive LRs from approximately 1.5–5 confer a small increase in the likelihood of the outcome, LRs between 5 and 10 confer a moderate increase in the likelihood of the outcome, and LRs greater than 10 confer a significant increase in the likelihood of the outcome. The absence of structural anomalies or additional soft markers likely decreases this risk, although formulas to assess the interaction of these risks are not readily available. Regardless of the screening strategy used, there is no one threshold value of posttest probability above which additional aneuploidy evaluation is routinely recommended, as risk estimates represent a continuum.

The approach to calculating posttest probability was particularly useful when patients desired aneuploidy

Perinatal Genetics. https://doi.org/10.1016/B978-0-323-53094-1.00010-2

screening and soft markers helped shape the "genetic sonogram" as another tool to further refine risk prediction. As data on soft markers have accumulated, variability in positive and negative LR estimates has been noted because of differences in patient populations studied, variability in the definition of a specific finding, and subjectivity in the detection rate as well as other causes.

When reviewed in aggregate, the current data suggest that the positive likelihood ratios for the common soft markers, with the exception of a thickened nuchal fold, are all exceedingly low (ranging from less than 1 to 6, in general). This low range suggests that if a positive likelihood ratio were to be incorporated into a patient's individual risk for aneuploidy, based on the available results from cfDNA or serum/integrated screening, there would not be a meaningful change in the estimate of absolute aneuploidy risk and thus would not warrant additional counseling or testing based solely on the identification of the isolated soft marker.[10] National recommendations from the Royal College of Obstetrics & Gynecology in the United Kingdom and from the Society of Obstetricians and Gynaecologists of Canada (SOGC) Genetics Committee and the Canadian College of Medical Geneticists (CCMG) suggest not adjusting a patient's a priori risk for trisomy 21 with the presence of any one soft marker, with the exception of a thickened nuchal fold.[11]

Moreover, if a woman has undergone diagnostic testing and the results indicate a normal karyotype, identification of a soft marker for the purposes of aneuploidy screening is insignificant and should be reported as such.

WHAT IS THE SIGNIFICANCE OF AN ECHOGENIC INTRACARDIAC FOCUS?

An EIF is defined as a small (<6 mm) echogenic area in either cardiac ventricle that is as bright as surrounding bone and visualized in at least two separate planes (Fig. 10.1).[12] EIFs may appear in either cardiac ventricle, although left-sided EIFs are more common, and are thought to represent microcalcifications of papillary muscles.[13,14] The pathogenesis of this finding is unclear.

EIFs are identified in 3%–5% of karyotypically normal fetuses, and significant ethnic variation exists.[15-18] In the largest analysis of 7480 ethnically diverse women having amniocentesis, the prevalence of EIF was 8.3% among Middle-Eastern women, 6.9% among Asian-American women, 6.7% among African-American women, 3.4% among Hispanic women, and 3.3% among Caucasian women, with lower prevalence among Asian-Indian and Native-American women.[18] Smaller studies have demonstrated a higher prevalence of EIF among women of Asian descent, with estimates up to 30%.[19,20]

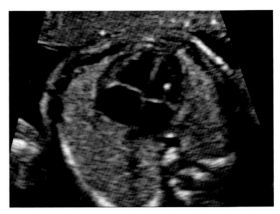

FIG. 10.1 Echogenic intracardiac focus. (Courtesy of Bryann Bromley, MD.)

EIFs do not represent a structural or functional cardiac abnormality, and they have not been associated with cardiac malformations in the fetus or newborn.[21-23] Fetal echocardiography and additional ultrasound imaging solely to serially follow an EIF are not recommended, and no postnatal follow-up is indicated. When isolated, an EIF should be considered a variant of normal.

Since the first descriptions of EIFs as a soft marker for trisomy 21, a subsequent large body of literature has demonstrated varying positive likelihood ratios for trisomy 21, depending on the population studied and whether the EIF was isolated or in combination with other soft markers.[8,16,17,24-27] Overall, however, the association between the presence of an EIF and trisomy 21 is weak. In the presence of an isolated EIF, the risk of trisomy 21 is not meaningfully altered, and therefore, an isolated EIF can be considered a variant of normal and additional aneuploidy evaluation is not indicated in women previously screened for aneuploidy. In the absence of any prior aneuploidy screening, the positive likelihood ratio for an EIF ranges between 1.4 and 1.8, with lower confidence bounds extending to or beyond 1, suggesting little to no increased risk.[25,28]

WHAT IS THE SIGNIFICANCE OF A CHOROID PLEXUS CYST?

A CPC is a small fluid-filled structure within the choroid of the lateral ventricles of the fetal brain (Fig. 10.2). Sonographically, CPCs appear as echolucent cysts within the echogenic choroid. CPCs may be single or multiple, unilateral or bilateral, and most often are less than 1 cm in diameter. CPCs are identified in approximately 1%–2% of fetuses in the second trimester and

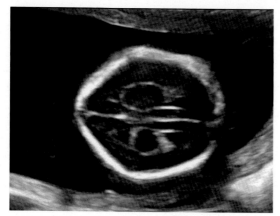

FIG. 10.2 Choroid plexus cyst. (Courtesy of Bryann Bromley, MD.)

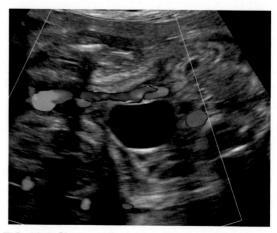

FIG. 10.3 Single umbilical artery. (Courtesy of Bryann Bromley, MD.)

are commonly isolated findings in euploid fetuses.[29,30] CPCs are present in 30%–50% of fetuses with trisomy 18 but in such cases are typically seen alongside multiple structural anomalies, including structural heart defects, clenched hands, talipes deformity of the feet, growth restriction, and polyhydramnios.

A CPC is not considered a structural or functional brain abnormality, and nearly all resolve by 28 weeks.[31] Patients may be counseled that neurodevelopmental outcomes in euploid children born after a prenatal diagnosis of choroid plexus cysts have not shown differences in neurocognitive ability, motor function, or behavior.[32–35] Consequently, no additional ultrasound imaging is recommended solely to serially follow an isolated CPC, and no postnatal follow-up is indicated. When isolated, in a population previously screened for aneuploidy, CPCs should be considered a variant of normal, and no additional aneuploidy testing is indicated. In a population that has not been screened for aneuploidy, positive LRs for trisomy 18 ranged from 0.9-5.6, with the vast majority suggesting little risk.[36–39] Based on the literature, the best estimate for the LR is less than 2. The presence of a choroid plexus cyst does not alter the risk of trisomy 21.[40]

WHAT IS THE SIGNIFICANCE OF A SINGLE UMBILICAL ARTERY?

The normal umbilical cord contains two arteries and one vein; single umbilical artery (SUA) is the result of atrophy or agenesis of one of the arteries. An SUA can be detected on cross section of the umbilical cord during a routine second-trimester ultrasound exam or using color-flow Doppler to examine the umbilical

arteries in the pelvis at an even earlier gestational age (Fig. 10.3).

The incidence of SUA is 0.25%–1% of all singleton pregnancies and up to 4.6% of twin gestations.[41–43] An isolated SUA should be distinguished from an SUA that is present with other abnormalities. Co-occuring structural abnormalities most commonly involve the cardiovascular and renal systems.[41] With an SUA and a structural abnormality, the frequency of associated aneuploidy ranges from 4% to 50%.[44] A thorough assessment of cardiac anatomy should be performed by a practitioner experienced in the detection of fetal cardiac anomalies, and if adequately visualized and normal, fetal echocardiogram is not routinely recommended.[45,46] For patients with an isolated SUA, there is no increased risk of aneuploidy.[44,47]

Isolated SUA has been associated in some studies with an increased risk of fetal growth restriction (FGR), although other studies suggest that an isolated SUA does not place the fetus at increased risk for FGR.[48–52] In a cohort of fetuses with isolated SUA, the observed incidence of growth restriction was not higher than that expected.[48] Similarly, in a cohort of fetuses with isolated SUA compared with those without isolated SUA, rates of SGA at birth did not differ between groups.[49] Moreover, a metaanalysis did not demonstrate a statistically significant difference in mean birthweight or a statistically significant increase in proportion of SGA births among fetuses with isolated SUA.[53] However, a cohort study with a larger control group of fetuses with a three-vessel cord did demonstrate an increased risk of FGR, polyhydramnios, oligohydramnios, placental abruption, cord prolapse, and perinatal mortality among those with isolated SUA, after controlling for other confounders.[52] This study was not included in the metaanalysis above. Given conflicting evidence, third-trimester ultrasound for evaluation of growth can be considered; antenatal testing is recommended only if fetal growth restriction or other indications develop.

At the time of delivery, pediatricians should be notified of the prenatal findings. Postnatal exam of infants with a prenatal diagnosis of isolated SUA revealed structural anomalies in up to 7% of fetuses in one study.[54]

WHAT IS THE SIGNIFICANCE OF ECHOGENIC BOWEL?

Echogenic bowel is diagnosed when the fetal bowel displays echogenicity equal to or greater than that of surrounding fetal bone, typically the iliac wing (Fig. 10.4). Transducer frequency can influence the diagnosis because higher frequency transducers tend to exaggerate the finding. Therefore, a lower frequency transducer (5 MHz or less) with harmonic imaging turned off and set at lower gain should be used to confirm the diagnosis.[55]

Echogenic bowel is observed in up to 1.8% of second-trimester ultrasound exams.[56-58] This finding is often isolated, but an increased incidence of structural anomalies, particularly renal and cardiac anomalies, has been demonstrated in fetuses with echogenic bowel.[59] Although isolated echogenic bowel can be a transient or idiopathic finding in approximately 0.5% of all fetuses, it can also be associated with a wide range of pathologic conditions such as cystic fibrosis, congenital viral infection, primary gastrointestinal pathology,

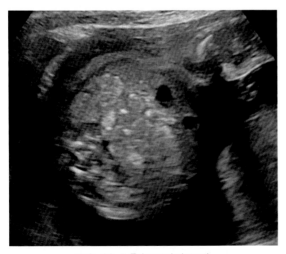

FIG. 10.4 Echogenic bowel.

intraamniotic bleeding, and growth restriction. The estimated incidence of each possible etiology varies because of small sample size studies and the subjectivity in the diagnosis.

Echogenic bowel has also been associated with trisomy 21 and less commonly with other karyotypic abnormalities.[59-62] Echogenic bowel is present as an isolated finding in 4%–25% of fetuses with aneuploidy.[59,61] Hypoperistalsis due to mechanical or functional bowel obstruction with subsequent dehydration of meconium is the proposed mechanism causing this finding in fetuses with abnormal karyotype. Among fetuses with isolated echogenic bowel, the positive LR for trisomy 21 depends on the population studied but ranges between 6 and 8.[24,25,46]

Studies have also demonstrated the development of echogenic bowel following invasive procedures such as intrauterine fetal transfusions, secondary to fetal swallowing of blood from the amniotic cavity.[63] It has been demonstrated that this finding may persist for 2–4 weeks following intrauterine transfusion.

Cystic fibrosis is associated with echogenic bowel, as abnormal pancreatic enzyme secretion leads to thickened meconium, and subsequent meconium ileus is observed in some newborns with cystic fibrosis. The risk for cystic fibrosis ranges from 0% to 13%.[59,60,64,65] The finding of dilated loops of bowel in addition to echogenic bowel may increase this risk to as high as 17%.[66] For all fetuses with isolated echogenic bowel, evaluation for cystic fibrosis is recommended. Parental cystic fibrosis carrier screening is the first step and should be determined if not previously assessed in the current or prior pregnancy. If both parents are found to be carriers, genetic counseling should be undertaken to discuss the risks and benefits of invasive testing for fetal genotyping. Racial and ethnic limitations of current cystic fibrosis screening panels should be taken into consideration when interpreting test results.

Congenital infection also has been associated with isolated echogenic bowel. Different mechanisms underlie the findings of echogenicity: (1) direct damage to the fetal intestinal wall with subsequent paralytic ileus; (2) intestinal perforation resulting in meconium peritonitis and focal calcification at the perforation sites; or (3) ascites secondary to hydrops leading to echogenicity on ultrasound. Cytomegalovirus (CMV) is the most commonly observed infection, but toxoplasmosis, rubella, herpes, varicella, and parvovirus also have been reported.[55,56,59] Although the majority of studies report a 2%–4% incidence of congenital infection in fetuses with echogenic bowel, rates up to 10% have been reported.[56,64] In a series of 650 cases with maternal primary CMV infection, seven fetuses with CMV infection had isolated echogenic bowel as the sole ultrasound finding.[67]

For all fetuses with echogenic bowel, evaluation for CMV infection is recommended. Although symptomatic maternal infection is uncommon, a history should be taken to evaluate for possible timing of symptoms of CMV. CMV IgG and IgM titers should be considered, with IgG avidity testing as applicable. If results are suggestive of primary infection, then amniocentesis should be considered, with other counseling and evaluation as appropriate.[68] Without a history of exposure or other clinical risk factors, the chance of positive results for other congenital infections, such as varicella, herpes, parvovirus, or toxoplasmosis, is very low.[69] Therefore, routine testing for these other infections may not be useful; however, the utility of testing should be determined based on the clinical scenario, differential diagnosis, and potential exposures.

Primary gastrointestinal pathology such as bowel obstruction, atresia, meconium peritonitis, and perforation also may cause an echogenic appearance of the fetal bowel, usually in association with other findings. In cases of obstruction and atresia, decreased meconium fluid content is the proposed cause for the increase in echogenicity.[55] The presence of meconium outside the intestinal lumen is likely responsible for the echogenic appearance in cases of bowel perforation.

Lastly, isolated echogenic bowel is associated with increased likelihood of growth restriction.[58-60] The pathophysiology of this finding is presumably due to areas of ischemia resulting from redistribution of blood flow away from the gut. Third-trimester ultrasound for the evaluation of growth and appearance of bowel among fetuses with isolated echogenic bowel is therefore recommended.

Although isolated echogenic bowel is associated with a sevenfold increased odds of intrauterine fetal demise, with a mean gestational age in the second trimester, the majority of fetuses with isolated echogenic bowel have normal outcomes.[58,64,70] The utility of antenatal fetal testing in this scenario is of unproven benefit. Partial or complete resolution of isolated echogenic bowel is reassuring, and normal fetal outcomes are likely.[71] Normal fetal outcomes have been demonstrated in fetuses with persistence of echogenic bowel as well; thus, persistent echogenicity should not be viewed as a marker for adverse outcome.[59,72] At the time of delivery, pediatricians should be made aware of the antenatal finding of echogenic bowel and prenatal workup performed, so that appropriate neonatal evaluation may be pursued.

WHAT IS THE SIGNIFICANCE OF URINARY TRACT DILATION?

UTD was previously described with variable terminology, including pyelectasis, pelviectasis, and hydronephrosis. In 2014, a consensus statement defined norms for antenatal UTD based on anterior-posterior renal pelvis diameter (APRPD), with less than 4 mm being normal between 16 and 27 weeks' gestation and less than 7 mm being normal between 28 weeks' gestation and delivery (Fig. 10.5).[73] To fully assess and classify UTD, additional ultrasound features to be evaluated include presence of calyceal dilation, parenchymal thickness and appearance, ureteral dilation, bladder abnormalities, and amniotic fluid volume. The complete evaluation of the urinary tract results in classification of A1 (low risk) versus A2-3 (increased risk) UTD, which guides antenatal management as well as postnatal follow-up (Table 10.1).

UTD occurs in 1%–2% of pregnancies and is most commonly a transient finding that is a variant of normal.[73] UTD less than 7–8 mm in the second trimester resolves in approximately 80% of cases.[73] However, in a minority of cases, UTD has a pathologic cause. Common pathologic causes include vesicoureteral reflux (the most common etiology), ureteropelvic junction obstruction, ureterovesical junction obstruction, multicystic dysplastic kidneys, and posterior urethral valves. Although some conditions can be diagnosed antenatally, in most cases a diagnosis is made postnatally.[73] After initial diagnosis of UTD, subsequent antenatal evaluation depends on classification (see Table 10.1).

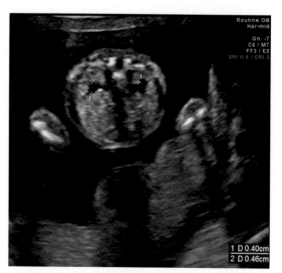

FIG. 10.5 Urinary tract dilation. (Courtesy of Bryann Bromley, MD.)

TABLE 10.1
Urinary Tract Dilation (UTD): Antenatal Classification of Findings

Ultrasound Findings	UTD A1	UTD A2-3
AP RPD	16–27w: 4–<7 mm	16–27w: ≥7 mm
	≥28w: 7–<10 mm	≥28w: ≥10 mm
Calyceal dilation	None or central	None, central, or peripheral
Parenchymal thickness	Normal	Normal or abnormal
Parenchymal appearance	Normal	Normal or abnormal
Ureters	Normal	Normal or abnormal
Bladder	Normal	Normal or abnormal
Unexplained oligohydramnios	Absent	Absent or present
Prenatal follow-up	Third-trimester ultrasound	Ultrasounds every 4–6 weeks + consultation with pediatric nephrology/urology

AP RPD, anterior-posterior renal pelvis diameter.
Reproduced from: Nguyen HT, Benson CB, Bromley B, Campbell JB, Chow J, Coleman B, et al. Multidisciplinary consensus on the classification of prenatal and postnatal urinary tract dilation (UTD classification system). *J Pediatr Urol.* 2014;10(6):982–998.

At the time of delivery, prenatal diagnosis of UTD A1 or A2-3 should be communicated to the pediatrician; resolved UTD A1, however, requires no postnatal follow-up.[73]

The association between trisomy 21 and UTD has been well described in several series, and the finding of UTD confers a positive LR of 1.5.[25] Among patients already screened for aneuploidy, additional aneuploidy evaluation with a finding of UTD may not be necessary, as the increase in risk, if any, is very low.

WHAT IS THE SIGNIFICANCE OF SHORTENED LONG BONES?

A shortened humerus and shortened femur have been variably defined in the literature. These include measurements below the fifth percentile for gestational age; biparietal diameter (BPD) to femur length (FL) ratio and BPD to humeral length (HL) ratio > 1.5 multiples of the median for gestational age; observed to expected ratio of FL (based on BPD) less than 0.92; and observed to expected ratio of HL (based on BPD) less than 0.90.[74]

Racial and ethnic variation in the normal distribution of femoral length in the midtrimester has been described in some studies, with long bones being shorter among Asian-American patients and longer among African-American patients.[75,76] Similar variation has not been described for midtrimester humeral lengths, and race/ethnicity-specific definitions of foreshortened long bones do not improve diagnostic test characteristics.[77,78] Parental race and ethnicity can lead to constitutionally short bones and should be considered in the differential diagnosis.

The finding of shortened long bones is also associated with skeletal dysplasia. In general, bone lengths in fetuses with skeletal dysplasias fall less than the third percentile for measurements in the second trimester, with the exception of achondroplasia, which may not manifest until the third trimester.[79]

Isolated shortened long bones are additionally associated with growth restriction.[80,81] In all fetuses with isolated shortened long bones, a third-trimester ultrasound for reassessment and evaluation of growth should be considered, but no additional evaluation for aneuploidy is needed.

The presence of either short femurs or short humeri has been associated with trisomy 21, with minimal elevation in risk. For shortened femurs, the positive LR from metaanalyses ranges from 1.5 to 2.7, with the confidence interval of the lower estimate crossing 1, suggesting minimal elevated risk.[25,26] For shortened humeri, the positive LR from metaanalyses ranges from 5.1 to 7.5.[25,26]

WHAT IS THE SIGNIFICANCE OF A THICKENED NUCHAL FOLD MEASUREMENT?

The nuchal fold is imaged in the transverse plane of the fetal head, angled caudally to capture the cerebellum and occipital bone, and calipers are placed between the outer edge of the skin and the outer edge of the occipital bone (Fig. 10.6). A thickened nuchal fold is defined as greater than 6 mm between 15 and 20 weeks' gestation.[82] Thickened nuchal fold was one of the first ultrasound markers of trisomy 21 identified and is one of the most specific signs to date.[82,83]

After the initial report, several prospective series of consecutive amniocenteses confirmed the association between an isolated thickened nuchal fold and trisomy 21, with rare false-positive cases.[1,3,83] The positive likelihood ratio ranges widely, between 3.8 and 17, suggesting a moderate to significant risk.[10,25,26]

For women with negative serum analyte or cfDNA screening results and isolated thickened nuchal fold, it is reasonable to pursue no further aneuploidy evaluation. However, given the high specificity of this marker, it is reasonable to offer diagnostic testing via amniocentesis or cfDNA screening (if not already completed) depending on other clinical circumstances and patient preference.

Regardless of the evaluation, serial ultrasounds of the evolution of the thickened nuchal fold are not indicated. Conflicting evidence exists regarding the association between a thickened nuchal fold and congenital heart disease; however, if cardiac anatomy has been performed by a practitioner experienced in the detection of fetal cardiac anomalies, and was adequately visualized and appears normal, and no further imaging is necessary.[7]

CONCLUSION

With significant advances in prenatal screening for fetal aneuploidy, the relative importance of ultrasound soft markers in assessing risk for aneuploidy has decreased greatly. With the exception of a thickened nuchal fold, when an isolated soft marker is identified after negative screening results, patients may be reassured that the risks of fetal aneuploidy remain low. These recommendations are in line with recent recommendations from several other leading societies, given improvements in aneuploidy screening as well as ultrasound technology.[11,84,85] In some cases, the positive likelihood ratios associated with the finding of an isolated soft marker are helpful in counseling, and further testing may be useful. Evaluation for associated conditions that are unrelated to fetal aneuploidy remains important when soft markers are identified.

REFERENCES

1. Benacerraf BR, Frigoletto FD, Cramer DW. Down syndrome: sonographic sign for diagnosis in the second-trimester fetus. *Radiology.* 1987;163(3):811–813.
2. Lockwood C, Benacerraf B, Krinsky A, et al. A sonographic screening method for Down syndrome. *Am J Obstet Gynecol.* 1987;157(4 Pt 1):803–808.
3. Benacerraf BR, Gelman R, Frigoletto FD. Sonographic identification of second-trimester fetuses with Down's syndrome. *N Engl J Med.* 1987;317(22):1371–1376.
4. Benacerraf BR, Mandell J, Estroff JA, Harlow BL, Frigoletto FD. Fetal pyelectasis: a possible association with Down syndrome. *Obstet Gynecol.* 1990;76(1):58–60.
5. Malone FD, Canick JA, Ball RH, et al. First-trimester or second-trimester screening, or both, for Down's syndrome. *N Engl J Med.* 2005;353(19):2001–2011.
6. Cell-free DNA. *Screening for Fetal Aneuploidy - ACOG [Internet];* 2017. Available from: http://www.acog.org/Resources-And-Publications/Committee-Opinions/Committee-on-Genetics/Cell-free-DNA-Screening-for-Fetal-Aneuploidy.
7. Reddy UM, Abuhamad AZ, Levine D, Saade GR. Fetal imaging workshop invited participants. Fetal imaging: executive summary of a joint Eunice Kennedy Shriver National institute of child Health and human development, society for maternal-fetal Medicine, American institute of ultrasound in Medicine, American College of Obstetricians and Gynecologists, American College of radiology, society for pediatric radiology, and society of radiologists in ultrasound fetal imaging workshop. *Obstet Gynecol.* 2014;123(5):1070–1082.

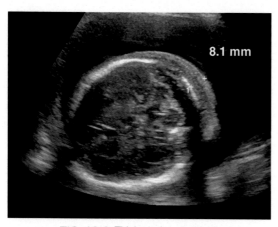

8.1 mm

FIG. 10.6 Thickened nuchal fold.

8. Nyberg DA, Luthy DA, Resta RG, Nyberg BC, Williams MA. Age-adjusted ultrasound risk assessment for fetal Down's syndrome during the second trimester: description of the method and analysis of 142 cases. *Ultrasound Obstet Gynecol Off J Int Soc Ultrasound Obstet Gynecol.* 1998;12(1):8–14.

9. Norton ME. Follow-up of sonographically detected soft markers for fetal aneuploidy. *Semin Perinatol.* 2013;37(5):365–369.

10. Agathokleous M, Chaveeva P, Poon LCY, Kosinski P, Nicolaides KH. Meta-analysis of second-trimester markers for trisomy 21. *Ultrasound Obstet Gynecol Off J Int Soc Ultrasound Obstet Gynecol.* 2013;41(3):247–261.

11. National Institute for Health and Care Excellence. *Antenatal care for uncomplicated pregnancies | Guidance and guidelines. [Internet]*; 2017. Available from: https://www.nice.org.uk/guidance/cg62/chapter/1-Guidance#screening-for-fetal-anomalies.

12. Rodriguez R, Herrero B, Bartha JL. The continuing enigma of the fetal echogenic intracardiac focus in prenatal ultrasound. *Curr Opin Obstet Gynecol.* 2013;25(2):145–151.

13. Winn VD, Sonson J, Filly RA. Echogenic intracardiac focus: potential for misdiagnosis. *J Ultrasound Med Off J Am Inst Ultrasound Med.* 2003;22(11). 1207–1214–1217.

14. Bromley B, Lieberman E, Shipp TD, Richardson M, Benacerraf BR. Significance of an echogenic intracardiac focus in fetuses at high and low risk for aneuploidy. *J Ultrasound Med Off J Am Inst Ultrasound Med.* 1998;17(2):127–131.

15. Shanks AL, Odibo AO, Gray DL. Echogenic intracardiac foci: associated with increased risk for fetal trisomy 21 or not? *J Ultrasound Med Off J Am Inst Ultrasound Med.* 2009;28(12):1639–1643.

16. Bromley B, Lieberman E, Laboda L, Benacerraf BR. Echogenic intracardiac focus: a sonographic sign for fetal Down syndrome. *Obstet Gynecol.* 1995;86(6):998–1001.

17. Sotiriadis A, Makrydimas G, Ioannidis JPA. Diagnostic performance of intracardiac echogenic foci for Down syndrome: a meta-analysis. *Obstet Gynecol.* 2003;101(5 Pt 1):1009–1016.

18. Tran SH, Caughey AB, Norton ME. Ethnic variation in the prevalence of echogenic intracardiac foci and the association with Down syndrome. *Ultrasound Obstet Gynecol Off J Int Soc Ultrasound Obstet Gynecol.* 2005;26(2):158–161.

19. Shipp TD, Bromley B, Lieberman E, Benacerraf BR. The frequency of the detection of fetal echogenic intracardiac foci with respect to maternal race. *Ultrasound Obstet Gynecol Off J Int Soc Ultrasound Obstet Gynecol.* 2000;15(6):460–462.

20. Rebarber A, Levey KA, Funai E, Monda S, Paidas M. An ethnic predilection for fetal echogenic intracardiac focus identified during targeted midtrimester ultrasound examination: a retrospective review. *BMC Pregnancy Childbirth.* 2004;4(1):12.

21. Wax JR, Donnelly J, Carpenter M, et al. Childhood cardiac function after prenatal diagnosis of intracardiac echogenic foci. *J Ultrasound Med Off J Am Inst Ultrasound Med.* 2003;22(8):783–787.

22. Facio MC, Hervías-Vivancos B, Broullón JR, Avila J, Fajardo-Expósito MA, Bartha JL. Cardiac biometry and function in euploid fetuses with intracardiac echogenic foci. *Prenat Diagn.* 2012;32(2):113–116.

23. Perles Z, Nir A, Gavri S, Golender J, Rein AJJT. Intracardiac echogenic foci have no hemodynamic significance in the fetus. *Pediatr Cardiol.* 2010;31(1):7–10.

24. Brown DL, Roberts DJ, Miller WA. Left ventricular echogenic focus in the fetal heart: pathologic correlation. *J Ultrasound Med Off J Am Inst Ultrasound Med.* 1994;13(8):613–616.

25. Nyberg DA, Souter VL, El-Bastawissi A, Young S, Luthardt F, Luthy DA. Isolated sonographic markers for detection of fetal Down syndrome in the second trimester of pregnancy. *J Ultrasound Med Off J Am Inst Ultrasound Med.* 2001;20(10):1053–1063.

26. Smith-Bindman R, Hosmer W, Feldstein VA, Deeks JJ, Goldberg JD. Second-trimester ultrasound to detect fetuses with Down syndrome: a meta-analysis. *J Am Med Assoc.* 2001;285(8):1044–1055.

27. Coco C, Jeanty P, Jeanty C. An isolated echogenic heart focus is not an indication for amniocentesis in 12,672 unselected patients. *J Ultrasound Med Off J Am Inst Ultrasound Med.* 2004;23(4):489–496.

28. Bromley B, Lieberman E, Shipp TD, Benacerraf BR. The genetic sonogram: a method of risk assessment for Down syndrome in the second trimester. *J Ultrasound Med Off J Am Inst Ultrasound Med.* 2002;21(10). 1087–1096–1098.

29. Morcos CL, Platt LD, Carlson DE, Gregory KD, Greene NH, Korst LM. The isolated choroid plexus cyst. *Obstet Gynecol.* 1998;92(2):232–236.

30. DeRoo TR, Harris RD, Sargent SK, Denholm TA, Crow HC. Fetal choroid plexus cysts: prevalence, clinical significance, and sonographic appearance. *AJR Am J Roentgenol.* 1988;151(6):1179–1181.

31. Chitkara U, Cogswell C, Norton K, Wilkins IA, Mehalek K, Berkowitz RL. Choroid plexus cysts in the fetus: a benign anatomic variant or pathologic entity? Report of 41 cases and review of the literature. *Obstet Gynecol.* 1988;72(2):185–189.

32. DiPietro JA, Cristofalo EA, Voegtline KM, Crino J. Isolated prenatal choroid plexus cysts do not affect child development. *Prenat Diagn.* 2011;31(8):745–749.

33. DiPietro JA, Costigan KA, Cristofalo EA, et al. Choroid plexus cysts do not affect fetal neurodevelopment. *J Perinatol Off J Calif Perinat Assoc.* 2006;26(10):622–627.

34. Bernier FP, Crawford SG, Dewey D. Developmental outcome of children who had choroid plexus cysts detected prenatally. *Prenat Diagn.* 2005;25(4):322–326.

35. Digiovanni LM, Quinlan MP, Verp MS. Choroid plexus cysts: infant and early childhood developmental outcome. *Obstet Gynecol.* 1997;90(2):191–194.

36. Goetzinger KR, Stamilio DM, Dicke JM, Macones GA, Odibo AO. Evaluating the incidence and likelihood ratios for chromosomal abnormalities in fetuses with common central nervous system malformations. *Am J Obstet Gynecol.* 2008;199(3):285.e1–e6.

37. Cho RC, Chu P, Smith-Bindman R. Second trimester prenatal ultrasound for the detection of pregnancies at increased risk of Trisomy 18 based on serum screening. *Prenat Diagn.* 2009;29(2):129–139.

38. Ouzounian JG, Ludington C, Chan S. Isolated choroid plexus cyst or echogenic cardiac focus on prenatal ultrasound: is genetic amniocentesis indicated? *Am J Obstet Gynecol.* 2007;196(6):595.e1–e3; discussion 595.e3.

39. Coco C, Jeanty P. Karyotyping of fetuses with isolated choroid plexus cysts is not justified in an unselected population. *J Ultrasound Med Off J Am Inst Ultrasound Med.* 2004;23(7):899–906.

40. Yoder PR, Sabbagha RE, Gross SJ, Zelop CM. The second-trimester fetus with isolated choroid plexus cysts: a meta-analysis of risk of trisomies 18 and 21. *Obstet Gynecol.* 1999;93(5 Pt 2):869–872.

41. Hua M, Odibo AO, Macones GA, Roehl KA, Crane JP, Cahill AG. Single umbilical artery and its associated findings. *Obstet Gynecol.* 2010;115(5):930–934.

42. Heifetz SA. Single umbilical artery. A statistical analysis of 237 autopsy cases and review of the literature. *Perspect Pediatr Pathol.* 1984;8(4):345–378.

43. Murphy-Kaulbeck L, Dodds L, Joseph KS, Van den Hof M. Single umbilical artery risk factors and pregnancy outcomes. *Obstet Gynecol.* 2010;116(4):843–850.

44. Dagklis T, Defigueiredo D, Staboulidou I, Casagrandi D, Nicolaides KH. Isolated single umbilical artery and fetal karyotype. *Ultrasound Obstet Gynecol Off J Int Soc Ultrasound Obstet Gynecol.* 2010;36(3):291–295.

45. DeFigueiredo D, Dagklis T, Zidere V, Allan L, Nicolaides KH. Isolated single umbilical artery: need for specialist fetal echocardiography? *Ultrasound Obstet Gynecol Off J Int Soc Ultrasound Obstet Gynecol.* 2010;36(5):553–555.

46. Gossett DR, Lantz ME, Chisholm CA. Antenatal diagnosis of single umbilical artery: is fetal echocardiography warranted? *Obstet Gynecol.* 2002;100(5 Pt 1):903–908.

47. Lubusky M, Dhaifalah I, Prochazka M, et al. Single umbilical artery and its siding in the second trimester of pregnancy: relation to chromosomal defects. *Prenat Diagn.* 2007;27(4):327–331.

48. Wiegand S, McKenna DS, Croom C, Ventolini G, Sonek JD, Neiger R. Serial sonographic growth assessment in pregnancies complicated by an isolated single umbilical artery. *Am J Perinatol.* 2008;25(3):149–152.

49. Bombrys AE, Neiger R, Hawkins S, et al. Pregnancy outcome in isolated single umbilical artery. *Am J Perinatol.* 2008;25(4):239–242.

50. Predanic M, Perni SC, Friedman A, Chervenak FA, Chasen ST. Fetal growth assessment and neonatal birth weight in fetuses with an isolated single umbilical artery. *Obstet Gynecol.* 2005;105(5 Pt 1):1093–1097.

51. Mailath-Pokorny M, Worda K, Schmid M, Polterauer S, Bettelheim D. Isolated single umbilical artery: evaluating the risk of adverse pregnancy outcome. *Eur J Obstet Gynecol Reprod Biol.* 2015;184:80–83.

52. Burshtein S, Levy A, Holcberg G, Zlotnik A, Sheiner E. Is single umbilical artery an independent risk factor for perinatal mortality? *Arch Gynecol Obstet.* 2011;283(2):191–194.

53. Voskamp BJ, Fleurke-Rozema H, Oude-Rengerink K, et al. Relationship of isolated single umbilical artery to fetal growth, aneuploidy and perinatal mortality: systematic review and meta-analysis. *Ultrasound Obstet Gynecol Off J Int Soc Ultrasound Obstet Gynecol.* 2013;42(6):622–628.

54. Chow JS, Benson CB, Doubilet PM. Frequency and nature of structural anomalies in fetuses with single umbilical arteries. *J Ultrasound Med Off J Am Inst Ultrasound Med.* 1998;17(12):765–768.

55. Nadel A. Ultrasound evaluation of the fetal gastrointestinal tract and Abdominal wall. In: *Callen's Ultrasonography in Obstetrics and Gynecology.* 6th ed. Elsevier; 2017.

56. Simon-Bouy B, Muller F. French Collaborative Group. Hyperechogenic fetal bowel and Down syndrome. Results of a French collaborative study based on 680 prospective cases. *Prenat Diagn.* 2002;22(3):189–192.

57. Hurt L, Wright M, Dunstan F, et al. Prevalence of defined ultrasound findings of unknown significance at the second trimester fetal anomaly scan and their association with adverse pregnancy outcomes: the Welsh study of mothers and babies population-based cohort. *Prenat Diagn.* 2016;36(1):40–48.

58. Goetzinger KR, Cahill AG, Macones GA, Odibo AO. Echogenic bowel on second-trimester ultrasonography: evaluating the risk of adverse pregnancy outcome. *Obstet Gynecol.* 2011;117(6):1341–1348.

59. Strocker AM, Snijders RJ, Carlson DE, et al. Fetal echogenic bowel: parameters to be considered in differential diagnosis. *Ultrasound Obstet Gynecol Off J Int Soc Ultrasound Obstet Gynecol.* 2000;16(6):519–523.

60. Nyberg DA, Dubinsky T, Resta RG, Mahony BS, Hickok DE, Luthy DA. Echogenic fetal bowel during the second trimester: clinical importance. *Radiology.* 1993;188(2):527–531.

61. MacGregor SN, Tamura R, Sabbagha R, Brenhofer JK, Kambich MP, Pergament E. Isolated hyperechoic fetal bowel: significance and implications for management. *Am J Obstet Gynecol.* 1995;173(4):1254–1258.

62. Aagaard-Tillery KM, Malone FD, Nyberg DA, et al. Role of second-trimester genetic sonography after Down syndrome screening. *Obstet Gynecol.* 2009;114(6):1189–1196.

63. Sepulveda W, Reid R, Nicolaidis P, Prendiville O, Chapman RS, Fisk NM. Second-trimester echogenic bowel and intraamniotic bleeding: association between fetal bowel echogenicity and amniotic fluid spectrophotometry at 410 nm. *Am J Obstet Gynecol.* 1996;174(3):839–842.

64. Mailath-Pokorny M, Klein K, Klebermass-Schrehof K, Hachemian N, Bettelheim D. Are fetuses with isolated echogenic bowel at higher risk for an adverse pregnancy outcome? Experiences from a tertiary referral center. *Prenat Diagn.* 2012;32(13):1295–1299.

65. Dicke JM, Crane JP. Sonographically detected hyperechoic fetal bowel: significance and implications for pregnancy management. *Obstet Gynecol.* 1992;80(5):778–782.

66. Muller F, Simon-Bouy B, Girodon E, et al. Predicting the risk of cystic fibrosis with abnormal ultrasound signs of fetal bowel: results of a French molecular collaborative study based on 641 prospective cases. *Am J Med Genet.* 2002;110(2):109–115.

67. Guerra B, Simonazzi G, Puccetti C, et al. Ultrasound prediction of symptomatic congenital cytomegalovirus infection. *Am J Obstet Gynecol.* 2008;198(4):380.e1–e7.

68. Society for Maternal-Fetal Medicine (SMFM), Hughes BL, Gyamfi-Bannerman C. Diagnosis and antenatal management of congenital cytomegalovirus infection. *Am J Obstet Gynecol.* 2016;214(6):B5–B11.

69. Sepulveda W, Sebire NJ. Fetal echogenic bowel: a complex scenario. *Ultrasound Obstet Gynecol Off J Int Soc Ultrasound Obstet Gynecol.* 2000;16(6):510–514.

70. Al-Kouatly HB, Chasen ST, Karam AK, Ahner R, Chervenak FA. Factors associated with fetal demise in fetal echogenic bowel. *Am J Obstet Gynecol.* 2001;185(5):1039–1043.

71. Ronin C, Mace P, Stenard F, et al. Antenatal prognostic factor of fetal echogenic bowel. *Eur J Obstet Gynecol Reprod Biol.* 2017;212:166–170.

72. Buiter HD, Holswilder-Olde Scholtenhuis MAG, Bouman K, van Baren R, Bilardo CM, Bos AF. Outcome of infants presenting with echogenic bowel in the second trimester of pregnancy. *Arch Dis Child Fetal Neonatal Ed.* 2013;98(3):F256–F259.

73. Nguyen HT, Benson CB, Bromley B, et al. Multidisciplinary consensus on the classification of prenatal and postnatal urinary tract dilation (UTD classification system). *J Pediatr Urol.* 2014;10(6):982–998.

74. Goetzinger K, Odibo AO. Ultrasound evaluation of fetal aneuploidy in the first and second trimesters. In: *Callen's Ultrasonography in Obstetrics and Gynecology.* 6th ed. Elsevier; 2017.

75. Shipp TD, Bromley B, Mascola M, Benacerraf B. Variation in fetal femur length with respect to maternal race. *J Ultrasound Med Off J Am Inst Ultrasound Med.* 2001;20(2):141–144.

76. Borgida AF, Zelop C, Deroche M, Bolnick A, Egan JFX. Down syndrome screening using race-specific femur length. *Am J Obstet Gynecol.* 2003;189(4):977–979.

77. Zelop CM, Borgida AF, Egan JFX. Variation of fetal humeral length in second-trimester fetuses according to race and ethnicity. *J Ultrasound Med Off J Am Inst Ultrasound Med.* 2003;22(7):691–693.

78. Harper LM, Gray D, Dicke J, Stamilio DM, Macones GA, Odibo AO. Do race-specific definitions of short long bones improve the detection of down syndrome on second-trimester genetic sonograms? *J Ultrasound Med Off J Am Inst Ultrasound Med.* 2010;29(2):231–235.

79. Hernandez-Andrade E, Yeo L, Goncalves L, Luewan S, Garcia M, Romero R. Skeletal dysplasias. In: *Callen's Ultrasonography in Obstetrics and Gynecology.* Elsevier; 2017.

80. Goetzinger KR, Cahill AG, Macones GA, Odibo AO. Isolated short femur length on second-trimester sonography: a marker for fetal growth restriction and other adverse perinatal outcomes. *J Ultrasound Med Off J Am Inst Ultrasound Med.* 2012;31(12):1935–1941.

81. Kaijomaa M, Ulander V-M, Ryynanen M, Stefanovic V. Risk of adverse outcomes in euploid pregnancies with isolated short fetal femur and humerus on second-trimester sonography. *J Ultrasound Med Off J Am Inst Ultrasound Med.* 2016;35(12):2675–2680.

82. Benacerraf BR. The history of the second-trimester sonographic markers for detecting fetal Down syndrome, and their current role in obstetric practice. *Prenat Diagn.* 2010;30(7):644–652.

83. Benacerraf BR, Frigoletto FD, Laboda LA. Sonographic diagnosis of Down syndrome in the second trimester. *Am J Obstet Gynecol.* 1985;153(1):49–52.

84. Salomon LJ, Alfirevic Z, Audibert F, et al. ISUOG consensus statement on the impact of non-invasive prenatal testing (NIPT) on prenatal ultrasound practice. *Ultrasound Obstet Gynecol Off J Int Soc Ultrasound Obstet Gynecol.* 2014;44(1):122–123.

85. Audibert F, De Bie I, Johnson J-A, et al. No. 348-Joint SOGC-CCMG guideline: update on prenatal screening for fetal aneuploidy, fetal anomalies, and adverse pregnancy outcomes. *J Obstet Gynaecol Can JOGC J Obstet Gynecol Can JOGC.* 2017;39(9):805–817.

CHAPTER 11

Genetic Evaluation of Fetal Sonographic Abnormalities

P. KAITLYN EDELSON, MD • LORRAINE DUGOFF, MD • BRYANN BROMLEY, MD

INTRODUCTION

Structural malformations, many of which can be diagnosed antenatally, are present in approximately 2%–3% of live births.[1–3] Fetuses with structural malformations are at increased risk for an underlying genetic disorder, even in the setting of a normal karyotype. The clinical prognosis is highly variable depending on the presence of a genetic syndrome, the specific type of anomaly that is present, as well as whether the anomaly is isolated or part of a spectrum of malformations involving other organ systems.

WHAT IS THE ROLE OF ULTRASOUND IN IDENTIFYING FETAL ANOMALIES?

Fetal assessment by ultrasound is a standard component of prenatal care. The American College of Obstetricians and Gynecologists (ACOG) recommends that all obstetric patients be offered ultrasound evaluation at least once during pregnancy.[4] The average number of ultrasounds performed in the United States has increased from 1.5 per pregnancy in 1995 to between four and five scans in low-risk patients in 2011.[5,6]

Screening for congenital anomalies by ultrasound is the primary indication for second-trimester anatomic imaging and has been demonstrated to improve the detection of major fetal anomalies before 24 weeks (RR 3.46 [95% CI: 1.67–7.14]).[7] Factors that influence detection rates include the setting in which the ultrasound is performed (community based vs. tertiary care), the fetal gestational age at the time of the study, and technical imaging challenges such as obesity.[8,9] Adherence to a systematic imaging protocol improves prenatal diagnosis of anomalies.[10] In pregnancies where a malformation is identified and termination is chosen, there is over 98% confirmation of the primary diagnosis.[11]

WHAT IS THE DIFFERENCE BETWEEN A STANDARD AND DETAILED ANATOMIC SCAN?

The American Institute of Ultrasound in Medicine (AIUM) and ACOG distinguish between standard second-trimester examinations and detailed examinations.[4,12,13] A standard examination is utilized to evaluate fetal anatomy in a population at low risk for congenital anomalies. A more comprehensive or detailed obstetrical ultrasound examination is performed for women at increased risk for a congenital malformation based on medical history, results of laboratory evaluations, or concerns identified on a standard obstetrical ultrasound examination. Detailed fetal anatomic imaging is performed by a provider with additional training and expertise in obstetrical imaging and dysmorphology assessment.[13] It is important to recognize that despite optimal imaging and diagnostic testing, there is a residual risk of an undetected abnormality.[14–16] Additionally, false-positive findings may occur. These may be structural anomalies that are suspected but not confirmed after birth, "markers" of aneuploidy[15] (see Chapter 10) or conditions such as ventriculoseptal defects or mild ventriculomegaly that may resolve during the course of pregnancy.[17,18]

WHAT IS THE IMPACT OF GESTATIONAL AGE IN IDENTIFYING FETAL ANOMALIES?

The Late First-Trimester Scan: 11⁰–13⁶ Weeks

A late first-trimester ultrasound is performed primarily to measure the nuchal translucency (NT) as a component of first-trimester risk assessment for aneuploidy[19] (see Chapter 8). Although a thickened nuchal translucency confers an increased risk of aneuploidy, it is also a marker for increased risk of structural anomalies and other genetic conditions.[20–22] Imaging the fetus at this

Perinatal Genetics. https://doi.org/10.1016/B978-0-323-53094-1.00011-4

gestational age provides the first opportunity to perform an anatomic assessment of the fetus.[23] Although this is not currently standard practice in the United States, it is feasible by dedicated sonographers and sonologists.[24–26]

Estimates of detection rates for major anomalies between 11 weeks 0 days and 13 weeks 6 days vary from 18% to 84%, with most authors reporting a sensitivity of approximately 50% for major anomalies. The detection rate depends on the anatomic area that is being evaluated.[10,20,25,27–31]

A systematic review of 78,002 fetuses that underwent ultrasound examination between 11–14 weeks found that the detection rate of nuchal defects was 92%, whereas only 34% of limb, face, and genitourinary tract anomalies were detected.[10] In addition, there was a higher detection rate in fetuses evaluated between 13 and 14 weeks than those examined between 11 and 12 weeks. Detection rates are higher in those with multiple abnormalities compared with a single finding, and in high-risk populations (61%) compared with low-risk populations (32%). The adherence to an imaging protocol improves detection rates as does the use of transvaginal imaging.[10,31] With experience and recognition of additional markers, detection rates may improve.[32–34]

Some anomalies, such as anencephaly, alobar holoprosencephaly, body stalk anomalies, omphalocele, and major disruption of fetal contour, should almost always be detected during this gestational age window. Others, such as cardiac defects, spina bifida, and facial clefts, are more challenging to diagnose. Finally, some anomalies, such as those involving the corpus callosum and congenital lung malformations, are not detectable at this early gestational age, partly because of timing of embryologic development.[25,28,30] As with all obstetrical imaging, the natural history of some diagnosed abnormalities may not be fully understood or may change with advancing gestation.[17]

The early anatomic evaluation of the fetus allows patients to consider the implications of the condition detected and pursue expert consultation and diagnostic testing. Detection of structural anomalies between 11 and 14 weeks allows those patients who choose to terminate to do so at an earlier gestational age, when the procedure is safer.[35] For those who continue their pregnancy, a follow-up ultrasound examination at 18–22 weeks is necessary to better elucidate the abnormality.

It is important that patients understand that a "normal" first-trimester ultrasound does not exclude all major or lethal anomalies and this imaging window does not replace the standard second-trimester anatomic assessment of the fetus.

Second-Trimester Anatomic Survey

The gold standard for prenatal anomaly screening by ultrasound in the United States is an ultrasound examination performed between 18 and 22 weeks of gestation. Anatomic imaging should be performed in accordance with a contemporary imaging protocol. This may be a standard scan performed in patients at "low risk" for congenital anomalies or a detailed scan in those who are at "increased risk."[4,12,13]

The majority of literature on routine screening for congenital anomalies in unselected populations was performed several decades ago with wide variations in reported detection rate of anomalies.[36] The Eurofetus study, performed in 61 obstetric centers between 1990 and 1993 reported a prenatal detection of 61.4% of fetuses with an anomaly and 56.2% of all malformations. The detection of major anomalies was 73.7% compared with 45.7% of minor anomalies. Overall, 55% of major anomalies were detected before 24 weeks. The sensitivity of anomaly detection was 88.3% for the central nervous system and 84.8% for the genitourinary tract, as compared with 38.8% for the heart and great vessels.[37]

In more contemporary literature evaluating first and second-trimester anatomic imaging, approximately 75%–95% of structural malformations may be suspected or detected.[15,20,38–40] Detection rates will vary with the population studied, the follow-up available, the experience and skill of the imager, the imaging protocol utilized, and imaging conditions such as obesity, which may preclude an optimal anatomic evaluation.[8,41]

Third-Trimester Scans

Routine ultrasound in the third trimester is not currently standard practice. However, there are certain anomalies that are not usually diagnosed until this advanced gestational age, such as microcephaly, lissencephaly, or achondroplasia (Fig. 11.1A and B). The contribution of a third-trimester scan was demonstrated in a prospective study of 8074 fetuses who had previously had a normal first and second-trimester ultrasound and were reexamined between 28 and 32 weeks. At the third-trimester ultrasound, an additional 15% of the total anomalies were diagnosed despite two prior normal ultrasounds. The anomalies diagnosed in the third trimester were primarily urogenital, cardiovascular, and central nervous system anomalies.[40] Overall, 90% of anomalies in the cohort were detected prenatally, whereas 10% were not detected until after birth.[40]

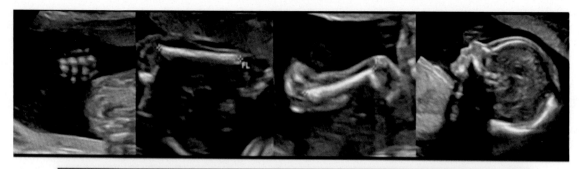

2D Measurements	AUA	Value	m1	m2	m3	Meth.	GP		Age
EFW (Hadlock)			Value		Range	Age	Range	GP	Williams
AC/BPD/FL									N/A
BPD (Hadlock)	✓	4.95 cm	4.94	4.99	4.93	avg.	├──┼──┤	66.4%	21w0d
FL (Hadlock)	✓	3.28 cm	3.21	3.35		avg.	├──┼─┤	30.2%	20w2d
HL (Jeanty)	✓	3.10 cm	3.11	3.09		avg.	├──┼─┤	38.4%	20w2d

A

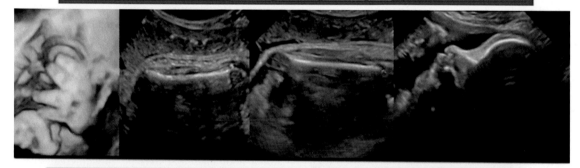

2D Measurements	AUA	Value	m1	m2	m3	Meth.	GP	Age
BPD (Hadlock)	✓	9.90 cm	9.95	9.80	9.96	avg.	├────┼─┤	96.3%	40w4d
FL (Hadlock)	■	6.04 cm	6.02	6.33	5.77	avg.	┤├───┼──┤	<2.3%	31w3d
HL (Jeanty)	■	5.51 cm	5.49	5.61	5.43	avg.	┤├───┼──┤	<5.0%	32w0d

B

FIG. 11.1 Achondroplasia. **(A)** Second-trimester fetal anatomic evaluation demonstrating normal morphology and biometry. **(B)** The same fetus imaged at 39 weeks shows severe shortening of the long bones and a trident hand raising the suspicion of achondroplasia, which was confirmed with genetic testing after birth.

WHAT IS THE IMPORTANCE OF A SYSTEMATIC ULTRASOUND EVALUATION USING PATTERN RECOGNITION?

If a fetal anomaly is identified, it is incumbent on the sonologist to formulate a differential diagnosis. The sonologist must be a detective, using a deliberate stepwise approach of observation and deductive reasoning.[42] With pattern recognition of genetic syndromes in mind, a structured systematic and thoughtful evaluation of other organ systems, looking for sentinel features, will allow the sonologist to narrow the differential diagnosis.[42,43]

As an example, a required anatomic component of the standard fetal ultrasound includes evaluation of the upper lip.[4,12] Facial clefts are relatively prevalent, occurring in about 15 per 10,000 live births in the United States.[1] Contemporary reports suggest that approximately 69%–80% of cleft lip with or without cleft palate is diagnosed before 24 weeks' gestation.[44,45] In nearly two-thirds of fetuses in which a cleft lip is identified, there will be an associated cleft palate.[1,44] Cleft palate without a disrupted lip is most often not diagnosed prenatally.[44,46] In 77% of cases, a facial cleft is an isolated finding; however, in 16% of cases, they are associated with malformations in other organ systems and approximately 7% of cases occur as part of a recognized genetic syndrome.[45,47]

Once a facial cleft is identified, it is critical to determine the extent of the clefting. How much of the lip does it involve? Does it extend to the nares or even up the face to the orbits? Does it involve the palate? Is it unilateral, bilateral, or central? The risk of associated anomalies increases with more severe degrees of clefting.[46,47]

There are numerous chromosomal abnormalities and genetic syndromes associated with facial clefting, and an attempt to uncover sentinel features by detailed anatomic evaluation will narrow the differential diagnosis of a potentially nonisolated condition.[42] If the fetus has a central or median cleft, an examination of the central nervous system and cardiac anatomy should be performed. Additionally, the hands should be evaluated for postaxial polydactyly, which would lead to a suspicion of trisomy 13, or if a facial cleft is associated with choroid plexus cysts and clenched hands, trisomy 18 would be suspected (Fig. 11.2). If the median cleft is associated with polysyndactyly or a bifid hallux, one must consider oro-facial-digital syndrome as an etiology.[48] If the cleft is associated with ectrodactyly of the

hands (split or cleft hand), ectrodactyly-ectodermal dysplasia-clefting (EEC) syndrome would be the most likely diagnosis. Facial clefting may be associated with skeletal dysplasias, and an evaluation of the ribs, long bones, and hands may lead to a suggestion of Roberts syndrome or Majewski syndrome.[42,48,49] If the anatomic evaluation reveals that the cleft does not follow an expected embryologic sequence and other asymmetric defects such as transverse limb defects are present, the sonologist should look for evidence of amniotic bands. In some rare cases, the cleft may extend up the face and involve the orbits (Tessier cleft). Even in cases of presumed isolated clefting, family history is important to potentially differentiate a sporadic event from the autosomal dominant Van der Woude syndrome. Once a facial cleft is identified and the differential diagnosis narrowed, genetic counseling and diagnostic testing is recommended.

WHAT IS THE ROLE OF PATTERN RECOGNITION IN COMMON ANEUPLOIDY SYNDROMES?

Each of the common autosomal trisomies presents with a relatively distinct constellation of findings that allows a tentative prenatal diagnosis based on imaging. Detailed anatomic assessment with attention to pattern recognition including evaluation of the fetal hands helps narrow the suspected diagnosis. Other chromosomal anomalies that may be encountered, such as monosomy X and triploidy, also have distinct features that often can be recognized on prenatal sonographic evaluation. These conditions may be diagnosed by karyotype.

Trisomy 21 (Down Syndrome)

Trisomy 21 is the most common chromosomal abnormality resulting in a live birth, occurring in approximately 1 in 700 pregnancies.[50] Prenatal sonography evaluating the nuchal translucency and/or second-trimester "markers" of aneuploidy in conjunction with standard analyte screening can identify at least 85%–90% of affected fetuses.[51-53] Sonography alone is useful in identifying 50%–80% of affected fetuses based on "markers" and to a lesser extent structural anomalies.[51,53] Please see Chapter 10 for further discussion of ultrasound markers of aneuploidy. Approximately 20%–30% of fetuses with trisomy 21 will have a structural malformation. The major structural anomalies identified in fetuses with trisomy 21 include cardiac anomalies such as atrioventricular canal defects, tetralogy of Fallot, and ventriculoseptal defects.[54,55]

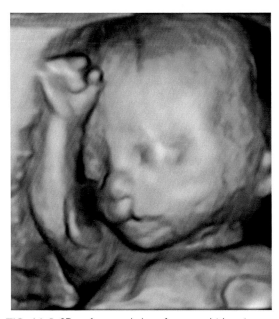

FIG. 11.2 3D surface rendering of a second-trimester fetus with trisomy 18 demonstrating a facial cleft and persistently clenched hands. This fetus also had choroid plexus cysts and a major cardiac defect.

Noncardiac abnormalities include mild ventriculomegaly, duodenal atresia, and esophageal atresia. Fetuses with trisomy 21 may also have abnormal fluid collections, such as a pericardial or pleural effusions, or nonimmune hydrops.[56]

Trisomy 18 (Edwards Syndrome)

Trisomy 18 is the second most common autosomal trisomy in live-born infants, occurring in 1 in 3134 pregnancies.[50] Fetuses with trisomy 18 have multiple congenital abnormalities that are identifiable by prenatal sonography, resulting in a detection rate of 98%–100% by imagers using protocols that involve a detailed evaluation of the fetal heart and hands.[57-59] Lower detection rates are reported before 18 weeks' gestation.[59]

Structural abnormalities of the central nervous system that are often identified in affected fetuses include neural tube defects, agenesis of the corpus callosum, and posterior fossa abnormalities, including cerebellar hypoplasia.[57-59] Other anomalies that may be seen in affected fetuses are micrognathia, omphalocele, diaphragmatic hernia, and cystic renal dysplasia. Examination of the extremities, particularly the fetal hands, is critical in making a presumptive diagnosis of trisomy 18, as fetuses with this condition may have radial ray defects (usually unilateral). The sentinel features of this syndrome are clenched hands and overlapping index fingers, which are identified in 95% of affected fetuses (Fig. 11.2). Other abnormalities of the extremities include clubbed and rocker-bottom feet.[58]

Fetal growth restriction is seen in 50% of affected fetuses in the second trimester, and the unusual combination of intrauterine growth restriction and polyhydramnios in the third trimester is highly suspicious for this condition.[60] Although choroid plexus cysts are seen in 50% of fetuses with trisomy 18, they are rarely (if ever) seen as an isolated finding in affected fetuses. Similarly, a strawberry-shaped skull or a single umbilical artery may be seen in affected fetuses but again, not characteristically, as an isolated finding.[57,58] Survival with trisomy 18 is limited, with many fetuses dying before birth and few surviving past the first year of life.[61] Those that do survive have significant developmental and medical challenges. In pregnancies where prenatal cytogenetic confirmation is obtained, termination rates are 84%.[62] In those that are live-born, survival to 5 years is 12%.[63]

Trisomy 13 (Patau Syndrome)

Trisomy 13 is also seen in live-born infants, although less commonly than trisomy 18 or 21, occurring in 1 in 7000 pregnancies. It is associated with severe intellectual disability and numerous congenital anomalies.[50] Prenatal detection by ultrasound is 90%–100% in the second trimester.[64] Abnormal findings include holoprosencephaly, agenesis of the corpus callosum, cerebellar malformations, and neural tube defects. Affected individuals will often have severe craniofacial defects such as hypotelorism, micro- or anophthalmia, midface hypoplasia, and proboscis (Fig. 11.3). Bilateral cleft lip and palate and midline clefts are common. Affected fetuses also often have major congenital heart defects. Omphalocele and enlarged echogenic kidneys may be associated with this syndrome, and postaxial polydactyly also suggests the diagnosis of trisomy 13 when associated with other major anomalies. Fetal growth restriction is common. Many affected fetuses die in utero and in those that are live-born, survival to 5 years is less than 10%.[63] In pregnancies where prenatal cytogenetic confirmation is obtained, termination rates are 89%.[62]

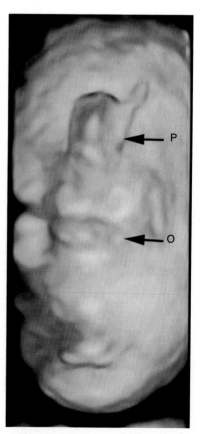

FIG. 11.3 3D surface rendering of the face in a fetus with trisomy 13 demonstrating a single orbit ("O" arrow) and a proboscis ("P"arrow).

Monosomy X (Turner Syndrome)

Monosomy X occurs due to complete or partial absence of the X chromosome. The prevalence in live-born females is reported as 1 in 2000; however, the majority of affected fetuses are spontaneously aborted.[65] The classic features of 45,X on second-trimester sonography are a female fetus with a large septated cystic hygroma involving the posterior and lateral neck with skin thickening and lymphedema that may extend down the trunk. Abnormal fluid collections characteristic of nonimmune hydrops may be seen. Cardiovascular abnormalities are identified in 10%–40% of fetuses, most commonly left-sided cardiac anomalies such as coarctation of the aorta or hypoplastic left heart syndrome.[66] Renal malformations including a horseshoe kidney and collecting system malformations have been identified in approximately 25%–40% of cases.[67] Prenatal detection by ultrasound is reported to be in 68% overall, and sonographic findings are evident in 92% of those with complete monosomy X and 56% of those with mosaicism for monosomy X.[65] In some cases, prenatal detection is in the later third-trimester because of the recognition of congenital cardiac anomalies.[68] In cases where the diagnosis of monosomy X is associated with congenital anomalies, termination rates of 78% are reported.[68]

Triploidy

In triploidy, there is a complete extra set of haploid chromosomes as a consequence of fertilization of a diploid ovum (digynic) or fertilization by two sperm (dispermy) or a diploid sperm (diandric). Triploidy is reported to occur in 1%–3% of clinically recognized pregnancies, and most fetuses with this condition are spontaneously aborted by midpregnancy.[69] Two distinct phenotypes have been reported and sonographically identified in 80% of fetuses with this condition.[70] Fetuses with diandric triploidy tend to have enlarged cystic placentas and may have symmetrical growth restriction (Fig. 11.4A). Those with digynic triploidy have a small placenta and severe fetal growth restriction with relative macrocephaly and oligohydramnios (Fig. 11.4B).

Sonographic abnormalities are identified in 85%–92% of second-trimester fetuses with triploidy.[69,71] Massalska et al. reported on the sonographic findings of 67 fetuses with triploidy by karyotype and noted structural anomalies in 60% of affected fetuses. The majority of structural anomalies reported in this condition are not unique and include abnormalities of the central nervous system, including ventriculomegaly, neural tube defects, and abnormalities of the posterior fossa. Fetuses also may have major congenital heart anomalies and craniofacial deformities. Abnormalities of the placenta are seen in 25% of affected fetuses, and fetal growth restriction is almost universal, with characteristic features including severe early growth restriction with relative macrocephaly.[69,70] A sentinel hand feature of this condition is syndactyly of the third and fourth fingers.[72] Fetal survival to birth is very rare.[70,73]

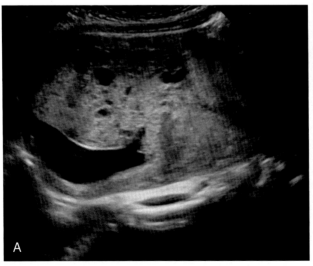 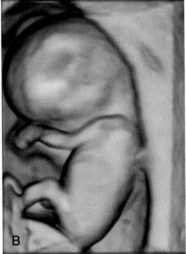

FIG. 11.4 **(A)** Anterior thick cystic placenta fetus with triploidy at 13 weeks' gestation. **(B)** 3D surface rendering of the body of a different fetus with triploidy at 13 weeks. The fetus is growth restricted and has a large head compared with the small size of the body.

Early prenatal diagnosis is important as the presence of this condition is associated with maternal complications including severe hyperemesis and early-onset preeclampsia.[71]

WHAT IS THE ROLE OF PATTERN RECOGNITION IN OTHER GENETIC SYNDROMES?

Although sonographically one may suspect a condition based on a constellation of findings, genetic counseling or consultation with a geneticist is critical to narrowing the differential diagnosis and choosing the optimal testing strategy.

22q11.2 Deletion Syndrome (DiGeorge Syndrome/Velocardiofacial Syndrome)

The 22q11.2 deletion syndrome is caused by a hemizygous (only one copy of the 22q region) deletion on the chromosomal region of 22q11.2 and is associated with broad phenotypic variability. Before the identification of the genetic deletion, different groupings of overlapping and similar conditions had a variety of different names, including DiGeorge syndrome, velocardiofacial (Shprintzen) syndrome, and others, which are now known collectively as 22q11.2 deletion syndrome.

The syndrome is characterized by variable phenotypic findings that range from mild to severe. The most common findings are related to cardiac abnormalities, reported in 45%–74% of affected individuals.[74] Noncardiac findings include cleft palate or palatal insufficiency, thymic hypoplasia with immune deficiency, and parathyroid hypoplasia with hypocalcemia. Developmental and language delay, autism spectrum disorder, and an increase in schizophrenia are associated with this syndrome.[75] Specific deletions in genes within the region known as TBX1 may be related to physical features of the syndrome, whereas deletion in the COMT gene is suspected to play a role in the increased risk of neuropsychiatric and behavior issues.[76]

The prevalence is approximately 1 in 4000 births, although it may be underdiagnosed because of mild features.[74] Prenatal detection has been reported based on thickened nuchal translucency in the first trimester; it is the most common pathogenic copy number variant reported in fetuses with normal karyotype and abnormal microarray findings.[22,77]

In the second trimester, prenatal suspicion of 22q11.2 deletion syndrome is largely based on the detection of cardiac abnormalities, most commonly conotruncal abnormalities such as tetralogy of Fallot and truncus arteriosus. These major anomalies can be detected by standard sonographic assessment of the fetal heart, which includes evaluation of the great vessels. Subtle cardiac findings such as right-sided and interrupted aortic arch are also associated with this syndrome but require a more detailed evaluation of the fetal heart.[78] The presence of a congenital heart defect is the most common indication for genetic testing in affected individuals.[74] In a registry-based series of prenatally detected cases of 22q11.2 deletion in France, 84% of affected individuals had a congenital heart defect; in 62%, the cardiac defect was an isolated finding.[74] Evaluation of the thymus for hypoplasia/aplasia may improve the detection of this condition and is optimally visualized in the three-vessel trachea view. However, this is challenging with less than 10% identified in a recent prenatal series.[74,79]

Other prenatal abnormalities potentially detectable by ultrasound include cleft palate, which may be suspected by the presence of micrognathia. Evaluation of the face for evidence of hypertelorism and a broad nasal bridge may contribute to the suspicion of this syndrome. Renal anomalies may also be identified by prenatal sonography. In prenatally diagnosed cases, these features are often associated with other abnormalities, most notably congenital heart defects.[74]

Routine prenatal karyotype is usually normal, given the small size of the microdeletion, and is not useful for detecting this condition. The primary diagnostic study should be a microarray based on family history, abnormal ultrasound findings, or a positive cell-free DNA test. The use of FISH (fluorescent in situ hybridization) as an initial test is not recommended as other microdeletions associated with congenital heart defects may be present; therefore, chromosomal microarray is recommended in cases of fetal congenital heart defects. The use of FISH as an initial test is not recommended because smaller deletions may be missed. Testing by FISH may be used in cases in which an affected parent is known to have a 22q11.2 deletion.[80] Preimplantation genetic evaluation is possible for families in which a pathogenic variant has been identified. Although cell-free DNA screening for 22q11 is commercially available, it is not recommended by professional societies because its sensitivity and positive predictive value are unknown.[80]

Noonan Syndrome

Noonan syndrome (NS) is an autosomal dominant disorder (de novo mutation is common) with a prevalence of 1 in 1000 to 1 in 2500.[81] Postnatally, the condition is characterized by distinctive facial features including a broad forehead and hypertelorism, right-sided cardiac defects, hypertrophic cardiomyopathy, musculoskeletal abnormalities, short stature, and intellectual disability.[82]

Noonan syndrome can be recognized using clinical criteria, and although affected individuals have normal chromosomes, molecular genetic testing reveals a pathogenic variant in over 75% of cases.[81] Individuals with Noonan syndrome may have a pathogenic variant in the *PTPN11, SOS1, MAP2K1, RAF1, RIT1,* and *KRAS* genes.[81]

Prenatal sonographic signs associated with NS are nonspecific but are often related to lymphatic dysplasia. Affected individuals may have a thickened nuchal translucency, nuchal jugular lymphatic sacs, cystic hygromas, and/or pleural effusions. The prenatal lymphatic features do not predict adverse postnatal outcomses, although structural anomalies are associated with developmental delay and hematologic abnormalities.[83,84]

Other prenatal sonographic findings include hypertelorism, hemivertebrae, right-sided heart defects such as pulmonary stenosis, hypertrophic cardiomyopathy, hydrops, and polyhydramnios.[82,84,85] Prenatal sonography has been poor in detection of cardiac anomalies in fetuses with Noonan syndrome. A recent study of 50 patients with NS reported cardiac defects in 87%; however, less than 10% were identified prenatally.[84]

NS is the most common single-gene disorder in patients with an increased NT and normal karyotype. Approximately 7%–10% of fetuses with an increased NT and normal karyotype have NS identified by gene sequencing.[21] In the absence of abnormal karyotype, NS should be considered if prenatal ultrasound demonstrates an abnormality in lymphatic development such as cystic hygroma, thickened NT, ascites, or pleural effusions as well as those with congenital heart defects.

Beckwith-Wiedemann Syndrome

Beckwith-Wiedemann Syndrome (BWS) is an overgrowth syndrome in which the hallmark features include macroglossia and omphalocele, although there is wide clinical heterogeneity. The condition is associated with an increased risk of embryonal malignancy such as Wilms tumor.[86] BWS has an estimated incidence of 1 in 14,000 and usually occurs sporadically, although familial transmission occurs in 15% of cases.[86] There is an increased frequency in monozygotic twins,[86] and assisted reproductive technologies are associated with a 10-fold increased risk of BWS.[87]

The structural findings seen in some affected individuals with BWS are amenable to prenatal imaging. Sonographically, BWS has been associated with an increased nuchal translucency measurement and omphalocele.[77] Detection of omphalocele is excellent in the 11–14 weeks-window.[10] In a prenatal series of isolated omphalocele without other major structural anomalies or autosomal trisomy, 20% of fetuses were demonstrated to have

BWS[88] (Fig. 11.5). Placental mesenchymal dysplasia in which the placenta appears enlarged and hydropic with multiple cysts (similar to a molar appearance) has been associated with BWS.[89]

Macroglossia is a hallmark feature of BWS and can often be detected by prenatal sonography, although in some cases it may not be apparent until later in gestation or even after birth (Fig. 11.6). When present,

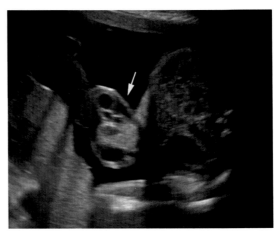

FIG. 11.5 Axial image through the umbilical cord insertion into the fetal abdomen demonstrating a bowel containing omphalocele (arrow) in a fetus with Beckwith-Wiedemann syndrome.

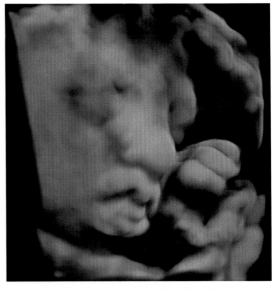

FIG. 11.6 3D surface rendering of the fetal face in the third trimester showing macroglossia, a finding may be seen in some fetuses with Beckwith Wiedemann syndrome.

macroglossia may lead to disordered swallowing and polyhydramnios.[90] The generalized overgrowth of the fetus results in a large abdominal circumference because of the combination of nephromegaly (large kidneys with normal architecture) and hepatomegaly, contributing to the diagnosis of macrosomia,[90] although the growth pattern may vary by molecular subtype.[87]

As with other conditions, the possibility of a syndromic etiology should be considered when a structural abnormality is detected. If an omphalocele is identified prenatally, a detailed anatomic scan should be performed to exclude other structural anomalies suggestive of an autosomal trisomy (cardiac defects, clenched hands, postaxial polydactyly). If the karyotype is normal or the omphalocele is seemingly isolated, the sonologist should consider BWS and carefully examine the fetal face for macroglossia and size of the internal organs for organomegaly.

BWS is caused by alterations in the imprinted genes on chromosome 11p15.5, which may be identified in 80% of affected individuals. A number of different mechanisms including loss or gain in methylation and paternal uniparental disomy have been reported.[86,87,91] Genetic testing may be performed by chorionic villus sampling or amniocentesis, although amniocentesis may be more reliable because of variation in methylation of chorionic villi.[92] Genetic testing approaches can include DNA methylation studies, chromosomal microarray, single-gene testing, copy number analysis for sequences within 11p15.5, karyotype, and use of multigene panels that include genes in the BWS critical region.

CHARGE Syndrome

CHARGE syndrome is an autosomal dominant condition characterized by multiple congenital malformations; this disorder is primarily reported in children and adults, and the phenotype in these individuals is not necessarily reflective of the antenatal presentation.[93] The prevalence of CHARGE is 1 in 8500 to 15,000 live births.[94] The majority of cases are de novo.

The acronym recognizes a cluster of findings that may be seen in affected individuals, including Coloboma of the eye, Heart defects, Choanal Atresia, Growth Restriction, Genital malformations, and Ear abnormalities. Other anomalies that have been described in association with CHARGE include orofacial clefts and trachea-esophageal malformations.[95] The condition is variably expressed so that not all affected individuals will have the same features, and the severity of findings also differs. Findings such as heart defects and genital malformations overlap with other syndromes.

Identifying a prenatal constellation of structural abnormalities leading to a presumptive diagnosis of CHARGE syndrome is challenging, underscoring the importance of a meticulous detailed ultrasound by a provider experienced in evaluating dysmorphic fetuses. A study of 40 fetuses (38 of whom terminated) with abnormal sonographic features and a CHD7 variant consistent with CHARGE sequence reflects the most severe end of the CHARGE spectrum.[93] Features that may be identified on prenatal ultrasound include major congenital cardiac abnormalities, abnormalities of the central nervous system, orofacial clefts, esophageal abnormalities, and abnormal genitalia. However, these anomalies are not specific to CHARGE. Microophthalmia raises the suspicion of CHARGE in a fetus with a nonspecific major congenital abnormality. The evaluation of the nose is of diagnostic importance, as the finding of abnormal nares raises the suspicion for choanal atresia, especially if associated with polyhydramnios.[93,95] Arhinencephaly, which is complete absence of the olfactory tract formation, and abnormalities of the semicircular canals should raise the suspicion of CHARGE. An abnormal shape to the external ear is a constant feature of CHARGE in the fetus. The external ear appearance can be evaluated with prenatal ultrasound imaging, utilizing color Doppler and 3D imaging.[93–96] Evaluation of the inner ear and olfactory sulcus using MRI in the prenatal diagnosis of CHARGE has been reported.[93]

CHARGE syndrome is caused by a mutation in the chromodomain helicase DNA-binding protein-7 (CHD7) gene on chromosome 8. Postnatal diagnosis of CHARGE syndrome is based on a combination of major and minor diagnostic criteria. Molecular testing for CHD7 will confirm the diagnosis in the majority of cases. The CHD7 variant is found in 90%–95% of affected individuals and mostly occurs de novo.[97] Some individuals with a CHARGE phenotype may have a 22q11.2 deletion or other cytogenetic abnormalities. In contrast, 10%–20% individuals with a clinical diagnosis will not have an identified abnormal gene sequence. Prenatal suspicion for CHARGE is made in the presence of multiple congenital anomalies that overlap with other syndromes. Prenatal diagnostic testing may include CVS or amniocentesis. Workup may include karyotype and microarray analysis that will help exclude other syndromes with overlapping features. If chromosomal microarray analysis is nondiagnostic, CHD7 gene sequencing is recommended. If gene sequencing is negative, deletion/duplication analysis can be performed. If the CHD7 analysis is nondiagnostic, whole-exome sequencing may be considered.[97]

Smith-Lemli-Opitz Syndrome

SLOS is an autosomal recessive disorder caused by a variant in the *DHCR7* gene, which encodes the enzyme 7-dehydrocholesterol reductase (7-DHC). Affected individuals have elevated serum 7-DHC levels and low levels of serum cholesterol. Many fetuses with SLOS die in utero resulting in a live birth incidence of 1 in 20,000 to 60,000.[98,99]

The disorder results in multiple structural malformations, although the phenotypic spectrum is broad. Affected individuals may have congenital heart defects, micrognathia and cleft palate, upturned nares, and ptosis. Other anomalies characteristic of SLOS include abnormalities of the extremities, such as postaxial polydactyly and syndactyly of second and third toes, as well as abnormal genitalia. Growth restriction, microcephaly, and developmental delay, which may range from mild to severe, are common in affected individuals.[99]

Sonographically, SLOS has been associated with an increased nuchal translucency measurement, although this is a nonspecific finding.[100] Prenatal anatomic imaging may detect cardiac abnormalities, most notably atrioventricular canal defects and septal defects. Additional abnormalities reported with SLOS include holoprosencephaly, agenesis of the corpus callosum and cerebellar hypoplasia, hypertelorism, and micrognathia. These major anomalies are not unique to SLOS but should prompt the sonologist to evaluate the genitals, looking for hypospadias or ambiguous genitalia. Correlation with known karyotype is useful in cases where the genitalia appears female. Evaluation of the distal extremities to detect postaxial polydactyly and 2–3 syndactyly of the toes may increase the suspicion of SLOS. Growth restriction has been reported to be present in 30% of affected fetuses between 20 and 22 weeks and in 70% between 30 and 34 weeks.[101] The combination of growth restriction and genital anomalies should prompt consideration of the diagnosis of SLOS. Microcephaly, although a common postnatal finding, may not be present at the time anatomic imaging is performed, and antenatal detection of microcephaly in SLOS has been poor.[101] Although affected fetuses may be noted to have some of the features noted above on prenatal ultrasound, it is also possible for an affected fetus to have a normal fetal ultrasound evaluation.

A low maternal serum unconjugated estriol concentration on second-trimester maternal serum screening for aneuploidy in a fetus should raise suspicion of SLOS in a fetus with a normal karyotype.[102] Steroid measurement in maternal urine may be useful in diagnosis of

SLOS.[103] In addition, amniotic fluid and chorionic villi contain high levels of 7-DHC in affected fetuses.[104] Mutation analysis from amniotic fluid or chorionic villi can be used for prenatal diagnosis if a proband in the family has previously been identified with a *DHCR7* gene mutation. For pregnancies with no family history of SLOS, where the diagnosis is suspected based on ultrasound findings, abnormal maternal serum screening, or both, measurement of 7-DHC levels in amniotic fluid or tissue obtained from CVS is an alternative to sequence analysis of the *DHCR7* gene.[105]

VACTERL

VACTERL sequence includes Vertebral, Anal atresia, Cardiac, Tracheoesophageal fistula with Esophageal atresia, Renal anomalies, and Limb defects (primarily radial ray). At least three features should be present to consider this diagnosis as well as the absence of other conditions.[16,106] In 90% of cases, VACTERL is sporadic although there is a small subset of patients with a first-degree relative with similar anomalies, suggesting that there may be an inherited component.[107] VACTERL occurs in approximately 1 in 10,000 to 1:40,000 live births.[16,106]

VACTERL may be suspected on prenatal sonography, although some clinical features are difficult to identify on routine prenatal ultrasound. In a registry-based study of 19 cases of VACTERL, approximately 50% were identified by prenatal sonography and cases detected prenatally had more malformations than those diagnosed postnatally[16] (Fig. 11.7A and B). Renal, limb, and vertebral anomalies are the most amenable to prenatal diagnosis. Renal anomalies associated with VACTERL include renal agenesis (unilateral or bilateral), cystic or dysplastic kidneys as well as renal fusion abnormalities.[106] Major limb anomalies are also amenable to prenatal detection; however, an astute sonologist must be aware to look for more subtle abnormalities such as isolated thumb anomalies.

Vertebral anomalies can be subtle; although evaluation of the fetal spine is part of a routine anatomic evaluation, only two-thirds of cases of hemivertebrae are detected prenatally.[108,109] Other vertebral anomalies may be even more elusive.

Cardiac findings in VACTERL may be subtle and include vascular anomalies such as right-sided aortic arch and anomalous venous structures, which require more detailed imaging of the fetal cardiac anatomy. Tracheoesophageal fistula with esophageal atresia may be suspected on antenatal ultrasound by the combination of polyhydramnios and a small or absent stomach bubble. Anal atresia is also potentially

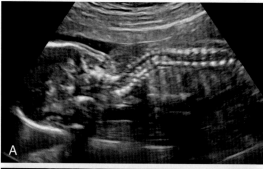

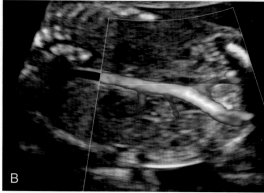

FIG. 11.7 **(A)** Modified coronal view through the fetal spine demonstrating hemivertebra and scoliosis. **(B)** This fetus also had unilateral renal agenesis and corresponding absent renal artery demonstrated by Doppler color flow. These findings are seen in some fetuses with VACTERL syndrome.

diagnosable by dilated loops of bowel or intensely echogenic foci in the bowel lumen that may result from the combination of meconium and urine in a fistula between the gastrointestinal and genitourinary tracts.[110,111] A single umbilical artery not only is often a normal variant in prenatal imaging but has also been associated with VACTERL.

The diagnosis of VACTERL is based on the presence of at least three associated malformations (although there is controversy among experts as to the relative emphasis that should be placed on certain features). The differential diagnosis is broad, as many of the individual features overlap with numerous other syndromes including trisomy 18 and CHARGE sequence.

The diagnosis of VACTERL is made by clinical examination. Many features overlap with other conditions amenable to prenatal genetic testing, and these should be excluded. CVS and/or amniocentesis should be offered with chromosomal microarray analysis in cases with fetal structural abnormalities.

WHAT IS THE ROLE OF ADJUNCTIVE IMAGING IN PRENATAL EVALUATION OF FETAL ANOMALIES?

MRI

Ultrasound remains the primary screening modality for fetal anomalies. Fetal magnetic resonance imaging (MRI) is an important adjunct to imaging some fetal anomalies, as it confers the benefit of increased soft-tissue contrast resolution. The American College of Radiology (ACR) and the Society for Pediatric Radiology (SPR) recommend MRI in the setting of uncertain or incompletely evaluated anomalies and to assist in counseling, guiding treatment, and delivery planning.[112]

MRI is indicated in cases of suspected brain and spine anomalies, vascular abnormalities of the brain, and congenital abnormalities of the spine.[112] In the MERIDIAN trial, the use of fetal MRI improved the diagnostic accuracy of brain anomalies by 23%–29% depending on gestational age and provided additional diagnostic information in 49% of cases.[113] A recent metaanalysis of fetal MRI use for brain anomalies found that fetal MRI correctly diagnosed 91% of brain anomalies, which resulted in a 16% increase in correct diagnosis above ultrasound alone.[114] MRI may be useful in cases of thoracic pathology, specifically congenital lung malformations, congenital diaphragmatic hernia, and volumetric assessment of fetal lung parenchyma. MRI may be utilized in cases of face and neck masses to better assess airway obstruction and delivery planning. Additionally, MRI may be helpful when an abnormality is diagnosed that may benefit from fetal surgery to confirm the diagnosis, plan the operative approach, and rule out additional pathology.[112] MRI is widely viewed as safe in pregnancy, and to date, there are no known harmful effects to the developing fetus.[112]

Fetal Echocardiography

Fetal echocardiography is an adjunctive diagnostic tool in the evaluation of fetal anomalies. Congenital heart disease affects 6–12 in 1000 live births and accounts for 42% of infant deaths.[115] Many noncardiac structural abnormalities have associated cardiac anomalies. Adequate identification and characterization of fetal heart anomalies before delivery is crucial to allow for the opportunity of prenatal genetic testing, delivery planning, and timing of postnatal interventions.[116]

Fetal echocardiography differs from routine cardiac evaluation during the routine fetal anatomic survey and has been shown in systematic reviews to be more sensitive and specific at identifying cardiac anomalies than routine anatomic survey evaluation.[116,117] The routine evaluation of the heart relies on standard views of the four chambers and the right and left outflow tracts.[12] Detailed obstetrical imaging includes the four-chamber view and outflow tracts as well as an evaluation of the three vessels and trachea views, aortic arch, and superior and inferior vena cava.[13] Fetal echocardiography involves the sequential analysis of atria, ventricles, and great arteries as well as an evaluation of the venous system. The evaluation of cardiac rhythm, structure, and function is integral to the evaluation of cardiac anomalies.[78] The added benefit of a fetal echocardiogram after a *normal* detailed evaluation by a maternal-fetal medicine expert is low.[118] However, echocardiography is helpful to better delineate a suspected heart defect and allow assessment of the prognosis.

WHAT ABNORMALITIES ARE SPECIFIC TO TWINS?

The number of twin gestations has increased over the past several decades, largely because of advanced reproductive technologies and older maternal age at conception.[119] In 2009, 1 of every 30 infants born was a twin.[120] The majority of this increase is attributable to dizygotic twinning.

The prevalence of nonchromosomal congenital anomalies is increased in twins compared with singletons.[121] Overall, 3.5% of twins have an abnormality compared with 2.7% of singletons. The increased risk is most notable in monochorionic twins where there is a twofold increase in prevalence compared with singletons.[122] Recently, it has been reported that the rates of chromosomal anomalies appear to be less in twins than singletons.[121,123,124]

In twin gestations with a nonchromosomal abnormality, only one twin is affected in 88% of cases. In those twins where both twins have an anomaly, only 10%–20% have the same malformation.[121] Additionally, there are some anomalies that are intrinsic to monozygotic twinning such as conjoined twins, changes that may occur after demise of one twin, and twin reversed arterial perfusion (TRAP) sequence.

It is critical to accurately assess chorionicity and amnionicity in twin gestations, as these findings have major implications for genetic risk. Ultrasound determination of amnionicity and chorionicity is optimal in the first trimester and decreases in accuracy with advancing gestational age.[125] Therefore, all multiples should have determination of amnionicity and chorionicity by an experienced provider at the time of their first imaging study. Chorionicity and amnionicity characteristics are critical to the management of twin gestations and is accurate in 96.7% of twins overall (100% in the first trimester) when evaluated at a tertiary care center compared with 46.1% from a referring facility.[126]

Prenatal diagnosis of anomalies is more challenging in twins. In a recent systematic review of first-trimester ultrasound detection of congenital anomalies, 27.3% of anomalies were identified in twins compared with a detection rate of approximately 50% in singletons.[10,127] The second-trimester detection rate may also be lower, although this is not consistently reported, with many specialist centers reporting sensitivities of 88% and specificity of 100% for detection of an anomaly in twins.[121,128,129]

The most common congenital anomalies in twins are congenital heart defects, central nervous system abnormalities, genitourinary anomalies, and musculoskeletal abnormalities.[122] Congenital heart defects are more common in twins (2.5%) than in singletons (0.7%) and are substantially higher in monochorionic twins (4%). Monochorionic twins have an almost fourfold increased risk of severe CHD compared with singletons, and therefore screening for CHD is warranted.[130] Monochorionic twins are uniquely at increased risk for other obstetrical complications such as twin to twin transfusion syndrome and intrauterine demise of one twin.

Monozygotic twins are presumed to be genetically identical, although this is not always the case. Numerous discordances for chromosomal abnormalities, single-gene disorders, mitochondrial diseases, and genetic imprinting abnormalities have been reported.[131] The perinatal outcome of a twin gestation in which one twin has a congenital anomaly has been controversial. Some studies report an increased risk of prematurity and fetal growth restriction, whereas others do not show an increased risk.[121,132,133]

In patients who request selective termination after detection of an abnormality in one twin, determination of amnionicity and chorionicity is critical in determining which procedure is most appropriate.[134] Dichorionic twins have separate placentation, and selective reduction may be performed by intracardiac injection of potassium chloride. Monochorionic twins have vascular connections between their placentas, and a variety of occlusive techniques have been described.

WHAT IS THE APPROPRIATE EVALUATION FOR A FETUS WITH A SUSPECTED STRUCTURAL ANOMALY?

Once a structural anomaly has been identified and characterized by detailed prenatal sonography and if warranted, MRI and/or fetal echocardiography, a multispecialty provider team should be assembled. The first step is counseling by a genetic counselor or physician with expertise in the complexities of prenatal genetic testing. It is important to obtain a thorough genetic/family history which may provide relevant information that may help to establish a diagnosis.

Providers should provide nondirective pre- and posttest counseling and recognize the importance of patient values and preferences (see Chapter 3).[135] The field of prenatal diagnosis is rapidly evolving with new modalities and genetic tests increasingly available to establish or refine a genetic diagnosis. Before selecting a testing strategy, pretest counseling should identify the risks, benefits, and limitations of each testing strategy. Obtaining this additional genetic information also comes with ethical issues pertaining to disclosure to patients. Reporting "abnormal" genetic information that is of uncertain clinical significance may have profound consequences to parental decision-making as to whether to continue a pregnancy, or in the attachment to a child who may be labeled as having a genetic disease that may in fact be a normal variant.[136-138]

Patients with a fetal structural abnormality should be offered diagnostic testing including chromosomal microarray. In twin gestations, testing of each fetus is generally performed (see Chapter 14) although many patients with a monochorionic gestation elect to only test one fetus.

The most commonly used diagnostic modalities are chorionic villus sampling (CVS), which can be performed between 10 and 13 weeks of gestation, and amniocentesis, which can be performed after 15 weeks of gestation. The fetal loss rate for both procedures is between 1 in 300 and 1 in 1000.[137] Following such diagnostic procedures, karyotype, fluorescent in situ hybridization (FISH), chromosomal microarray (see Chapter 12), and gene sequencing (see Chapter 13) can be performed.

Once a diagnostic test result becomes available, patients should be given the opportunity to discuss the results with a genetic counselor and/or a geneticist, and a multidisciplinary team should be convened to discuss the implications of the structural abnormalities. The members of the team depend on the nature of the diagnosis suspected but generally should consist of the genetic testing specialist, an obstetrician and/or maternal fetal medicine specialist, social work and/or psychologist, and pediatrician or pediatric surgery subspecialist as appropriate, as well as faith-based support in an interested patient. Multiple studies have shown increased patient satisfaction and decreased anxiety after counseling by large multidisciplinary teams.[139-141] The discussion should focus on the significance of the findings and underlying genetic etiology for the health of the fetus, range of possible postnatal outcomes, and anticipated prognosis. Not all genetic conditions will be identified, despite a comprehensive assessment, and some evaluations will uncover information of uncertain significance or of significance to the extended family.

Karyotype and Fluorescent In Situ Hybridization

Karyotype abnormalities are seen in up to 50% of fetuses with some structural malformation(s) and is the standard to evaluate chromosomal abnormalities.[142,143] A G-banded karyotype has a resolution of 5–10 Mb. If an abnormal sonographic examination is suspicious for a major trisomy, for example, a fetus with alobar holoprosencephaly, midline facial cleft, and postaxial polydactyly in whom trisomy 13 is the leading suspected diagnosis, diagnostic testing can begin with a karyotype that may or may not include FISH. FISH can be used on uncultured cells and can be used for rapid and accurate detection of chromosome 21, 13, 18, X, and Y abnormalities, with results in 24–28 hours. If the FISH result is normal, the laboratory should be instructed to perform a chromosomal microarray instead of a karyotype. Limitations of FISH are that it cannot determine whether a translocation is present, and normal FISH results should always be confirmed by G-banded karyotype so as not to miss other aneuploidies. Karyotype requires cultured cells and typically takes between 10 and 12 days to complete. If a karyotype evaluation is normal, chromosomal microarray should be performed in cases with structural abnormalities.

Chromosomal Microarray Analysis

Chromosomal microarray analysis (CMA) detects small gains and losses of genetic material at a higher resolution of genetic information (10–100 kb) than traditional karyotype. CMA is recommended as the first-line diagnostic test in fetuses with a structural abnormality and should be offered to any patient (regardless of the presence of a fetal anomaly) who is undergoing diagnostic testing.[137,138]

Several studies have evaluated the use of CMA after normal karyotype results and found that CMA adds significant diagnostic value.[144,145] Donnelly evaluated 1082 pregnancies with known anomalies and found that 8% of patients with normal karyotypes had clinically significant copy number variants (CNVs) that would have been undetected by karyotype alone.[146] De Wit performed a metaanalysis and reported that in a fetus with identified anomalies but a normal karyotype, CMA detected a clinically significant CNV or diagnosis in 3%–8% of cases with a single identified anomaly and in 10% of cases with two or more anomalies.[147]

Limitations of CMA include limited detection of low-level tissue mosaicism, and an inability to detect balanced chromosome rearrangements and some triploidies, although the use of SNP-based arrays improves detection of these conditions.[144] Additionally, because of the high resolution of genetic data generated by CMA, some tests yield variants of uncertain significance (VUS), which are not associated with a known clinical diagnosis or syndrome. This information proves to be very difficult for providers and patients alike because of the lack of understanding of clinical significance, prognosis, and penetrance, underscoring the importance of pretest genetic counseling.[148]

Benefits of CMA include that it can be performed on tissue that is no longer viable, so it is useful in cases of fetal demise and a rapid turnaround time of 5–7 days (see Chapter 12).

Targeted Gene Sequencing

In fetuses in whom sonographic findings may be associated with a specific gene or one of a limited number of genes, targeted gene testing may be available. The availability of tests and their sensitivity for the detection of the condition being sought will vary and requires expert pre-test and post-test counseling by medical providers specializing in genetic testing.

Targeted gene testing may be prompted by sonographic findings such as an increased nuchal translucency in a fetus with a normal microarray, suggesting Noonan syndrome or with a suspected skeletal dysplasia for which there are specialized gene panels.[21]

Whole-Exome Sequencing

Exomes are regions of the genome that are known to encode proteins and include approximately 1%–2% of the genome but are thought to contain approximately

85% of disease-causing variants. WES may be useful in detecting genetic disorders when karyotype and microarray have been unrevealing. Pangalos et al. evaluated 14 euploid fetuses with major anomalies and found that WES identified a genetic diagnosis in 43% of cases.[149] Despite promising results, at the time of this publication, ACOG and SMFM do not recommend routine use of WES because of paucity of data on use in prenatal diagnosis.[137,150]

Determining the underlying genetic etiology for structural abnormalities, if one exists, can give patients and providers valuable information about prognosis, care planning, and recurrence risk. However, despite the importance of diagnosis, only a minority of children with congenital and developmental disorders have a formal genetic diagnosis[151] (see Chapter 13).

Cell-Free DNA

For patients who decline genetic diagnostic testing, additional screening tests can be performed to refine risk, although it is crucial that the patient understands that a negative screening test does not rule out genetic pathology.

Cell-free DNA (cfDNA) is a noninvasive screening test that evaluates cell-free DNA in maternal blood to assess risk of aneuploidy. It has been used increasingly in prenatal genetic screening for major autosomal trisomies.[152]

Multiple studies have shown a gap in genetic diagnosis when cfDNA is performed compared with the yield of diagnostic testing (karyotype, CMA), in cases when a fetus has been identified as having an anomaly on ultrasound. Benachi et al. performed both cfDNA and karyotype on 900 high-risk patients and determined that cfDNA alone missed 8% of cases of aneuploidy, triploidy, or sex chromosome pathology.[153] Other studies have estimated that in cases of congenital anomalies, cfDNA misses up to 10% of chromosome abnormalities, in addition to the residual risk of genetic disease detectable only by CMA (copy number variants)[154,155] (see Chapter 9).

Regardless of choices for prenatal testing, patients should have consultation with a multidisciplinary specialty team to discuss the clinical implications of the anatomic and genetic findings. A plan for pregnancy management made should include options for pregnancy termination, prenatal monitoring during the gestation, as well as timing and location of delivery. Referral to support groups or perinatal palliative care should also be available.[156]

CONCLUSION

When a structural abnormality is identified by prenatal sonography, a detailed evaluation of the fetus is critical with meticulous attention to pattern recognition, which will help refine a differential diagnosis. If clinically relevant, additional evaluation of the fetus with MRI and fetal echocardiography may be contributory for optimal prenatal consultation and pregnancy planning. Once fetal imaging has characterized the features identified, genetic counseling by a provider experienced in this field is critical to discuss options for diagnostic testing. Assembling a team of multidisciplinary providers who are experts in prenatal diagnosis and postnatal management of the condition is warranted. Patients should have as much information as possible to make decisions about their pregnancy management options and postnatal expectations and care.

REFERENCES

1. St Louis AM, Kim K, Browne ML, et al. Prevalence trends of selected major birth defects: a multi-state population-based retrospective study, United States, 1999 to 2007. *Birth Defects Res.* 2017;109(18):1442–1450.
2. Boyle B, Addor MC, Arriola L, et al. Estimating Global Burden of Disease due to congenital anomaly: an analysis of European data. *Arch Dis Child Fetal Neonatal Ed.* 2018;103(1):F22–F28.
3. Parker SE, Mai CT, Canfield MA, et al. Updated National Birth Prevalence estimates for selected birth defects in the United States, 2004–2006. *Birth Defects Res A Clin Mol Teratol.* 2010;88(12):1008–1016.
4. Practice bulletin No. 175: ultrasound in pregnancy. *Obstet Gynecol.* 2016;128(6):e241–e256.
5. Siddique J, Lauderdale DS, VanderWeele TJ, Lantos JD. Trends in prenatal ultrasound use in the United States: 1995 to 2006. *Med Care.* 2009;47(11):1129–1135.
6. O'Keeffe DF, Abuhamad A. Obstetric ultrasound utilization in the United States: data from various health plans. *Semin Perinatol.* 2013;37(5):292–294.
7. Whitworth M, Bricker L, Mullan C. Ultrasound for fetal assessment in early pregnancy. *Cochrane Database Syst Rev.* 2015;(7):CD007058.
8. Dashe JS, McIntire DD, Twickler DM. Effect of maternal obesity on the ultrasound detection of anomalous fetuses. *Obstet Gynecol.* 2009;113(5):1001–1007.
9. Pasko DN, Wood SL, Jenkins SM, Owen J, Harper LM. Completion and sensitivity of the second-trimester fetal anatomic survey in obese gravidas. *J Ultrasound Med.* 2016;35(11):2449–2457.
10. Rossi AC, Prefumo F. Accuracy of ultrasonography at 11–14 weeks of gestation for detection of fetal structural anomalies: a systematic review. *Obstet Gynecol.* 2013;122(6):1160–1167.
11. Struksnaes C, Blaas HG, Eik-Nes SH, Vogt C. Correlation between prenatal ultrasound and postmortem findings in 1029 fetuses following termination of pregnancy. *Ultrasound Obstet Gynecol.* 2016;48(2):232–238.
12. American Institute of Ultrasound in M. AIUM practice guideline for the performance of obstetric ultrasound examinations. *J Ultrasound Med.* 2013;32(6):1083–1101.
13. Wax J, Minkoff H, Johnson A, et al. Consensus report on the detailed fetal anatomic ultrasound examination: indications, components, and qualifications. *J Ultrasound Med.* 2014;33(2):189–195.
14. Lemyre E, Infante-Rivard C, Dallaire L. Prevalence of congenital anomalies at birth among offspring of women at risk for a genetic disorder and with a normal second-trimester ultrasound. *Teratology.* 1999;60(4):240–244.
15. Boyd PA, Rounding C, Chamberlain P, Wellesley D, Kurinczuk JJ. The evolution of prenatal screening and diagnosis and its impact on an unselected population over an 18-year period. *BJOG.* 2012;119(9):1131–1140.
16. Debost-Legrand A, Goumy C, Laurichesse-Delmas H, et al. Prenatal diagnosis of the VACTERL association using routine ultrasound examination. *Birth Defects Res A Clin Mol Teratol.* 2015;103(10):880–886.
17. Volpe P, De Robertis V, Campobasso G, Tempesta A, Volpe G, Rembouskos G. Diagnosis of congenital heart disease by early and second-trimester fetal echocardiography. *J Ultrasound Med.* 2012;31(4):563–568.
18. Baffero GM, Crovetto F, Fabietti I, et al. Prenatal ultrasound predictors of postnatal major cerebral abnormalities in fetuses with apparently isolated mild ventriculomegaly. *Prenat Diagn.* 2015;35(8):783–788.
19. Santorum M, Wright D, Syngelaki A, Karagioti N, Nicolaides KH. Accuracy of first-trimester combined test in screening for trisomies 21, 18 and 13. *Ultrasound Obstet Gynecol.* 2017;49(6):714–720.
20. Souka AP, Pilalis A, Kavalakis I, et al. Screening for major structural abnormalities at the 11- to 14-week ultrasound scan. *Am J Obstet Gynecol.* 2006;194(2):393–396.
21. Ali MM, Chasen ST, Norton ME. Testing for Noonan syndrome after increased nuchal translucency. *Prenat Diagn.* 2017;37(8):750–753.
22. Grande M, Jansen FA, Blumenfeld YJ, et al. Genomic microarray in fetuses with increased nuchal translucency and normal karyotype: a systematic review and meta-analysis. *Ultrasound Obstet Gynecol.* 2015;46(6):650–658.
23. Salomon LJ, Alfirevic Z, Bilardo CM, et al. ISUOG practice guidelines: performance of first-trimester fetal ultrasound scan. *Ultrasound Obstet Gynecol.* 2013;41(1):102–113.
24. Timor-Tritsch IE, Bashiri A, Monteagudo A, Arslan AA. Qualified and trained sonographers in the US can perform early fetal anatomy scans between 11 and 14 weeks. *Am J Obstet Gynecol.* 2004;191(4):1247–1252.
25. Bromley B, Shipp TD, Lyons J, Navathe RS, Groszmann Y, Benacerraf BR. Detection of fetal structural anomalies in a basic first-trimester screening program for aneuploidy. *J Ultrasound Med.* 2014;33(10):1737–1745.

26. Reddy UM, Abuhamad AZ, Levine D, Saade GR. Fetal imaging workshop invited P. Fetal imaging: executive summary of a joint eunice Kennedy Shriver National Institute of child health and Human development, society for maternal-fetal medicine, American Institute of ultrasound in medicine, American College of obstetricians and Gynecologists, American College of Radiology, society for pediatric Radiology, and society of radiologists in ultrasound fetal imaging workshop. *Am J Obstet Gynecol.* 2014;210(5):387–397.

27. Becker R, Wegner RD. Detailed screening for fetal anomalies and cardiac defects at the 11–13-week scan. *Ultrasound Obstet Gynecol.* 2006;27(6):613–618.

28. Syngelaki A, Chelemen T, Dagklis T, Allan L, Nicolaides KH. Challenges in the diagnosis of fetal non-chromosomal abnormalities at 11–13 weeks. *Prenat Diagn.* 2011;31(1):90–102.

29. Borrell A, Robinson JN, Santolaya-Forgas J. Clinical value of the 11- to 13+6-week sonogram for detection of congenital malformations: a review. *Am J Perinatol.* 2011;28(2):117–124.

30. Grande M, Arigita M, Borobio V, Jimenez JM, Fernandez S, Borrell A. First-trimester detection of structural abnormalities and the role of aneuploidy markers. *Ultrasound Obstet Gynecol.* 2012;39(2):157–163.

31. Karim JN, Roberts NW, Salomon LJ, Papageorghiou AT. Systematic review of first-trimester ultrasound screening for detection of fetal structural anomalies and factors that affect screening performance. *Ultrasound Obstet Gynecol.* 2017;50(4):429–441.

32. Liao YM, Li SL, Luo GY, et al. Routine screening for fetal limb abnormalities in the first trimester. *Prenat Diagn.* 2016;36(2):117–126.

33. Chaoui R, Benoit B, Mitkowska-Wozniak H, Heling KS, Nicolaides KH. Assessment of intracranial translucency (IT) in the detection of spina bifida at the 11-13-week scan. *Ultrasound Obstet Gynecol.* 2009;34(3):249–252.

34. Chaoui R, Orosz G, Heling KS, Sarut-Lopez A, Nicolaides KH. Maxillary gap at 11–13 weeks' gestation: marker of cleft lip and palate. *Ultrasound Obstet Gynecol.* 2015;46(6):665–669.

35. Chasen ST, Kalish RB. Can early ultrasound reduce the gestational age at abortion for fetal anomalies? *Contraception.* 2013;87(1):63–66.

36. Health NCCfWsaCs. *Antenatal care: routine care for the healthy pregnant woman;* 2008.

37. Grandjean H, Larroque D, Levi S. The performance of routine ultrasonographic screening of pregnancies in the Eurofetus Study. *Am J Obstet Gynecol.* 1999;181(2):446–454.

38. Pilalis A, Basagiannis C, Eleftheriades M, et al. Evaluation of a two-step ultrasound examination protocol for the detection of major fetal structural defects. *J Matern Fetal Neonatal Med.* 2012;25(9):1814–1817.

39. Becker R, Schmitz L, Kilavuz S, Stumm M, Wegner RD, Bittner U. 'Normal' nuchal translucency: a justification to refrain from detailed scan? Analysis of 6858 cases with special reference to ethical aspects. *Prenat Diagn.* 2012;32(6):550–556.

40. Manegold G, Tercanli S, Struben H, Huang D, Kang A. Is a routine ultrasound in the third trimester justified? Additional fetal anomalies diagnosed after two previous unremarkable ultrasound examinations. *Ultraschall der Med.* 2011;32(4):381–386.

41. Hildebrand E, Selbing A, Blomberg M. Comparison of first and second trimester ultrasound screening for fetal anomalies in the southeast region of Sweden. *Acta Obstet Gynecol Scand.* 2010;89(11):1412–1419.

42. Benacerraf BB. The Sherlock Holmes approach to diagnosing fetal syndromes by ultrasound. *Clin Obstet Gynecol.* 2012;55(1):226–248.

43. Miller L. Sherlock Holmes' methods of deductive reasoning applied to medical diagnostics. *West J Med.* 1985;142(3):413–414.

44. Offerdal K, Jebens N, Syvertsen T, Blaas HG, Johansen OJ, Eik-Nes SH. Prenatal ultrasound detection of facial clefts: a prospective study of 49,314 deliveries in a non-selected population in Norway. *Ultrasound Obstet Gynecol.* 2008;31(6):639–646.

45. Fleurke-Rozema JH, van de Kamp K, Bakker MK, Pajkrt E, Bilardo CM, Snijders RJ. Prevalence, diagnosis and outcome of cleft lip with or without cleft palate in The Netherlands. *Ultrasound Obstet Gynecol.* 2016;48(4):458–463.

46. Gillham JC, Anand S, Bullen PJ. Antenatal detection of cleft lip with or without cleft palate: incidence of associated chromosomal and structural anomalies. *Ultrasound Obstet Gynecol.* 2009;34(4):410–415.

47. Group IW. Prevalence at birth of cleft lip with or without cleft palate: data from the international perinatal database of typical oral clefts (IPDTOC). *Cleft Palate Craniofac J.* 2011;48(1):66–81.

48. Benacerraf BB. Ultrasound of fetal syndromes. In: Benacerraf BB, ed. *Ultrasound of Fetal Syndromes.* Philadelphia: Elsevier Health Sciences; 2008.

49. Benacerraf BR. Prenatal sonographic diagnosis of short rib-polydactyly syndrome type II, Majewski type. *J Ultrasound Med.* 1993;12(9):552–555.

50. Mai CT, Kucik JE, Isenburg J, et al. Selected birth defects data from population-based birth defects surveillance programs in the United States, 2006 to 2010: featuring trisomy conditions. *Birth Defects Res A Clin Mol Teratol.* 2013;97(11):709–725.

51. Bromley B, Lieberman E, Shipp TD, Benacerraf BR. The genetic sonogram: a method of risk assessment for Down syndrome in the second trimester. *J Ultrasound Med.* 2002;21(10):1087–1096.

52. Aagaard-Tillery KM, Malone FD, Nyberg DA, et al. Role of second-trimester genetic sonography after Down syndrome screening. *Obstet Gynecol.* 2009;114(6):1189–1196.

53. Agathokleous M, Chaveeva P, Poon LC, Kosinski P, Nicolaides KH. Meta-analysis of second-trimester markers for trisomy 21. *Ultrasound Obstet Gynecol.* 2013;41(3):247–261.

54. Devore GR. Genetic sonography: the historical and clinical role of fetal echocardiography. *Ultrasound Obstet Gynecol.* 2010;35(5):509–521.

55. Morlando M, Bhide A, Familiari A, et al. The association between prenatal atrioventricular septal defects and chromosomal abnormalities. *Eur J Obstet Gynecol Reprod Biol.* 2017;208:31–35.

56. Bromley B, Benacerraf BB. Chromosomal abnormalities. In: Rumack CM, Levine D, eds. *Diagnostic Ultrasound.* 5th ed. Philadelphia: Elsevier Health Sciences; 2018.

57. Watson WJ, Miller RC, Wax JR, Hansen WF, Yamamura Y, Polzin WJ. Sonographic findings of trisomy 18 in the second trimester of pregnancy. *J Ultrasound Med.* 2008;27(7):1033–1038.

58. Yeo L, Guzman ER, Day-Salvatore D, Walters C, Chavez D, Vintzileos AM. Prenatal detection of fetal trisomy 18 through abnormal sonographic features. *J Ultrasound Med.* 2003;22(6):581–590.

59. Bronsteen R, Lee W, Vettraino IM, Huang R, Comstock CH. Second-trimester sonography and trisomy 18: the significance of isolated choroid plexus cysts after an examination that includes the fetal hands. *J Ultrasound Med.* 2004;23(2):241–245.

60. Carlson DE, Platt LD, Medearis AL. The ultrasound triad of fetal Hydramnios, abnormal hand posturing, and any other anomaly predicts autosomal trisomy. *Obstet Gynecol.* 1992;79(5):731–734.

61. Morris JK, Savva GM. The risk of fetal loss following a prenatal diagnosis of trisomy 13 or trisomy 18. *Am J Med Genet A.* 2008;146A(7):827–832.

62. Tonks AM, Gornall AS, Larkins SA, Gardosi JO. Trisomies 18 and 13: trends in prevalence and prenatal diagnosis - population based study. *Prenat Diagn.* 2013;33(8):742–750.

63. Meyer RE, Liu G, Gilboa SM, et al. Survival of children with trisomy 13 and trisomy 18: a multi-state population-based study. *Am J Med Genet A.* 2016;170A(4):825–837.

64. Papp C, Beke A, Ban Z, Szigeti Z, Toth-Pal E, Papp Z. Prenatal diagnosis of trisomy 13: analysis of 28 cases. *J Ultrasound Med.* 2006;25(4):429–435.

65. Papp C, Beke A, Mezei G, Szigeti Z, Ban Z, Papp Z. Prenatal diagnosis of Turner syndrome: report on 69 cases. *J Ultrasound Med.* 2006;25(6):711–717.

66. McBride KL, Zender GA, Fitzgerald-Butt SM, et al. Linkage analysis of left ventricular outflow tract malformations (aortic valve stenosis, coarctation of the aorta, and hypoplastic left heart syndrome). *Eur J Hum Genet: EJHG.* 2009;17(6):811–819.

67. Carvalho AB, Guerra Junior G, Baptista MT, de Faria AP, Marini SH, Guerra AT. Cardiovascular and renal anomalies in Turner syndrome. *Rev Assoc Med Bras.* 2010;56(6):655–659.

68. Baena N, De Vigan C, Cariati E, et al. Turner syndrome: evaluation of prenatal diagnosis in 19 European registries. *Am J Med Genet A.* 2004;129A(1):16–20.

69. McWeeney DT, Munne S, Miller RC, et al. Pregnancy complicated by triploidy: a comparison of the three karyotypes. *Am J Perinatol.* 2009;26(9):641–645.

70. Massalska D, Bijok J, Ilnicka A, Jakiel G, Roszkowski T. Triploidy - variability of sonographic phenotypes. *Prenat Diagn.* 2017;37(8):774–780.

71. Jauniaux E, Brown R, Rodeck C, Nicolaides KH. Prenatal diagnosis of triploidy during the second trimester of pregnancy. *Obstet Gynecol.* 1996;88(6):983–989.

72. Toufaily MH, Roberts DJ, Westgate MN, Holmes LB. Triploidy: variation of phenotype. *Am J Clin Pathol.* 2016;145(1):86–95.

73. Lakovschek IC, Streubel B, Ulm B. Natural outcome of trisomy 13, trisomy 18, and triploidy after prenatal diagnosis. *Am J Med Genet A.* 2011;155A(11):2626–2633.

74. Besseau-Ayasse J, Violle-Poirsier C, Bazin A, et al. A French collaborative survey of 272 fetuses with 22q11.2 deletion: ultrasound findings, fetal autopsies and pregnancy outcomes. *Prenat Diagn.* 2014;34(5):424–430.

75. Bassett AS, Lowther C, Merico D, et al. Rare genome-wide copy number variation and expression of schizophrenia in 22q11.2 deletion syndrome. *Am J Psychiat.* 2017;174(11):1054–1063.

76. Arinami T. Analyses of the associations between the genes of 22q11 deletion syndrome and schizophrenia. *J Hum Genet.* 2006;51(12):1037–1045.

77. Souka AP, Von Kaisenberg CS, Hyett JA, Sonek JD, Nicolaides KH. Increased nuchal translucency with normal karyotype. *Am J Obstet Gynecol.* 2005;192(4):1005–1021.

78. American Institute of Ultrasound in M. AIUM practice guideline for the performance of fetal echocardiography. *J Ultrasound Med.* 2013;32(6):1067–1082.

79. Chaoui R, Heling KS, Lopez AS, Thiel G, Karl K. The thymic-thoracic ratio in fetal heart defects: a simple way to identify fetuses at high risk for microdeletion 22q11. *Ultrasound Obstet Gynecol.* 2011;37(4):397–403.

80. Dugoff L, Mennuti MT, McDonald-McGinn DM. The benefits and limitations of cell-free DNA screening for 22q11.2 deletion syndrome. *Prenat Diagn.* 2017;37(1):53–60.

81. Tartaglia M, Gelb BD, Zenker M. Noonan syndrome and clinically related disorders. *Best Practice & Research Clinical Endocrinology & Metabolism.* 2011;25(1):161–179.

82. Croonen EA, Nillesen W, Schrander C, et al. Noonan syndrome: comparing mutation-positive with mutation-negative Dutch patients. *Mol Syndromol.* 2013;4(5):227–234.

83. Gaudineau A, Doray B, Schaefer E, et al. Postnatal phenotype according to prenatal ultrasound features of Noonan syndrome: a retrospective study of 28 cases. *Prenat Diagn.* 2013;33(3):238–241.

84. Baldassarre G, Mussa A, Silengo M, Ferrero GB. Comment on "prenatal diagnosis and prognosis in Noonan syndrome". *Prenat Diagn.* 2013;33(13):1318–1320.

85. de Mooij YM, van den Akker NM, Bekker MN, Bartelings MM, van Vugt JM, Gittenberger-de Groot AC. Aberrant lymphatic development in euploid fetuses with

increased nuchal translucency including Noonan syndrome. *Prenat Diagn.* 2011;31(2):159–166.

86. Weksberg R, Shuman C, Beckwith JB. Beckwith-Wiedemann syndrome. *Eur J Hum Genet.* 2010;18(1):8–14.

87. Mussa A, Molinatto C, Cerrato F, et al. Assisted reproductive techniques and risk of beckwith-wiedemann syndrome. *Pediatrics.* 2017;140(1).

88. Wilkins-Haug L, Porter A, Hawley P, Benson CB. Isolated fetal omphalocele, Beckwith-Wiedemann syndrome, and assisted reproductive technologies. *Birth Defects Res A Clin Mol Teratol.* 2009;85(1):58–62.

89. H'Mida D, Gribaa M, Yacoubi T, et al. Placental mesenchymal dysplasia with beckwith-wiedemann syndrome fetus in the context of biparental and androgenic cell lines. *Placenta.* 2008;29(5):454–460.

90. Williams DH, Gauthier DW, Maizels M. Prenatal diagnosis of Beckwith-Wiedemann syndrome. *Prenat Diagn.* 2005;25(10):879–884.

91. Choufani S, Shuman C, Weksberg R. Molecular findings in Beckwith-Wiedemann syndrome. *Am J Med Genet Part C Semin Med Gen.* 2013;163C(2):131–140.

92. Eggermann T, Soellner L, Buiting K, Kotzot D. Mosaicism and uniparental disomy in prenatal diagnosis. *Trends Mol Med.* 2015;21(2):77–87.

93. Legendre M, Gonzales M, Goudefroye G, et al. Antenatal spectrum of CHARGE syndrome in 40 fetuses with CHD7 mutations. *J Med Genet.* 2012;49(11):698–707.

94. Busa T, Legendre M, Bauge M, et al. Prenatal findings in children with early postnatal diagnosis of CHARGE syndrome. *Prenat Diagn.* 2016;36(6):561–567.

95. Colin E, Bonneau D, Boussion F, et al. Prenatal diagnosis of CHARGE syndrome by identification of a novel CHD7 mutation in a previously unaffected family. *Prenat Diagn.* 2012;32(7):692–694.

96. Acanfora MM, Stirnemann J, Marchitelli G, Salomon LJ, Ville Y. Ultrasound evaluation of development of olfactory sulci in normal fetuses: a possible role in diagnosis of CHARGE syndrome. *Ultrasound Obstet Gynecol.* 2016;48(2):181–184.

97. Hefner MA, Fassi E. Genetic counseling in CHARGE syndrome: diagnostic evaluation through follow up. *Am J Med Genet Part C Semin Med Gen.* 2017;175(4):407–416.

98. Lazarin GA, Haque IS, Evans EA, Goldberg JD. Smith-Lemli-Opitz syndrome Carrier frequency and estimates of in utero mortality rates. *Prenat Diagn.* 2017;37(4):350–355.

99. Ryan AK, Bartlett K, Clayton P, et al. Smith-Lemli-Opitz syndrome: a variable clinical and biochemical phenotype. *J Med Genet.* 1998;35(7):558–565.

100. Hyett JA, Clayton PT, Moscoso G, Nicolaides KH. Increased first trimester nuchal translucency as a prenatal manifestation of Smith-Lemli-Opitz syndrome. *Am J Med Genet.* 1995;58(4):374–376.

101. Goldenberg A, Wolf C, Chevy F, et al. Antenatal manifestations of Smith-Lemli-Opitz (RSH) syndrome: a retrospective survey of 30 cases. *Am J Med Genet A.* 2004;124A(4):423–426.

102. Craig WY, Haddow JE, Palomaki GE, et al. Identifying Smith-Lemli-Opitz syndrome in conjunction with prenatal screening for Down syndrome. *Prenat Diagn.* 2006;26(9):842–849.

103. Jezela-Stanek A, Ciara E, Malunowicz E, et al. Differences between predicted and established diagnoses of Smith-Lemli-Opitz syndrome in the Polish population: underdiagnosis or loss of affected fetuses? *J Inher Metab Dis.* 2010;33(suppl 3):S241–S248.

104. Kratz LE, Kelley RI. Prenatal diagnosis of the RSH/Smith-Lemli-Opitz syndrome. *Am J Med Genet.* 1999;82(5):376–381.

105. Prenatal testing for DHCR7 gene variants: Smith-Lemli-Opitz syndrome. *GeneDx Prenatal Test Inf Sheet.* 2016.

106. Solomon BD, Baker LA, Bear KA, et al. An approach to the identification of anomalies and etiologies in neonates with identified or suspected VACTERL (vertebral defects, anal atresia, tracheo-esophageal fistula with esophageal atresia, cardiac anomalies, renal anomalies, and limb anomalies) association. *J Pediatr.* 2014;164(3):451–457. e451.

107. Solomon BD. VACTERL/VATER association. *Orphanet J Rare Dis.* 2011;6:56.

108. Wax JR, Watson WJ, Miller RC, et al. Prenatal sonographic diagnosis of hemivertebrae: associations and outcomes. *J Ultrasound Med.* 2008;27(7):1023–1027.

109. Basude S, McDermott L, Newell S, et al. Fetal hemivertebra: associations and perinatal outcome. *Ultrasound Obstet Gynecol.* 2015;45(4):434–438.

110. Perlman S, Bilik R, Leibovitch L, Katorza E, Achiron R, Gilboa Y. More than a gut feeling - sonographic prenatal diagnosis of imperforate anus in a high-risk population. *Prenat Diagn.* 2014;34(13):1307–1311.

111. Pohl-Schickinger A, Henrich W, Degenhardt P, Bassir C, Huseman D. Echogenic foci in the dilated fetal colon may be associated with the presence of a rectourinary fistula. *Ultrasound Obstet Gynecol.* 2006;28(3):341–344.

112. Radiology ACo. *ACR–SPR Practice Parameter for the Safe and Optimal Performance of Fetal Magnetic Resonance Imaging (MRI);* 2015.

113. Griffiths PD, Bradburn M, Campbell MJ, et al. Use of MRI in the diagnosis of fetal brain abnormalities in utero (MERIDIAN): a multicentre, prospective cohort study. *Lancet.* 2017;389(10068):538–546.

114. Jarvis D, Mooney C, Cohen J, et al. A systematic review and meta-analysis to determine the contribution of mr imaging to the diagnosis of foetal brain abnormalities in Utero. *Eur Radiol.* 2017;27(6):2367–2380.

115. Donofrio MT, Moon-Grady AJ, Hornberger LK, et al. Diagnosis and treatment of fetal cardiac disease: a scientific statement from the American Heart Association. *Circulation.* 2014;129(21):2183–2242.

116. Randall P, Brealey S, Hahn S, Khan KS, Parsons JM. Accuracy of fetal echocardiography in the routine detection of congenital heart disease among unselected and low risk populations: a systematic review. *BJOG.* 2005;112(1):24–30.

117. Zhang YF, Zeng XL, Zhao EF, Lu HW. Diagnostic value of fetal echocardiography for congenital heart disease: a systematic review and meta-analysis. *Medicine.* 2015;94(42):e1759.

118. Tasha I, Brook R, Frasure H, Lazebnik N. Prenatal detection of cardiac anomalies in fetuses with single umbilical artery: diagnostic accuracy comparison of maternal-fetal-medicine and pediatric cardiologist. *J Pregnancy.* 2014;2014:265421.

119. Kulkarni AD, Jamieson DJ, Jones Jr HW, et al. Fertility treatments and multiple births in the United States. *N Engl J Med.* 2013;369(23):2218–2225.

120. Martin JA, Hamilton BE, Osterman MJ. Three decades of twin births in the United States, 1980–2009. *NCHS Data Brief.* 2012;(80):1–8.

121. Boyle B, McConkey R, Garne E, et al. Trends in the prevalence, risk and pregnancy outcome of multiple births with congenital anomaly: a registry-based study in 14 European countries 1984–2007. *BJOG.* 2013;120(6):707–716.

122. Glinianaia SV, Rankin J, Wright C. Congenital anomalies in twins: a register-based study. *Hum Reprod.* 2008;23(6):1306–1311.

123. Boyle B, Morris JK, McConkey R, et al. Prevalence and risk of Down syndrome in monozygotic and dizygotic multiple pregnancies in Europe: implications for prenatal screening. *BJOG.* 2014;121(7):809–819; discussion 820.

124. Sparks TN, Norton ME, Flessel M, Goldman S, Currier RJ. Observed rate of down syndrome in twin pregnancies. *Obstet Gynecol.* 2016;128(5):1127–1133.

125. Maruotti GM, Saccone G, Morlando M, Martinelli P. First-trimester ultrasound determination of chorionicity in twin gestations using the lambda sign: a systematic review and meta-analysis. *Eur J Obstet Gynecol Reprod Biol.* 2016;202:66–70.

126. Wan JJ, Schrimmer D, Tache V, et al. Current practices in determining amnionicity and chorionicity in multiple gestations. *Prenat Diagn.* 2011;31(1):125–130.

127. D'Antonio F, Familiari A, Thilaganathan B, et al. Sensitivity of first-trimester ultrasound in the detection of congenital anomalies in twin pregnancies: population study and systematic review. *Acta Obstet Gynecol Scand.* 2016;95(12):1359–1367.

128. Edwards MS, Ellings JM, Newman RB, Menard MK. Predictive value of antepartum ultrasound examination for anomalies in twin gestations. *Ultrasound Obstet Gynecol.* 1995;6(1):43–49.

129. Zhang XH, Qiu LQ, Huang JP. Risk of birth defects increased in multiple births. *Birth Defects Res A Clin Mol Teratol.* 2011;91(1):34–38.

130. Best KE, Rankin J. Increased risk of congenital heart disease in twins in the North of England between 1998 and 2010. *Heart.* 2015;101(22):1807–1812.

131. Rustico MA, Baietti MG, Coviello D, Orlandi E, Nicolini U. Managing twins discordant for fetal anomaly. *Prenat Diagn.* 2005;25(9):766–771.

132. Harper LM, Odibo AO, Roehl KA, Longman RE, Macones GA, Cahill AG. Risk of preterm delivery and growth restriction in twins discordant for structural anomalies. *Am J Obstet Gynecol.* 2012;206(1):e71–e75.

133. Linskens IH, Elburg RM, Oepkes D, Vugt JM, Haak MC. Expectant management in twin pregnancies with discordant structural fetal anomalies. *Twin Res Hum Genet.* 2011;14(3):283–289.

134. Bebbington M. Selective reduction in multiple gestations. *Best Pract Res Clin Obstet Gynaecol.* 2014;28(2):239–247.

135. Chard RL, Norton ME. Genetic counseling for patients considering screening and diagnosis for chromosomal abnormalities. *Clin Lab Med.* 2016;36(2):227–236.

136. Bernhardt BA, Soucier D, Hanson K, Savage MS, Jackson L, Wapner RJ. Women's experiences receiving abnormal prenatal chromosomal microarray testing results. *Genet Med.* 2013;15(2):139–145.

137. American College of O, Gynecologists' Committee on Practice B-O, Committee on G, Society for Maternal-Fetal M, et al. Practice bulletin No. 162: prenatal diagnostic testing for genetic disorders. *Obstet Gynecol.* 2016;127(5):e108–e122.

138. Society for Maternal-Fetal Medicine, Electronic address PSO, Dugoff L, Norton ME, Kuller JA. The use of chromosomal microarray for prenatal diagnosis. *Am J Obstet Gynecol.* 2016;215(4):B2–B9.

139. Bijma HH, van der Heide A, Wildschut HI. Decision-making after ultrasound diagnosis of fetal abnormality. *Reprod Health Matters.* 2008;16(suppl 31):82–89.

140. Han HH, Choi EJ, Kim JM, Shin JC, Rhie JW. The importance of multidisciplinary management during prenatal care for cleft lip and palate. *Arch Plast Surg.* 2016;43(2):153–159.

141. Aite L, Trucchi A, Nahom A, Zaccara A, La Sala E, Bagolan P. Antenatal diagnosis of surgically correctable anomalies: effects of repeated consultations on parental anxiety. *J Perinatol.* 2003;23(8):652–654.

142. Staebler M, Donner C, Van Regemorter N, et al. Should determination of the karyotype be systematic for all malformations detected by obstetrical ultrasound? *Prenat Diagn.* 2005;25(7):567–573.

143. Zhang S, Lei C, Wu J, et al. A retrospective study of cytogenetic results from amniotic fluid in 5328 fetuses with abnormal obstetric sonographic findings. *J Ultrasound Med.* 2017;36(9):1809–1817.

144. Wapner RJ, Martin CL, Levy B, et al. Chromosomal microarray versus karyotyping for prenatal diagnosis. *N Engl J Med.* 2012;367(23):2175–2184.

145. Bornstein E, Berger S, Cheung SW, et al. Universal prenatal chromosomal microarray analysis: additive value and clinical dilemmas in fetuses with a normal karyotype. *Am J Perinatol.* 2017;34(4):340–348.

146. Donnelly JC, Platt LD, Rebarber A, Zachary J, Grobman WA, Wapner RJ. Association of copy number variants with specific ultrasonographically detected fetal anomalies. *Obstet Gynecol.* 2014;124(1):83–90.

147. de Wit MC, Srebniak MI, Govaerts LC, Van Opstal D, Galjaard RJ, Go AT. Additional value of prenatal genomic array testing in fetuses with isolated structural ultrasound abnormalities and a normal karyotype: a systematic review of the literature. *Ultrasound Obstet Gynecol.* 2014;43(2):139–146.
148. Walser SA, Kellom KS, Palmer SC, Bernhardt BA. Comparing genetic counselor's and patient's perceptions of needs in prenatal chromosomal microarray testing. *Prenat Diagn.* 2015;35(9):870–878.
149. Pangalos C, Hagnefelt B, Lilakos K, Konialis C. First applications of a targeted exome sequencing approach in fetuses with ultrasound abnormalities reveals an important fraction of cases with associated gene defects. *PeerJ.* 2016;4:e1955.
150. Practice bulletin No. 163: screening for fetal aneuploidy. *Obstet Gynecol.* 2016;127(5):e123–e137.
151. Gergev G, Mate A, Zimmermann A, Rarosi F, Sztriha L. Spectrum of neurodevelopmental disabilities: a cohort study in Hungary. *J Child Neurol.* 2015;30(3):344–356.
152. Gil MM, Accurti V, Santacruz B, Plana MN, Nicolaides KH. Analysis of cell-free DNA in maternal blood in screening for aneuploidies: updated meta-analysis. *Ultrasound Obstet Gynecol.* 2017;50(3):302–314.
153. Benachi A, Letourneau A, Kleinfinger P, et al. Cell-free DNA analysis in maternal plasma in cases of fetal abnormalities detected on ultrasound examination. *Obstet Gynecol.* 2015;125(6):1330–1337.
154. Beulen L, Faas BHW, Feenstra I, van Vugt JMG, Bekker MN. Clinical utility of non-invasive prenatal testing in pregnancies with ultrasound anomalies. *Ultrasound Obstet Gynecol.* 2017;49(6):721–728.
155. Shani H, Goldwaser T, Keating J, Klugman S. Chromosomal abnormalities not currently detected by cell-free fetal DNA: a retrospective analysis at a single center. *Am J Obstet Gynecol.* 2016;214(6):729.e721–e729.e711.
156. Mariona F, Burnett M, Zoma M, Blake J, Khouri H. Early unexpected diagnosis of fetal life-limiting malformation; antenatal palliative care and parental decision. *J Matern Fetal Neonatal Med.* 2017:1–8.

CHAPTER 12

Chromosomal Microarray Analysis

JESSICA L. GIORDANO, MS, CGC • MELISSA STOSIC, MS, CGC •
BRYNN LEVY, PHD • RONALD WAPNER, MD

INTRODUCTION

For more than half a century, classical cytogenetics was the standard of care in the diagnosis of developmental disabilities and congenital anomalies. More recently, the introduction of microarray technology into clinical medicine has allowed the identification of subchromosomal abnormalities leading to the diagnosis of an increasing number of genetic conditions in both the fetus and the child. A chromosomal microarray analysis (CMA) is a high-resolution genomic technology with the ability to detect the same pathogenic chromosomal imbalances detectable via karyotype as well as smaller submicroscopic deletions and duplications, known as copy number variants (CNVs), which are often associated with congenital anomalies and intellectual disabilities.

In 2010, a consensus statement was published establishing CMA as the first-tier clinical diagnostic test in the pediatric setting for individuals with developmental disabilities, congenital anomalies, or dysmorphic features, given that CMA can identify the cytogenetic etiology in 15%–20% more patients than a G-banded karyotype.[1] Subsequent studies in the prenatal setting found that pathogenic CNVs were present in 1%–1.7% of structurally normal fetuses and 6%–7% of anomalous fetuses.[2–8]

In 2013, The American College of Obstetricians and Gynecologists (ACOG) and The Society for Maternal-Fetal Medicine (SMFM) jointly recommended that CMA should replace or supplement karyotype in the evaluation of a fetus with anomalies. It is also recommended that CMA be made available to any patient choosing prenatal diagnostic testing for any indication, including anxiety.[9] This recommendation confirms their opinion that all women be offered the option of prenatal diagnostic testing regardless of age and is based on the fact that CNVs occur with equal frequency at all ages. Notably, the rate of pathogenic CNVs is higher than the risk of Down syndrome in women under 36 years of age, and the risk for a pathogenic CNV is four times higher than the risk of trisomy 21 in a woman under 30 years of age.[10]

In the last decade, advances have occurred in aneuploidy screening, including use of cell-free DNA (cfDNA), as well as in the amount of genetic information available through diagnostic testing using CMA. These simultaneous occurrences have created new counseling challenges and the need for increased patient education.[11] Although our ability to reliably screen for a few common aneuploidies (i.e., trisomies 13, 18, 21) has dramatically improved, our ability to diagnose hundreds of additional conditions (e.g., DiGeorge syndrome, Prader–Willi syndrome, and cri-du-chat syndrome) by chorionic villus sampling (CVS) or amniocentesis has also dramatically improved. This has led to some laboratories incorporating a subset of CNVs into their cfDNA screening algorithms. Although this approach is not presently as accurate as diagnostic testing, it demonstrates the increasing emergence of molecular techniques into screening.

WHAT IS A MICROARRAY AND HOW DOES THE TECHNOLOGY COMPARE WITH A KARYOTYPE?

Karyotyping visualizes chromosomes under the microscope and allows detection of large structural alterations such as aneuploidy, large deletions and duplications, marker chromosomes, and rearrangements such as translocations and inversions. In clinical prenatal diagnostic analysis, the G-banded karyotype has a resolution of 7–10 million base pairs (MB). Diagnosis of smaller findings is limited, and there is variation between different pre- and postnatal preparations. In addition, interpretation may be somewhat subjective since the assessment is completed visually, creating a risk for discrepancy between laboratories. The karyotype also requires the use of living, cultured cells, which often take 2 weeks to grow and have a risk for culture failure.

Chromosomal microarray analysis (CMA) uses genomic technology to identify small subchromosomal gains and losses called CNVs. CMA has a much higher resolution than a karyotype, potentially detecting gains and losses as small as approximately

Perinatal Genetics. https://doi.org/10.1016/B978-0-323-53094-1.00012-6

50 kilobases (KB). CMA can be completed using extracted DNA from cultured or uncultured (direct) cells, giving it a quicker turnaround time (potentially 3–5 days), which is particularly important for patients pursuing prenatal diagnosis for pregnancy management decisions. The ability to run a microarray on uncultured cells also allows for testing nonviable tissues from an intrauterine demise or spontaneous loss. Lastly, the CMA is interpreted using computer algorithms in combination with laboratory director expertise, allowing a less subjective interpretation. Two different CMA technologies exist with many laboratories using both in combination.

Array comparative genomic hybridization (aCGH) arrays use short (25–50 base pairs) laboratory-made sequences of single-stranded DNA called oligonucleotides and are designed to detect copy number alterations (gains or losses of genetic information) compared with a reference control at specific genomic locations (see Fig. 12.1). In this method, patient and control DNA samples are cut into fragments, labeled with fluorescent colors (typically green and red), mixed together, and placed on an array, which contains millions of oligonucleotide probes from multiple human genome reference sequences. The mixture of DNAs hybridize (bind) to complimentary sequences on the array and

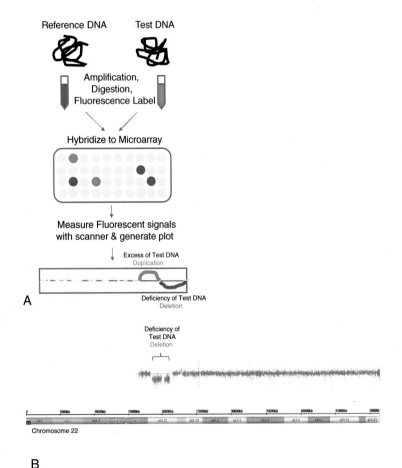

FIG. 12.1 Array comparative genomic hybridization process (aCGH)—Part A shows the aCGH process, which results in determination of the ratio of reference to test DNA at each oligonucleotide on the array. This ratio shows when there is an excess or deficiency of test DNA and is used to identify imbalances such as whole chromosome aneuploidy or microdeletions or duplications. Red signifies a loss of test DNA, and green signifies a gain of test DNA. Part B shows the actual generated image of the copy number plot from an aCGH platform on a case with approximately a 3-MB deletion of 22q11.2.

the intensity of fluorescence is measured, allowing for the detection of a gain or loss of genetic material in the sample compared with the control.[12]

Single-nucleotide polymorphism (SNP) arrays do not use a reference sequence; rather, they harness the power of polymorphisms in the genome. SNPs are differences in a single nucleotide within a stretch of DNA that are present in the population at a frequency of greater than 1% and are the most common form of genetic variation between individuals. An example of an SNP is the nucleotide thymine (T) replacing the nucleotide cytosine (C) at a specific location of DNA in a subset of the human population. Because SNPs occur normally in about every 300 nucleotides on average, and there are about 10 million SNPs in the human genome, they are an excellent target for the detection of gains or losses of genomic blocks of information (see Fig. 12.2).

The aCGH CMA is more limited than an SNP CMA because it can *only* detect gains and losses (CNVs), whereas SNPs allow the identification of a unique "genetic fingerprint," which is important for numerous reasons. Because each individual inherits a paternal and a maternal SNP at each location, a long contiguous stretch of homozygosity (LCSH), in which SNPs from only one parent are seen, can be identified and may represent either uniparental disomy (UPD) for a segment or a whole chromosome, or consanguinity. UPD is associated with genetic disease when an imprinted chromosome is involved (chromosomes 6, 7, 11, 14, 15) or if a pathogenic variant in a recessive disease gene is included in the region of homozygosity, so that the proband is then homozygous for that variant.[13] When an individual has consanguineous parents, the number of LCSHs will directly correlate with the degree of relationship. The use

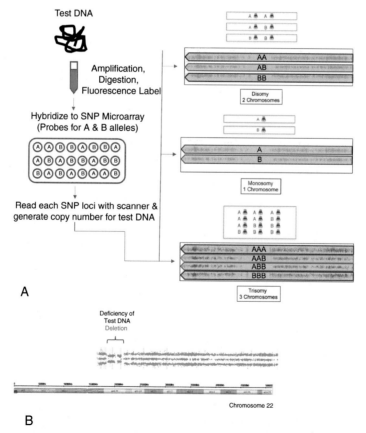

FIG. 12.2 Part A shows the SNP array process, which results in determination of the allele at each locus on the array. The alleles are then used to determine copy number to identify imbalances such as whole chromosome aneuploidy or microdeletions or duplications. Part B shows the actual generated image from an SNP array platform.

TABLE 12.1
Comparison of Detection of Diagnostic Technologies

Technology	Aneuploidy	Balanced Translocations and Inversions	Unbalanced Translocations	Triploidy	Long Contiguous Stretch of Homozygosity, Consanguinity, Zygosity, and Parentage	Copy Number Variants	Culture Required
G-banded karyotype	Yes	Yes	Yes	Yes	No	No	Yes
Comparative genomic hybridization array	Yes	No	Yes	No	No	Yes	No
SNP array	Yes	No	Yes	Yes	Yes	Yes	No

of SNPs also allows for the detection of triploidy, which is not detectable by aCGH as all chromosomes are duplicated. SNP microarrays can be used for the detection of parentage (maternity and paternity) compared with an alleged parents' DNA and can determine zygosity when testing samples from multiple gestations (see Table 12.1).

WHAT IS THE DIFFERENCE BETWEEN A TARGETED MICROARRAY AND A WHOLE GENOME MICROARRAY?

Many laboratories offer a "targeted" CMA and "whole genome" CMA, sometimes termed a "prenatal" versus a "postnatal" microarray, respectively. The ability of a CMA to identify CNVs depends on the number of unique probes on the array platform. Some laboratories use assays only targeting known genetic conditions and small CNVs that are known to be clinically relevant. Targeted arrays have probes restricted mainly to the genes known to be associated with those conditions. These targeted arrays will often have additional coverage (called the backbone) with probes spread equidistant across the genome (most commonly every 1 MB) in addition to more closely placed probes in the targeted regions. Incorporation of the backbone allows detection of larger and potentially significant deletions or duplications regardless of where they occur. Others have chosen to use whole genome arrays with dense coverage for a wider range of known conditions and a denser backbone to detect CNVs that may be clinically relevant because of size and/or Online Mendelian Inheritance in Man (OMIM) gene disease content, even if the CNV is not part of a well-described microdeletion/microduplication

syndrome. Some labs perform the same density array in all cases but may mask some portions of the data for prenatal interpretation in an attempt to reduce findings of uncertain significance. Although there are no standardized guidelines governing prenatal cases, many laboratories will maintain a CNV minimum size cutoff for reporting variants of uncertain significance (VUSs) (i.e., 1 MB or greater) and some may limit reporting of LCSH regions to imprinted chromosomes. The clinician should be familiar with the difference in assays and/or reporting standards for their laboratory of choice and, at times, be prepared to discuss the differences with a patient.

The American College of Medical Genetics and Genomics (ACMG) guidelines recommend that whole genome microarrays have a minimum detection of gains and losses of 400 kb or larger and an enrichment of probes in regions with known dosage-sensitive genes with strong correlation to congenital anomalies or neurocognitive impairment.[14] A whole genome array was previously thought to increase the likelihood for a laboratory to report a VUS, but studies assessing this have shown this not to be the case.[15]

WHAT CAN A MICROARRAY DETECT THAT A KARYOTYPE CANNOT?

CMA has a higher resolution than a karyotype, allowing for the detection of smaller CNVs in addition to aneuploidies and large chromosomal deletions and duplications. (See Table 12.2 for a list of common microdeletion/duplication syndromes). When a cryptic result is reported on a karyotype, such as a marker chromosome, CMA may be used to discern the origin; this

TABLE 12.2
Common Microdeletion and Duplication Syndromes and Frequency of Occurrence

Condition; Genomic Location	Incidence	Major Phenotypic Features
16p11.2 duplication	1/1900	Normal to DD, ASD, ADHD, microcephaly, psychiatric conditions
16p11.2 deletion	1/2300	ID/DD, ASD, ADHD, macrocephaly, psychiatric conditions
16p13.11 deletion	1/2300	ID/DD, seizures, schizophrenia
1q21.1 duplication	1/3300	Normal to motor skill and articulation difficulty, ID/DD, ASD, ADHD, scoliosis, abnormal gait, macrocephaly, short stature, psychiatric conditions (schizophrenia, anxiety, depression), CHD (especially Tetralogy of Fallot)
22q11.2 deletion syndrome (DiGeorge, VCFS)	1/4000	CHD (most commonly conotruncal), palate abnormalities, characteristic facies, ID/DD, immune deficiency, hypocalcemia, psychiatric conditions in early adulthood (schizophrenia, depression, bipolar disorder)
22q11.2 duplication	1/4000	Normal to ID/DD, growth retardation, hypotonia
1p36 deletion syndrome	1/5000	ID/DD, hypotonia, seizures, structural brain abnormalities, CHD, vision and hearing issues, skeletal anomalies, characteristic facies
Charcot–Marie–Tooth type 1A; 17p12 duplication	1/5000–1/10,000	Slowly progressive neuropathy causing distal muscle weakness and atrophy, sensory loss, and slow nerve conduction velocity first noticeable in the first or second decade
X-linked ichthyosis; Xp22.31 deletion	1/6000	ID/DD, ichthyosis, Kallmann syndrome, short stature, ocular albinism
Williams syndrome; 7q11.23 deletion	1/7500	ID/DD, cardiovascular disease, characteristic facies, connective tissue abnormalities, specific personality, growth anomalies, endocrine abnormalities
7q11.23 duplication	1/7500	DD, normal to ID intellectually, speech problems, hypotonia, problems with movement and walking, behavioral abnormalities, seizures, aortic enlargement
Prader–Willi syndrome; 15q11.2 paternal deletion	1/10,000	ID/DD, hypotonia and feeding difficulties in infancy, excessive eating, obesity, behavioral difficulties, hypogonadism, short stature
Angelman syndrome; 15q11.2 maternal deletion	1/12,000	ID/DD, severe speech impairment, gait ataxia, inappropriate happy affect, microcephaly, seizures
17q12 deletion	1/14,500	Kidney/urinary abnormalities, diabetes, ID/DD, ASD, psychiatric conditions
Sotos syndrome; 5q35 deletion	1/15,000	ID/DD, overgrowth, characteristic facies
Smith–Magenis syndrome; 17p11.2 deletion	1/15,000–1/25,000	ID/DD, characteristic facies, sleep disturbances, behavioral issues including self-injury and self-hugging and aggression, characteristic facies, reduced sensitivity to pain and temperature
Cri-du-chat; 5p15 deletion	1/15,000–1/50,000	High-pitched cry, microcephaly, hypotonia, characteristic facies, ID/DD, CHD
Koolen de Vries; 17q21 deletion	1/16,000	ID/DD, sociable personality, hypotonia, seizures, distinct facial features, CHD, kidney anomalies, foot deformities
Potocki–Lupski syndrome; 17p11.2 duplication	1/20,000	ID/DD, ASD, hypotonia, CHD

ADHD, attention deficit hyperactivity disorder; *ASD*, autism spectrum disorder; *CHD*, congenital heart defect; *DD*, developmental delay; *ID*, intellectual disability.

can be helpful in determining the clinical significance and prognosis. CMA can also be used when apparently balanced rearrangements are identified on a karyotype to determine if it is balanced or if there is a small deletion or duplication at the breakpoint(s). As outlined above and in Table 12.1, the SNP CMA additionally has the power to detect regions of homozygosity highlighting consanguinity and UPD, which may present an increased risk for recessive disease. SNP arrays can also determine parentage and in the case of twins, zygosity.

A benefit of microarray over traditional karyotype is that tissue culture is not required. DNA extracted from both uncultured (direct) or cultured villi and amniotic fluid are acceptable as is DNA from cord blood, stillbirth tissue samples, and products of conception. Some laboratories require a maternal specimen for maternal cell contamination studies. Parental specimens may also be requested to evaluate the inheritance of a CNV, for further evaluation of UPD, or other additional workup.

WHAT CAN A KARYOTYPE DETECT THAT A MICROARRAY CANNOT?

The G-banded karyotype remains the gold standard for the detection of balanced rearrangements, for example, Robertsonian or reciprocal translocations and paracentric or pericentric inversions. These are not detectable through CMA because the technology only identifies gains and losses of information, not balanced rearrangements. Karyotype is able to identify tetraploidy (92 chromosomes), whereas CMA cannot. In addition, karyotype may be better at identifying mosaicism. CMA can typically detect mosaicism down to approximately 15% or 20%, whereas karyotype with 15 cells counted can detect 15% mosaicism at 90% confidence, 19% mosaicism at 95% confidence, or 27% mosaicism at 99% confidence.[16] The clinical relevance of lower level mosaicism is questionable at times; but in some instances, this information can prove beneficial in the full evaluation of risk for genetic disease in a fetus.

HOW IS MICROARRAY DIFFERENT FROM TARGETED GENE TESTING AND WHOLE EXOME/GENOME SEQUENCING?

Microarray analysis is a genome-wide scan identifying deletions and duplications of at least 200–400 kb or larger, which usually contain multiple genes. CMA does not specifically sequence genes, that is, it cannot determine a change in a specific base pair within a gene. It will not diagnose single gene disorders such as cystic fibrosis and sickle cell disease and therefore

should not replace carrier screening in the prenatal setting. Alternatively, whole exome and whole genome sequencing (WES/WGS), which evaluate the genome at a single base pair level, are emerging technologies in pediatrics and now in perinatal medicine for the evaluation of undiagnosed developmental delays and congenital anomalies.[17,18] WES uses next-generation techniques to evaluate the protein-coding areas of the genome (exons), which compose 1%–1.5% of the genome. WGS evaluates both the introns and exons. These technologies create an abundance of genomic data that requires careful curation using bioinformatics and knowledge of clinical genetics.

WES has been demonstrated to identify single gene disorders in approximately 25%–30% of suspected pediatric disorders undiagnosed by karyotype and CMA.[19] A joint statement from the International Society of Prenatal Diagnosis (ISPD), SMFM, and Perinatal Quality Foundation (PQF) indicates that fetal WES/WGS could be considered when fetal anomalies are present and suggest a specific syndromic pattern or single gene disorder and CMA either does not solve the case or cannot be performed. This consensus group also indicates WES/WGS could be considered for parents who have a history of an undiagnosed fetus for which no sample is available from the affected proband. Although CMA is available to all women choosing prenatal diagnosis, there is no evidence to support offering WES/WGS as part of diagnostic testing in the absence of structural anomalies.[20]

In the prenatal setting, there are targeted sequencing panels that analyze groups of genes commonly associated with a specific syndrome or phenotype, such as Noonan syndrome when there is an increased nuchal translucency, or a skeletal dysplasia panel. Use of such panels should be completed in cases with suggestive findings either concurrently with microarray or as a reflex after a normal microarray result. With the expansion of carrier screening for recessive disorders and the expanding ability to diagnose pediatric conditions, the use of targeted gene variant testing has increased. However, as the cost of WES decreases, panels may be replaced by sequencing because panels are limited in the genes incorporated and may not include all genes associated with the phenotype.

ARE MICRODELETIONS AND MICRODUPLICATIONS DETECTABLE THROUGH CELL-FREE DNA SCREENING?

Given the omnipresent concern for procedure-related pregnancy loss associated with CVS and amniocentesis (albeit this risk is very small in experienced centers at approximately 1 in 700 to 1 in 1000), there has been a push to increase the yield of existing cfDNA screening by the inclusion of common microdeletion syndromes.[21] Laboratories offering CNV analysis as part of cfDNA screening usually include 1–7 well-described microdeletion syndromes, with 22q11.2 deletion being the most commonly offered (as this is the most frequently occurring). Such tests do not cover the majority of CNVs detectable via CMA, however. In a recent study of 2779 fetuses that compared the proportion of CMA pathogenic results that would not be detectable with cfDNA, the overall rate of a CMA pathogenic/likely pathogenic result was 5.0%, of which 44.0% (95% CI 36.0–52.2) were not detectable by cfDNA.[22] In addition, the detection rates for CNVs via cfDNA analysis are not well delineated and the positive predictive values (PPVs—the likelihood that a woman with a high-risk result is actually carrying an affected fetus) tend to be low as these CNVs are individually quite rare. The current ACMG guidelines suggest that it is acceptable to offer a woman having cfDNA testing the option of screening for a selected group of microdeletions associated with well-described phenotypes if the sensitivity, specificity, negative predictive value, and PPV for each individual condition are included in the report interpretation.[23] However, SMFM states that routine screening for microdeletions with cfDNA is not recommended. Some commercial laboratories have expanded their cfDNA capabilities to include reporting of all microdeletions >7 Mb, similar to the resolution of a karyotype. However, the majority of the pathogenic CNVs identified with diagnostic testing are substantially smaller than this.

A patient interested in identifying whether her fetus has a pathogenic microdeletion should have diagnostic testing by CVS or amniocentesis. Although cfDNA can detect CNVs, the sensitivity and specificity in routine use has not been validated. Accordingly, all positive tests must be confirmed by a diagnostic test. A patient with an anomalous fetus should be offered diagnostic testing with CMA as the first-tier test because approximately 6% will have a pathogenic CNV. If a patient declines diagnostic testing, a provider may consider cfDNA screening as an alternative, but the patient should be made aware of its limitations and far lower diagnostic yield.

HOW ARE MICROARRAY RESULTS REPORTED?

ACMG and the Association for Molecular Pathology (AMP) published a joint statement establishing standardization in the reporting of CNVs. Variants are categorized as pathogenic, likely pathogenic, uncertain significance, likely benign, or benign.[24] Likely benign and benign variants are usually not reported to the ordering provider and are therefore not included in a clinical laboratory report.

For CNVs, the report will include cytogenetic location, whether it is a deletion or duplication, the size of the change with specific nucleotide coordinates, the genome build or reference genome (currently hg19), the laboratory interpretation based on guidelines (see categories below), genes involved, and the recommended clinical follow-up, as shown in Fig. 12.3. Additionally, if parental samples were also studied and inheritance is known, it will also list whether it is de novo (dn) or inherited from the mother (mat) or father (pat). Categories of positive results are as follows:

Pathogenic: These CNVs are usually well-described syndromes, that is, Wolf–Hirschhorn, Angelman, or cri-du-chat syndrome (see Table 12.2). The clinician can typically find a plethora of data to describe these conditions; however, there may remain some uncertainty regarding the specific outcome for an individual, similar to counseling for a prenatal diagnosis of Down syndrome. These conditions are typically de novo but in some instances can be inherited from a parent with a translocation or other complex rearrangement and therefore, further evaluation of parental DNA is usually recommended via karyotype and/or fluorescence in situ hybridization (FISH).

Some pathogenic findings are predisposition CNVs, meaning they are changes associated with a wide spectrum of phenotype, often showing variable expressivity and may be inherited or de novo. Most frequently, these are autism susceptibility regions with a known, but variable, neurocognitive impact. Some variants are more penetrant than others, and the data for each should be reviewed in detail before counseling a patient. For example, the 16p11.2 deletion syndrome, associated with developmental delay, intellectual disability, and autism spectrum disorders, is characterized by impaired communication, socialization skills, delayed speech, and sometimes seizures. However, these signs and symptoms can vary within a single family, and some individuals may not have any clear physical, intellectual, or behavioral signs. For this specific condition, literature suggests that individuals with the deletion have an intellect that is two standard deviations below the mean for their matched sibling controls.[25] In other words, those that come from families with a high IQ may not seem symptomatic as their IQ may still be well within the low–normal range, although the deletion is still causing a loss

EXAMPLE REPORT
Probe targets: 2,696,550
Array type: SNP
Human Genome Build: hg19
Gender: Male
Microarray result: arr[hg19] 2q12.2q13 (107,029,680-111,365,996) x1
Interpretation: VUS
Diagnosis:
Molecular cytogenetic studies identified a 4.336 Mb interstitial deletion in the long arm of chromosome 2. Deleted region includes 36 OMIM -annotated genes and 4 of which are associated with disease (SLC5A7, RANBP2, EDAR, NPHP1)....

The "microarray result" portion indicates the specific chromosomal breakpoints as well as the specific basepairs impacted. "x1" indicates a deletion (loss) and "x3" indicates a duplication (gain).

FIG. 12.3 An example microarray report language.

of some level of intellect. Discovery of a predisposition CNV in an otherwise healthy pregnancy can create difficulty in quantifying the risk to the fetus, and although penetrance estimates have been computed, they may underestimate the true risks.[26] Counseling for these is often confounded by the fact that it is common for these to be inherited from a presumably healthy parent, making it difficult for a family to digest, especially given the 50% recurrence risk in a future pregnancy.

Another type of pathogenic result is one of an adult onset condition. There are a small number of well-described adult onset diseases caused by CNVs. Charcot–Marie–Tooth (duplication in 17p12) and its reciprocal deletion causing hereditary neuropathy with liability to pressure palsies are both examples. These may cause the clinician and patient difficulty in decision-making and may also inform a currently unaffected parent of a presymptomatic test result.

VUS: These CNVs usually meet guidelines for reporting because of their size and/or their gene content (i.e., the deletion or duplication of known OMIM-associated genes). Usually, there is a dearth of information regarding the clinical significance of a VUS finding, challenging both the clinician and patient in terms of how to proceed. Testing additional family members, particularly the parents, can prove helpful because de novo variants are generally more concerning than those who were inherited from a phenotypically normal parent. However, that rule is not absolute, and patients should be advised as such.

Region of homozygosity (also known as LCSH): LCSH is only detectable via SNP array-based analysis and will indicate either segmental or whole chromosome UPD,

consanguinity, or a distant common ancestor. Clinical follow-up will depend on the specific region identified. When UPD is suspected in a region that includes imprinted genes (e.g., chromosomes 6, 7, 11, 14, 15), additional testing may be recommended, such as methylation studies for Prader–Willi/Angelman (chr 15), Beckwith–Wiedemann (chr 11) or UPD studies for other specific chromosomes. If an LCSH region is found, reviewing the patient's Mendelian carrier screening for variants in the region in question is important for the evaluation of the risk for a recessive disease to be unmasked.

Mosaicism: This phenomenon is most well known in aneuploidy counseling, and mosaicism for aneuploidy is usually detectable via CMA when it is above 15%–20%. Mosaicism for a CNV is also possible. Further clinical recommendations are usually contingent on the specimen used for testing, e.g., if chorionic villi, follow-up amniocentesis is recommended.

WHAT ARE THE CURRENT GUIDELINES AROUND MICROARRAY UTILIZATION IN PREGNANCY?

ACOG and SMFM recommend that all women be offered the option of diagnostic testing regardless of maternal age. In regards to CMA, they recommend that it replace karyotype for any patient carrying a fetus with one or more structural anomalies who has elected to pursue diagnostic testing or for any patient with a fetal demise. They state that either CMA or karyotype be performed for any patient having diagnostic testing. Providers should discuss the benefits and limitations of both tests with the patient.[18]

ARE THERE CERTAIN ANOMALIES FOR WHICH A COPY NUMBER VARIANT IS MORE OR LESS LIKELY?

Overall, several large-scale studies and subsequent metaanalysis have proven the incremental benefit of CMA over karyotype in the setting of structural anomalies. These studies indicate a 6%–7% risk for a pathogenic CNV in the setting of a structural anomaly and a normal karyotype.[18] When a single organ system is affected, the risk for pathogenic CNV drops slightly approximately to 5%. Notably for counseling patients, the organ systems most associated with pathogenic CNVs include cardiac, renal, skeletal, urogenital, and CNS.[27] Donnelly et al. found that isolated renal and cardiac anomalies have the largest association with pathogenic CNVs at 15% and 10.6%, respectively, and that fetuses with more than one anomalous organ system have a 13% risk for a pathogenic or likely pathogenic CNV.[27] Lower incremental diagnostic yields for isolated increased nuchal translucency have been found (4.0%), likely because many increased nuchal translucencies are due to whole chromosome aneuploidy.[28]

IN WHAT OTHER CLINICAL SCENARIOS IS MICROARRAY USEFUL?

Because genetic abnormalities have been associated with at least 6%–13% of stillbirths, consideration of CMA is recommended in this scenario. Reddy et al. found that microarray is more likely than karyotype to provide a genetic diagnosis in cases of stillbirth.[29] Because CMA can be performed on DNA extracted directly from any fetal tissue and does not require living cells, it is a useful tool in the evaluation of stillbirth, intrauterine fetal demise, and spontaneous loss, even when aneuploidy is suspected.

CMA can be helpful in cases where karyotype identifies a marker chromosome, a translocation or other rearrangement (including balanced translocations), or other cryptic result. (See "What can a microarray detect that a karyotype cannot" above).

WHAT OTHER TESTS SHOULD BE ORDERED ALONGSIDE A MICROARRAY?
Maternal Cell Contamination Testing

Because prenatal samples are typically obtained traversing the maternal habitus, there is a risk that maternal cells may be present in villi or amniotic fluid and this poses a risk for misdiagnosis. In particular, villi have a higher risk for contamination compared to amniotic fluid because of difficulty in thoroughly cleansing maternal decidua from fetal cells.[30] A maternal cell contamination study uses a maternal DNA sample and compares its polymorphic markers to the prenatal DNA sample. When the proportion of maternal DNA is below the detection limit of the molecular test (<10% for SNP oligonucleotide assays), then the result is likely to represent the fetal genotype. If the level is >10%, then the excess of maternal DNA may obfuscate the fetal DNA and prevent the diagnosis of a genetic condition, particularly if the genetic condition is a very small CNV or mosaic. When a pregnancy is conceived via egg donor and CMA is pursued, MCC studies can still be performed, but the laboratory should be notified so they are not surprised when there are no matching polymorphic markers.

Fluorescence In Situ Hybridization

In the context of prenatal diagnosis, FISH remains the technique of choice for confirmation of the common trisomies and sex aneuploidies (13, 18, 21, X, Y) within 24–48 h after a diagnostic procedure. FISH provides relatively quick information to patients who have a high a priori risk for the common aneuploidies due to abnormal ultrasound findings consistent with a specific chromosomal syndrome, serum screening, or positive cell-free fetal DNA results.[9] FISH does not replace the diagnostic accuracy of a karyotype, which should still be pursued and will also assess for mosaicism and translocations. In the event of an abnormal FISH result, confirmed by a karyotype, and consistent with ultrasound findings, most clinicians would not pursue CMA further unless the patient planned continuation of the pregnancy and wanted the additional information provided by CMA. Separately, when a mosaic aneuploidy is seen on karyotype, FISH is used to count additional cells to further refine the level of mosaicism. In such cases, FISH allows the geneticist to count potentially hundreds of cells with relative ease. However, as rapid sequencing techniques that provide information about all aneuploidies in 4 h or less become mainstream, FISH may lose its usefulness.[31]

When Should a Karyotype Be Ordered in Addition to a Microarray?

The karyotype is a useful tool both in the follow-up of CMA results and in the evaluation of certain family histories. When a CMA result is suggestive of an unbalanced translocation (e.g., in the presence of a gain and a loss of information involving the distal ends of two chromosomes), then follow-up parental testing via karyotype is essential to determine recurrence risks for a couple. If a couple presents with a personal or family history of recurrent pregnancy loss or trisomy, then a parental blood karyotype is also helpful for the same reasons and may prompt prenatal diagnosis if abnormal.

HOW SHOULD INFORMED CONSENT BE OBTAINED?

Multiple organizations (SMFM, ACOG) recommend pretest counseling be performed by those trained in the interpretation of CMA results, including genetic counselors, geneticists, and other specialized providers with knowledge of genetics. These providers should meet with the patient to obtain informed consent, and this should include the following:[9,18,32]

- CMA has a higher resolution than a traditional karyotype, detecting an additional pathogenic CNV in approximately 6% of fetuses with an ultrasound anomaly and about 1%–1.7% of fetuses with normal anatomy ultrasound.
- CMA will not detect all genetic disorders, and additional specialized testing may be warranted if the provider deems necessary.
- Some identifiable genetic changes are associated with variable expressivity or reduced penetrance, and it may not be possible to fully predict the phenotype of the fetus.
- Despite advances, VUSs will sometimes be detected and further testing of parents may assist in the interpretation. However, there are times when the clinical significance of particular variants may remain unknown, which may lead to increased anxiety and stress in the pregnancy.
- CMA may detect adult onset diseases in the fetus, and such a finding may also be present in an undiagnosed parent.
- CMA may reveal consanguinity or nonpaternity.

The provider should help the patient consider his/her individual risks, reproductive goals, and preferences from a moral, ethical, religious, and/or financial perspective before choosing screening versus diagnostic testing and, if diagnostic testing is chosen, CMA or no CMA.[9]

The patient's decision about microarray is usually made in the context of his/her choice to pursue diagnostic testing. Some questions a patient may consider are the following:

- Do you want to know for sure if your pregnancy is affected by a genetic condition that is detectable by current technologies?
- How will the information help with pregnancy management? Would you consider termination if a significant condition is found? Would you prefer time for you and your family to prepare for the birth of a child with a genetic condition or to consider alternative options such as adoption?
- How would you feel if a VUS or predisposition CNV were found? Provide specific examples to the patient.
- How would you feel if an adult onset disease were found? Provide specific examples with the patient.

MICROARRAY RESULTS ARE POSITIVE; NOW WHAT?

A positive result, whether a known pathogenic variant or a VUS, poses counseling challenges and will necessitate in-depth preparation before results disclosure, preferably done by a genetics specialist such as a genetic counselor or geneticist. A positive result for a well-described CNV via prenatal diagnosis, such as Miller–Dieker syndrome, should prompt the provider to inform the patient of the natural history and prognosis of the condition, the available medical literature and patient support groups, the recommended follow-up via ultrasound and echocardiogram, and the appropriate referrals and support for the patient's choice (continuation, termination of pregnancy, adoption, etc.) Even with well-described CNVs such as this, uncertainty will exist regarding the specific disease course for each patient. Regardless of the patient's decision about pregnancy management, the patient and her partner should be offered appropriate parental follow-up studies to determine recurrence risks. Most known pathogenic variants will be de novo; however, some may be caused by a parental rearrangement, and this risk varies by condition. For example, approximately 80% of individuals with Miller–Dieker syndrome have a de novo deletion in 17p13.3, but 20% inherit a deletion from a parent with a balanced chromosomal rearrangement. A parent with a chromosomal rearrangement will have a higher recurrence risk than those who have a child with a de novo CNV. When a pathogenic susceptibility CNV is found, such as a 16p11.2 deletion, follow-up parental testing should be offered with the clear discussion that a parent may also harbor the CNV, conferring a 50% recurrence risk in all pregnancies.

When a VUS is found, the provider may require additional time before results disclosure to fully review the available databases and medical literature. The provider should inform the patient specifically regarding case series or limited data available regarding the natural history and prognosis of the CNV, the available medical literature and patient support groups, the recommended follow-up via ultrasound and echocardiogram, and the appropriate referrals and support for the patient's choice (continuation, termination of pregnancy, adoption, etc.).

Parental follow-up studies will usually be recommended via a CMA if the CNV is isolated and small, whereas karyotype ± FISH will usually be recommended if the CMA reveals a distal gain and a distal loss indicative of an unbalanced translocation. If the CNV is relatively common and detectable via FISH or quantitative PCR (qPCR), such follow-up tests will be recommended. When uncertain, the provider can contact the resulting laboratory for further advice regarding appropriateness of specific follow-up tests.

MICROARRAY RESULTS ARE NEGATIVE; NOW WHAT?

It behooves the provider to remind the patient at the time of results disclosure that CMA does not rule out all genetic conditions or birth defects. If the patient has a normal fetal ultrasound, the provider can be more reassuring than if there is a structural anomaly. The provider should take care to review the patient's pregnancy and family history to highlight the limitations of the test. For example, if there is a family history of autism, the provider may highlight the value of a genetics evaluation for the affected individual and the limitation of CMA to rule out all causes of autism. If the patient receives CMA at the time of CVS, he/she should also remind the patient to recontact his/her genetics provider if a new finding is identified on a second trimester anatomy ultrasound as additional testing may be recommended. If the normal microarray results are in the context of a structurally abnormal ultrasound, the results disclosure should include further discussion about the residual risks for a genetic condition given the finding. Additional testing may be warranted such as a sequencing panel for genes associated with the anomaly(ies) identified. Specific data are limited in this area as research catches up with the broad use of CMA, but a literature search should be conducted on a case-by-case basis.

WHAT RESOURCES ARE AVAILABLE TO CLINICIANS TO ASSIST WITH INTERPRETATION OF RESULTS?

- Genetic counselors and geneticists
- The laboratory that performed the microarray
- Gene review for specific findings
- OMIM/PubMed
- ClinGen
- ClinVar
- UCSD genome browser: https://genome.ucsc.edu/
- Include others

WHAT RESOURCES ARE AVAILABLE TO PATIENTS TO ASSIST IN UNDERSTANDING RESULTS?

- Genetic counselors and geneticists: https://www.nsgc.org/findageneticcounselor
- Unique: http://www.rarechromo.org/html/home.asp
- Genetic Support Foundation: https://geneticsupportfoundation.org/archive/genetics-and-you/pregnancy-and-genetics/pregnancy-and-genetics-tests/prenatal-chromosomal-microarray-cma
- Support groups by condition
- Genetic Alliance: http://www.geneticalliance.org/

REFERENCES

1. Fan YS, Jayakar P, Zhu H, et al. Detection of pathogenic gene copy number variations in patients with mental retardation by genomewide oligonucleotide array comparative genomic hybridization. *Hum Mutat.* 2007;28(11):1124–1132.
2. Wapner RJ, Martin CL, Levy B, et al. Chromosomal microarray versus karyotyping for prenatal diagnosis. *N Engl J Med.* 2012;367(23):2175–2184.
3. Shaffer LG, Dabell MP, Fisher AJ, et al. Experience with microarray-based comparative genomic hybridization for prenatal diagnosis in over 5000 pregnancies. *Prenat Diagn.* 2012;32(10):976–985.
4. Scott F, Murphy K, Carey L, et al. Prenatal diagnosis using combined quantitative fluorescent polymerase chain reaction and array comparative genomic hybridization analysis as a first-line test: results from over 1000 consecutive cases. *Ultrasound Obstet Gynecol.* 2013;41(5):500–507.
5. Van Opstal D, de Vries F, Govaerts L, et al. Benefits and burdens of using a SNP array in pregnancies at increased risk for the common aneuploidies. *Hum Mutat.* 2015;36(3):319–326.
6. Callaway JL, Shaffer LG, Chitty LS, Rosenfeld JA, Crolla JA. The clinical utility of microarray technologies applied to prenatal cytogenetics in the presence of a normal conventional karyotype: a review of the literature. *Prenat Diagn.* 2013;33(12):1119–1123.
7. Srebniak MI, Diderich KE, Joosten M, et al. Prenatal SNP array testing in 1000 fetuses with ultrasound anomalies: causative, unexpected and susceptibility CNVs. *Eur J Hum Genet.* 2016;24(5):645–651.
8. Hillman SC, McMullan DJ, Hall G, et al. Use of prenatal chromosomal microarray: prospective cohort study and systematic review and meta-analysis. *Ultrasound Obstet Gynecol.* 2013;41(6):610–620.
9. Practice bulletin No. 162: prenatal diagnostic testing for genetic disorders. *Obstet Gynecol.* 2016;127(5):e108–e122.
10. Srebniak MI, Joosten M, Knapen M, et al. Frequency of submicroscopic chromosome aberrations in pregnancies without increased risk for structural chromosome aberrations: a systematic review of literature and meta-analysis. *Ultrasound Obstet Gynecol.* 2017.
11. Evans MI, Wapner RJ, Berkowitz RL. Noninvasive prenatal screening or advanced diagnostic testing: caveat emptor. *Am J Obstet Gynecol.* 2016;215(3):298–305.
12. Levy B, Wapner R. Prenatal diagnosis by chromosomal microarray analysis. *Fertil Steril.* 2018;109(2):201–212.
13. Shaffer LG, Agan N, Goldberg JD, Ledbetter DH, Longshore JW, Cassidy SB. American College of Medical Genetics statement of diagnostic testing for uniparental disomy. *Genet Med.* 2001;3(3):206–211.
14. South ST, Lee C, Lamb AN, Higgins AW, Kearney HM. ACMG Standards and Guidelines for constitutional cytogenomic microarray analysis, including postnatal and prenatal applications: revision 2013. *Genet Med.* 2013;15(11):901–909.

15. Coppinger J, Alliman S, Lamb AN, Torchia BS, Bejjani BA, Shaffer LG. Whole-genome microarray analysis in prenatal specimens identifies clinically significant chromosome alterations without increase in results of unclear significance compared to targeted microarray. *Prenat Diagn.* 2009;29(12):1156–1166.

16. Hook EB. Exclusion of chromosomal mosaicism: tables of 90%, 95% and 99% confidence limits and comments on use. *Am J Hum Genet.* 1977;29(1):94–97.

17. Points to consider in the clinical application of genomic sequencing. *Genet Med.* 2012;14(8):759–761.

18. Committee opinion No. 682: microarrays and next-generation sequencing technology: the use of advanced genetic diagnostic tools in obstetrics and gynecology. *Obstet Gynecol.* 2016;128(6):e262–e268.

19. Yang Y, Muzny DM, Reid JG, et al. Clinical whole-exome sequencing for the diagnosis of mendelian disorders. *N Engl J Med.* 2013;369(16):1502–1511.

20. Joint position statement from the International Society for Prenatal Diagnosis (ISPD), the Society for Maternal Fetal Medicine (SMFM), and the Perinatal Quality Foundation (PQF) on the use of genome-wide sequencing for fetal diagnosis. *Prenat Diagn.* 2018;38(1):6–9.

21. Akolekar R, Beta J, Picciarelli G, Ogilvie C, D'Antonio F. Procedure-related risk of miscarriage following amniocentesis and chorionic villus sampling: a systematic review and meta-analysis. *Ultrasound Obstet Gynecol.* 2015;45(1):16–26.

22. Sotiriadis A, Papoulidis I, Siomou E, et al. Non-invasive prenatal screening versus prenatal diagnosis by array comparative genomic hybridization: a comparative retrospective study. *Prenat Diagn.* 2017;37(6):583–592.

23. Gregg AR, Skotko BG, Benkendorf JL, et al. Noninvasive prenatal screening for fetal aneuploidy, 2016 update: a position statement of the American College of Medical Genetics and Genomics. *Genet Med.* 2016;18(10):1056–1065.

24. Richards S, Aziz N, Bale S, et al. Standards and guidelines for the interpretation of sequence variants: a joint consensus recommendation of the American College of medical genetics and genomics and the association for molecular Pathology. *Genet Med.* 2015;17(5):405–424.

25. Hanson E, Bernier R, Porche K, et al. The cognitive and behavioral phenotype of the 16p11.2 deletion in a clinically ascertained population. *Biol Psychiatry.* 2015;77(9):785–793.

26. Rosenfeld JA, Coe BP, Eichler EE, Cuckle H, Shaffer LG. Estimates of penetrance for recurrent pathogenic copy-number variations. *Genet Med.* 2013;15(6):478–481.

27. Donnelly JC, Platt LD, Rebarber A, Zachary J, Grobman WA, Wapner RJ. Association of copy number variants with specific ultrasonographically detected fetal anomalies. *Obstet Gynecol.* 2014;124(1):83–90.

28. Grande M, Jansen FA, Blumenfeld YJ, et al. Genomic microarray in fetuses with increased nuchal translucency and normal karyotype: a systematic review and meta-analysis. *Ultrasound Obstet Gynecol.* 2015;46(6):650–658.

29. Reddy UM, Page GP, Saade GR, et al. Karyotype versus microarray testing for genetic abnormalities after stillbirth. *N Engl J Med.* 2012;367(23):2185–2193.

30. Antoniadi T, Yapijakis C, Kaminopetros P, et al. A simple and effective approach for detecting maternal cell contamination in molecular prenatal diagnosis. *Prenat Diagn.* 2002;22(5):425–429.

31. Wei S, Williams Z. Rapid short-read sequencing and aneuploidy detection using MinION nanopore technology. *Genetics.* 2016;202(1):37–44.

32. Dugoff L, Norton ME, Kuller JA. The use of chromosomal microarray for prenatal diagnosis. *Am J Obstet Gynecol.* 2016;215(4):B2–B9.

CHAPTER 13

Exome and Genome Sequencing

IGNATIA B. VAN DEN VEYVER, MD

INTRODUCTION

Current standards for prenatal genetic screening and testing are highly focused on detection of aneuploidies that are compatible with live birth, including trisomy 21, which affects 1:600 newborns overall and is associated with long-term survival, and the less common and more severe trisomies 18 and 13, which respectively affect 1:5000 and 1:15,000 liveborn infants.[1,2] When an amniocentesis or other prenatal diagnostic procedure is performed for fetal structural abnormalities detected by fetal imaging (ultrasound and/or MRI), aneuploidy is found in fewer than 1% to 30%–40% of cases, depending on the type of anomalies and the presence of single versus multiple anomalies.[1] The addition of chromosomal microarray analysis (CMA) provides an incremental detection rate of clinically significant copy number variants in 6%–7% of fetuses with prenatally diagnosed congenital anomalies and of more than 10% when there are multiple fetal anomalies. When amniocentesis or chorionic villus sampling (CVS) is performed for other indications, such as advanced maternal age or positive aneuploidy screening, the incremental diagnostic yield of CMA is 1%–1.7%.[2,3] Although CMA therefore offers significant diagnostic improvements over karyotype analysis, this standard workup still leaves approximately 60% or more pregnancies with fetal anomalies without a genetic diagnosis,[4,5] in large part because testing does not include single gene disorders. Although single gene disorders are individually rare, their collective disease burden is highly significant with an estimated frequency of 0.36% of live births or 1% overall.[6,7] There are currently >6000 single gene disorders and traits caused by pathogenic variants in >3800 genes listed in the Online Mendelian Inheritance of Men (OMIM) database (https://omim.org/statistics/gene Map accessed April 3, 2018). Overall, autosomal recessive genetic disorders account for 6%–8% of pediatric hospital admissions, in contrast to only 0.4%–2.5% for chromosomal abnormalities. Single gene disorders are also responsible for 20% of infant mortality.[6,8] Despite these numbers, these conditions are not included in traditional prenatal testing paradigms, or in guidelines for prenatal genetic workup for fetuses with congenital anomalies, largely because until recently it was difficult and impractical to determine which specific gene(s) to assess. With the development of high-throughput next-generation sequencing (NGS) technology, an entire genome or exome can now be sequenced in days. This has simultaneously accelerated the pace of new disease gene discovery and the development and diagnostic use of multigene panels, as well as whole exome sequencing (WES), which analyzes the 1%–2% of the genome that codes for expressed RNAs and proteins, and whole genome sequencing (WGS). Diagnostic WES is being increasingly integrated into pediatric and adult genetic disease evaluation, where the incremental detection rates of disease-causing variants ranges from 25% to more than 50%, depending on the clinical indication. We review here WES technology, its applications, and the still limited experience with its use for prenatal genetic diagnosis. Although early data on the utility of fetal WES for prenatal diagnosis are promising and suggest its value, they also highlight some pitfalls that arise from detection of variants of uncertain significance (VUSs), secondary or incidental findings, and unanticipated diagnoses in family members. These can all result in complex pre- and posttest counseling situations.

HOW ARE NEXT-GENERATION SEQUENCING, WHOLE EXOME SEQUENCING, AND WHOLE GENOME SEQUENCING PERFORMED?

For NGS, genomic DNA is first sheared into small fragments of about 50 to up to a few hundred nucleotides, and adapters are linked to one or both ends of these fragments. In WGS, where the entire genome is sequenced, this pool of fragments is called the sequencing library (Fig. 13.1). In contrast, with WES, only the 1%–2% of the genome that contains the coding exons, which harbor up to 85% of all known disease-causing mutations, is sequenced. With WES, the DNA fragments that overlap with exons and their flanking introns are first purified from the entire library by hybridization to a collection of DNA baits of known sequence that are attached to magnetic beads to generate an enriched sequencing library. A similar enrichment strategy is used for high-throughput sequencing with disease-specific multigene panels. The obtained sequencing library is then immobilized on a solid surface, amplified in clusters, denatured, and then sequenced by synthesis of a new complementary strand. In this process, each nucleotide (A, C, G, T) that is incorporated has a different fluorescent tag, so that its insertion at a specific location in the sequenced fragment can be recorded.[9-11] This is repeated multiple times in "massively parallel sequencing" for each nucleotide present in the overlapping fragments, resulting in rapid, accurate identification of the incorporated nucleotide for each cluster. The obtained sequence reads are then aligned using bioinformatics tools to generate a consensus sequence that is compared with the human reference sequence.[9,10]

The quality of the obtained sequence varies, and two parameters used to describe the quality are the sequencing depth, which refers to the number of overlapping reads for each base pair, and the sequence coverage, which refers to the fraction of the sequence that is covered at sufficient depth. The American College of Medical Genetics and Genomics (ACMG) recommends that for diagnostic WES, ≥ 90%–95% of the sequence should be covered at least 10-fold and that the average depth should be ≥100-fold.[12] (see Fig. 13.1).

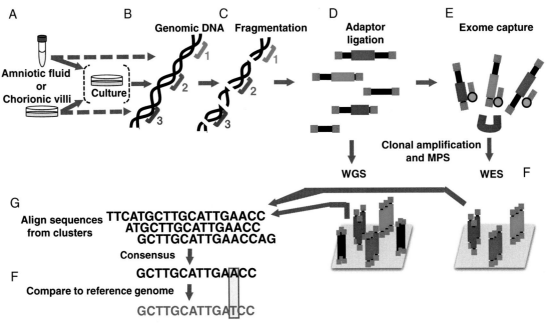

FIG. 13.1 **Next-generation Sequencing Methodology.** (A) Amniotic fluid and chorionic villi are obtained through an invasive prenatal diagnostic procedure. (B) Cell culture is initiated to grow fetal (trophoblast) cells for DNA. If sufficient material is available, genomic DNA can be prepared in parallel, while "back-up" cultures are growing. DNA is then sheared (C) into small fragments and ligated to adaptors (D) to prepare the sequencing library. (E) A capture step is added for whole exome sequencing to purify exons by hybridization to a collection of baits, which allows the targeted capture library to be purified from the rest of the genome. (F) This is followed by immobilization to a solid platform, amplification to form clusters that become the templates for massively parallel sequencing by incorporating labeled nucleotides that can be detected as they are added to the sequence that is generated from the templates. (G) Different overlapping sequences are aligned to form a consensus sequence. (F) The consensus is then compared to the reference sequence to detect difference; in the example in the figure there is a T > A change in the new sequence.

Unique Technical Considerations for Prenatal Genome Sequencing

Compared with its use for children or adults, genome-wide sequencing for prenatal diagnosis presents unique technical challenges.[13] Prenatally obtained samples, usually amniotic fluid or chorionic villus samples (CVS), are often smaller in volume with lower numbers of nucleated cells and may require a cell culture step before enough DNA can be made to prepare a sequencing library. Because the sample is obtained through an invasive procedure, there is also a small risk for contamination with maternal cells. In prenatal diagnosis, timing of the diagnostic test and rapid turnaround times are critical if the goal is to have results that can inform prenatal, perinatal, and postnatal management. Laboratories that offer prenatal genome-wide sequencing-based tests must therefore implement procedures to assure rapid turnaround times from sample submission to return of results. This is achieved by a combination of improvements of sequencing equipment, reagents and protocols, use of optimized workflows, including a trio-sequencing approach, wherein the fetal sample and parental samples are sequenced and analyzed in parallel to aid interpretation (see below).

HOW ARE GENOME-WIDE SEQUENCING DATA ANALYZED AND INTERPRETED?

Each sequenced human genome is unique and contains hundreds of thousands of sequence variations when compared with the reference genome, but the vast majority of these are benign and not associated with disease.[14] Although there are fewer variants, in the range of 20,000–50,000, identified with WES,[15] determining which of those are responsible for disease or a developmental phenotype is a highly complex process.

Diagnostic and research laboratories typically analyze sequence data in a stepwise approach using a combination of strategies, including comparison with databases of sequence variants found in healthy individuals and in various pathological states, together with bioinformatics tools that predict the functional impact of specific variants on the gene and its encoded protein. This allows filtering out of benign variants and prioritizing those that are most likely to be causative for the developmental phenotype or disease for which the sequencing was performed. In the United States, diagnostic laboratories offering WES abide by standards of variant interpretation and reporting developed by organizations such as the ClinGen Clinical Genome Resource (https://www.clinicalgenome.org/) and the ACMG[16,17] to classify variants into five categories: pathogenic, likely pathogenic, VUS, likely benign, and benign.[10,16,18]

The commonly used databases of genomic variants that are used to guide interpretation include the exome aggregation consortium (ExAc) database, genome aggregation database (gnomAD),[19] clinical variation database (ClinVar),[20] Human Gene Mutation Database (HGMD),[21] and Database of Chromosomal Imbalance and Phenotype in Humans Using Ensembl Resources (DECIPHER).[22] Sequence variants that are common in healthy individuals (single-nucleotide polymorphisms; SNPs) are more likely to be benign, whereas unique rare variants are more likely to be pathogenic and need to be further interpreted. Reports of other individuals with identical or other pathogenic variants in the same gene who have a known disorder or an overlapping phenotype strongly support pathogenicity, although there can be exceptions because of incomplete penetrance, variable expressivity, or misclassification of variants.

The functional consequence of a variant can also be predicted using bioinformatics tools[10,18] such as PolyPhen 2 (http://genetics.bwh.harvard.edu/pph2/), which classifies variants as probably damaging, possibly damaging, or benign[23]; SIFT (Sorting Intolerant from Tolerant; http://sift.jcvi.org/), which provides a score that indicates whether an amino acid change is predicted to be tolerated or damaging[24]; or MutationTaster2, which predicts if a sequence alteration is likely to be disease-causing or a benign polymorphism.[25] Typically, but not always, variants such as stop-gain (nonsense) or frameshift mutations that are predicted to lead to a complete absence of the produced protein are more likely to be pathogenic, whereas missense variants, which result in the substitution of one amino acid for another, can have variable effects.

The inheritance pattern of a rare variant in the family is also an important consideration. In inherited autosomal dominant disorders, the pathogenic or likely pathogenic variant is typically heterozygous and segregates in a family's pedigree with the inherited disease, but a "de novo" dominant variant is only found in the affected individual and not in either parent. For autosomal recessive disorders, the affected individual has a pathogenic or likely pathogenic variant on each allele of a gene, usually inherited "in trans" from each of the biological parents, who are carriers. Variants on the X chromosome cause X-linked inherited or de novo conditions. At times, supporting information from animal models or functional assays can be used to further refine the interpretation.

The final step, clinical interpretation, is critically important and requires collaboration and information sharing between the clinician and the diagnostic laboratory.

These combined approaches for variant interpretation rely greatly on publicly available data. Thus, because WES and WGS are emerging diagnostic and research tools for identifying the causes of birth defects and rare genetic disorders, data sharing in a manner that safeguards individual privacy has been formally recommended by professional societies[26,27] and is critical for advancing our understanding of pathogenicity and ability to most optimally apply WES or WGS for prenatal diagnosis.

Unique Interpretation Considerations for Prenatal Genome Sequencing

Although the databases, tools, and strategies outlined above are standardized for interpretation of any sequencing results, there are unique challenges in the prenatal setting that must be considered. All currently used databases are primarily populated with variant data originating from pediatric and adult presentations of genetic diseases and include very limited data from prenatal or fetal phenotypes. This is particularly challenging for prenatally lethal conditions that are not reported in neonates or children, as they may not survive to birth. An important aspect of WES interpretation is correlation of a discovered rare variant with an already known clinical phenotype that matches the phenotype of the sequenced proband. However, the proband's phenotype is often incompletely ascertained prenatally because of imaging limitations or because some features are not present until after birth or later in life. Early data from prenatal WES use have also revealed new unpredicted prenatal findings associated with known disease genes, resulting in "phenotypic expansion" of the features of known single gene disorders to include previously unascertained prenatal phenotypes.

An important current initiative in clinical genetics is the use of a standard phenotyping nomenclature, by using Human Phenotype Ontology (HPO)[28] terms, such that there is uniformity in phenotype descriptions in shared clinical data associated with specific variants from different centers. Like other databases, HPO terms also contain relatively limited clinically useful prenatal phenotypic descriptions. Initiatives are underway to include more prenatal phenotypes in clinical databases.

Because WES and WGS are genome-wide tests, pathogenic variants in genes that cause single gene disorders unrelated to the indication for prenatal testing can be found incidentally. If the identified single gene disorder usually presents after birth, in childhood, or even in adulthood, a fetus with such a "genotype first" result will not have clinical features of the disease until later in life. How to manage such findings is particularly challenging when the variant is a VUS or causes an adult-onset disorder. Laboratories and clinicians must therefore develop strategies for reporting such variants and informing parents about them.

WHAT TYPE OF GENETIC VARIANTS ARE DETECTED AND REPORTED?

Although NGS is a powerful tool in evaluating the human genome, this technology has limitations in which types of variants can be detected[1,5,11,18,29] (Table 13.1). It is well suited for detecting sequence variants that affect one or a few nucleotides (i.e., single-nucleotide variants; SNVs) in unique gene sequences, including missense mutations that result in a change in amino acid in the encoded protein; nonsense and frameshift mutations that cause premature stop codons (stop-gain mutations) resulting mostly in the absence of the protein; and splice-site mutations, which can disrupt exon-splicing, thereby altering the encoded protein. However, the final assembled sequence in NGS relies on the alignment of overlapping relatively short sequenced fragments, which does not work well for sequences with high homology to another sequence in the genome, such as duplicated genes or exons; pseudogenes; and highly homologous gene families. Repeat sequences, including endogenous repeats and triplet repeat amplification mutations, such as the CGG repeat expansion in the 5′ untranslated region of the *FMR1* gene that causes fragile X syndrome, are also difficult to detect by NGS. In addition, detection of structural chromosomal abnormalities or aneuploidy from WES is challenging and not currently feasible for clinical use; CMA remains the method of choice for clinical diagnosis of larger unbalanced chromosomal abnormalities[1,5,11,29,30] (see Chapter 12). In contrast, larger-size copy number changes, structural chromosomal abnormalities, and aneuploidy can be detected by low-coverage WGS, which can be used for detection of aneuploidy and for prenatal and preimplantation diagnosis.[31,32] Many of the currently used noninvasive cell-free DNA screening strategies for fetal aneuploidy rely on the principle of counting fragments sequenced through low-coverage WGS of maternal plasma cfDNA.[1] (see Chapter 9).

TABLE 13.1			
Types of Variants Detectable With Different NGS Applications			

	NGS METHOD		
Variant Type	**Multigene Panel**	**Whole Exome Sequencing**	**Whole Genome Sequencing**
Aneuploidy	–	–	++
Balanced chromosome rearrangements	–	–	+
Large CNV: >5 Mb	–	–	+
Intermediate CNV: 1–5 Mb	–	–	++
Small CNV: 0.1–1 Mb	++	+	++
Insertions/deletions <100 bp	+++	+++	+++
SNV in unique exons	+++	+++	+++
SNV at intron/exon boundary	+++	+++	+++
SNV in introns	–	–	+++
SNV in region of high homology	?	–	–
Mosaic SNV >15–20%[a]	++[a]	++[a]	++[a]
Trinucleotide repeat expansion	–	–	–

–, method not recommended; ?, can be detected depending on panel design; +, sometimes possible to detect; ++, adequately detected; +++ very well detected; *CNV*, copy number variant; *NGS*, next-generation sequencing; *SNV*, single-nucleotide variant.
[a]Algorithms for interpretation may need adjustment to detect mosaicism.

WES focuses on the 1%–2% of the genome that includes the coding sequences, whereas WGS has the potential to provide information on variants in other important regions, such as promoters and regulatory elements. For this reason, WGS has a higher diagnostic capacity, although it is more complex to confirm that a detected sequence variant truly causes the condition for which the sequencing was done, and often requires functional studies in cell lines or animal models. This is an important reason, in addition to higher cost, why diagnostic WGS is not currently routinely used by most laboratories.

Categories of Results, Incidental and Secondary Findings Found With Next-Generation Sequencing

The first category of results, which are always reported, is the pathogenic or likely pathogenic variants in genes that are (potentially) relevant to the indication for sequencing. In contrast, variants interpreted as benign or likely benign are usually not reported, as they have no clinical consequences. VUSs, for which pathogenicity is not established, are more complicated, as the benefit of reporting them must be weighed against the potential consequences of knowing such results,

including parental anxiety and decisions regarding prenatal and neonatal management being made based on uncertain information (Table 13.2A).

Another category involves results that are "incidental findings" (Table 13.2B), which are variants in genes that could cause a clinically significant disorder different from the original indication for sequencing. The ACMG has published guidelines stating that laboratories performing WES and WGS should actively search for pathogenic variants in 59 genes that cause largely adult-onset conditions such as a predisposition for cancer or cardiovascular disorders, for which a preventive or therapeutic action can improve health outcomes. They state that individuals undergoing genome-wide sequencing should be informed about this during pretest counseling and be given the option to "opt out" of receiving information on these "secondary findings" as part of their sequencing results. However, the ACMG guidelines specifically exclude recommendations regarding prenatally performed WES.[33-35] Specific guidance on reporting actionable findings in prenatal diagnosis is therefore still needed and must consider that variants in many of the 59 genes cause adult-onset disorders, that have until now largely been excluded from prenatal testing. Finally, variants that do not cause disease but confer carrier

TABLE 13.2
Classification of Sequence Variants

A. BY MUTATION PATHOGENICITY

- Pathogenic
- Likely pathogenic
- Variant of uncertain significance
- Likely benign
- Benign

B. BY RELEVANCE TO THE INDICATION FOR SEQUENCING

- In gene relevant to the phenotype
- In gene causing a different disease (incidental and secondary findings)

status for autosomal recessive or X-linked disorders, as well as pharmacogenetic variants, which may be relevant to response to certain medications or susceptibility to their side effects or toxicity, can be found with genome-wide sequencing and laboratories should have and communicate policies on whether and when they will report such variants.

WHAT IS THE DIFFERENCE BETWEEN PROBAND AND TRIO SEQUENCING?

When time is of the essence, such as in prenatal applications of diagnostic sequencing or for critically ill newborns with suspected genetic disorders,[36] a trio approach to sequencing is often used and is currently the recommended strategy for prenatal WES.[27] In trio WES, the DNA of the proband and both biological parents are sequenced in parallel. The sequence data from all three samples is then integrated to facilitate the analysis and interpretation of detected variants in the proband's (fetal) sequence. This allows for a more rapid determination of inheritance (de novo or inherited) and pathogenicity of variants. The challenges of trio sequencing are primarily related to informed consent and genetic counseling issues surrounding incidental and secondary findings in parents and are discussed in more detail under pre- and posttest counseling below.

WHAT HAS BEEN THE CLINICAL EXPERIENCE TO DATE WITH GENOME-WIDE SEQUENCING FOR PRENATAL DIAGNOSIS?

Diagnostic genome-wide sequencing, most commonly WES, is now regularly used for diagnosis of children and adults with suspected genetic disorders, birth defects, or other rare phenotypes of unknown cause. The reported diagnostic rate varies from 16% to 40% depending on the indication and population that was sequenced.[37–42] Even higher detection rates of more than 50% for some phenotypes and indications have been reported in recent studies on WES for critically ill neonates.[36,43] Based on these combined data, we have predicted that prenatal WES could potentially double the genetic diagnostic rate for fetal anomalies of unknown cause after standard workup with CMA and karyotype.

Early experience with prenatal WES consisted primarily of case reports and smaller series, some of which were embedded within larger postnatal series of diagnostic WES.[37,38,44–47] In a report on 30 cases of WES performed for prenatally detected fetal anomalies, the diagnostic rate was 10%, with an additional 17% in which variants of *potential* clinical significance were found.[48] Another study on 24 fetuses with ultrasound-detected abnormalities reported a 25% detection rate.[49] In 2017, a review of published and presented studies with more than five cases concluded that the diagnostic rate of WES was highly variable between 6.2% and 80%.[5] This suggests that there is high variability between the different studies in case selection and in which types of variants are considered pathogenic and therefore which are reported. Since then, Vora et al. reported a diagnosis or possible diagnosis in 7/15 (47%) in a small series of pregnancies with fetal anomalies.[50] Fu et al. performed WES on a research basis for 196 fetuses with normal CMA and karyotype, selected by the authors from >3900 cases with fetal anomalies, and reported a diagnostic rate of variants thought to be related to the clinical phenotype of 24%, with 6.1% having incidental findings and 12.8% identified with at least one VUS.[51] Data from the diagnostic laboratory affiliated with our institution[51a] show an overall diagnostic rate of WES for fetal anomalies of 32%. This series also contains a cohort of pregnancies that were still ongoing at the time of sequencing, with a similar diagnostic rate of 35%. Several larger prospective studies are planned and ongoing, which are anticipated to clarify the molecular diagnostic rate and clinical utility of WES for prenatally diagnosed fetal congenital anomalies in ongoing pregnancies.

A number of studies with mixed prenatal and neonatal samples have also begun to examine the benefit of WES for prenatally diagnosed fetal anomalies in specific organ systems. In one study, focusing on fetuses with congenital anomalies of the kidneys and urinary tract (CAKUT) with or without other associated abnormalities, pathogenic variants were found in 4/30 (14%)

cases where other tests were negative.[52] Chandler et al. reported an 81% (13/16) molecular diagnostic rate for skeletal dysplasias when rapid trio WES was done and variant interpretation focused on 240 relevant genes.[53] Other areas where early data indicate that WES will be effective is for prenatal lethal phenotypes,[45,54,55] or for cases with multiple affected pregnancies and suspicion for autosomal recessive inheritance.[55] In addition, in the absence of fetal DNA specimens, one report of WES of parental samples with integrated variant interpretation provided a diagnostic yield of >50%.[56]

WHAT ARE THE COMPONENTS OF PRETEST AND POSTTEST COUNSELING FOR PRENATAL NEXT-GENERATION SEQUENCING?

Counseling for genome-wide sequencing is typically lengthy and complicated because of the types and categories of results that will be reported, potential uncertainty of the findings, the implications for disease prediction, and prognosis for the sequenced proband and for family members. It is best done by expert professionals trained in genetics who can convey information in clear language understandable to lay persons. The individuals doing the genetic counseling should be trained in individual risk assessment and in nondirective guidance of parental decision-making regarding pregnancy management. This is especially challenging in the preconception and prenatal period, when testing is often pursued during a stressful time when parents are faced with recently discovered fetal anomalies. This counseling process begins before the test is performed and sometimes continues until well after the results are communicated.

WHO SHOULD RECEIVE COUNSELING AND PROVIDE INFORMED CONSENT?

To achieve timely and accurate results, the current approach to fetal genome-wide sequencing is to perform "trio sequencing." Thus, considering that information is obtained about three individuals, including the fetus (proband) and both biological parents, it is recommended that both parents receive pretest counseling and participate in the informed consent process. Practically, this usually occurs in a joint session with both parents. However, considering the possibility of discovering nonpaternity or an undisclosed close relationship between parents, some have recommended that the parents receive pretest counseling separately to allow the woman to decline the test independently in the event she is

concerned about revealing this information. If joint pretest counseling is performed with both parents, the biological mother should have an independent opportunity for a confidential individual conversation early in the process, during which the potential to discover nonpaternity is discussed and she is given the opportunity to decline testing if desired. Counseling for pregnancies conceived using gamete donors is more complex. Trio sequencing is not possible when anonymous donors are involved, and the potential risk of identifying the donor from the fetal sequence must be included in the pretest education. When known donors contribute gametes, they may have to be informed and included in the consent procedure when trio sequencing is used.

WHAT ARE THE ELEMENTS OF PRETEST EDUCATION AND INFORMED CONSENT?

It is recognized that detailed information about the technology and the conditions that can be detected will be too complex and potentially overwhelming for parents. This hinders understanding and retention of the most important information that parents need to make reasonably informed decisions. Thus, generalized information about the nature of the WES (or WGS) test along with opportunities for parents to ask questions and present their viewpoints is generally more effective and better received. Parents should be informed that until large studies are completed, experience with WES or WGS for prenatal diagnosis is still very limited, and that the true detection rate for a clinically significant result is not yet known and varies with the indication.[5]

As with all genetic testing, counseling should include the concept that testing is optional and not contingent on any management decisions parents might make with the results. Information should be provided about possible outcomes (definitive pathogenic variant, likely pathogenic variant, uncertain findings, incidental and secondary findings, negative result, no result), about the potential to uncover nonpaternity or close parentage (unknown parental consanguinity and in trios, also grand-parental consanguinity). Pretest counseling should include laboratory policies for reporting incidental findings, secondary findings, and VUS along with any options for parental choices and decisions regarding such information.[13,57] The estimated turnaround time from sample procurement to results should be communicated, including how sample volume and quality can affect reportable results and turnaround time. With a rapid trio WES, the turnaround time can be less than 2–3 weeks, but often the results take significantly longer.

Because the field is evolving so quickly, and our knowledge regarding variants is increasing rapidly, options and policies for future reinterpretation of the results should also be communicated.[27] Cost of testing, insurance coverage, and possible effects on future insurability should also be addressed.[58] Patients should be informed about the benefits and risks of sharing of variant information in public databases or research exchange services such as GeneMatcher,[59] and their consent for information sharing should be documented (Table 13.3A).[27]

WHAT ARE THE ELEMENTS OF RESULTS DISCLOSURE AND POSTTEST COUNSELING?

Prenatal genome-wide sequencing is complex, and all posttest counseling (Table 13.3B) is ideally performed in person, in a dedicated counseling session, during which all available information (including negative results) and their implication is conveyed. Parents should be given the opportunity to revisit their choices for receiving uncertain results and secondary findings and be given the opportunity to ask questions. Posttest counseling should also include a discussion about pregnancy and neonatal management options, including reproductive decisions based on the results. Fully addressing all of these may require more than one encounter with a genetics professional as well as a multidisciplinary team approach, depending on the results. The importance of results for parents and other family members should also be discussed along with resources and advice on best strategies to inform those who may benefit from knowing the results.

WHAT ARE CURRENT ETHICAL AND SOCIETAL CONSIDERATIONS?

Clinical implementation of new complex diagnostic tests such as exome sequencing should consider the four guiding medical ethics principles of autonomy, beneficence, nonmaleficence, and justice. To be

---

TABLE 13.3
Elements of Genetic Counseling for Prenatal Diagnostic Whole Exome Sequencing

A. PRETEST COUNSELING ELEMENTS

1. Both parents included because of trio sequencing
2. Independent consent option for mother, to address possible nonpaternity detection
3. Timeframe to results and possibility of no or late result (after birth)
4. Realistic expectations about diagnostic rate
5. Categories of results that can be identified
6. Possibility for variants of uncertain significance
7. Reporting policies and options for incidental and secondary findings, including adult-onset disorders and carrier status
8. Implications of results for parents and other family members
9. Potential for discovery of consanguinity
10. Importance of data sharing and reinterpretation
11. Expected cost

B. POSTTEST COUNSELING

1. Discloses results and implications for prognosis for the fetus after birth
2. Confirms choices and policies on incidental findings from pretest counseling
3. Addresses confirmatory testing
4. Addresses decisions about pregnancy, delivery and neonatal management
5. Addresses implications of results for parents and other family members
6. Facilitates multidisciplinary referral and care
7. Emotional support

able to exert their *autonomy* as decision-makers for their future children, parents have to understand sufficient general information about the test itself and the implications of test results. Thus, providers have to be knowledgeable enough to provide comprehensive pretest counseling adapted to the parents' level of understanding.[5,60] Such pretest counseling should cover all aspects, including disclosure of close parentage, nonpaternity, consanguinity, and the potential for actionable variants in parents when trio sequencing is done. Parental autonomy must be weighed against the future child's autonomy to decide whether he or she wishes to know genetic information about them.[61] This is especially relevant for adult-onset disorders, for which any incidental discovery during prenatal testing carries the same ethical difficulties as presymptomatic testing in children.[62-64] The contrasting ethical principles of *beneficence* and *nonmaleficence* drive guidance on reporting of secondary and incidental findings and VUS. The ACMG recommendation on reporting pathogenic variants in 59 actionable genes in exome data specifically excludes consideration of fetal diagnosis,[34,35] likely because the possible actions after such a finding differ between prenatal and postnatal testing, primarily because the option of pregnancy termination exists prenatally. For example, if a *BRCA1* mutation is found in a fetus, a decision to terminate a pregnancy can be contemplated, whereas if found in children or adults, screening for cancer and early treatment are the only option.

Likewise, receiving information on VUS in WES results can be very difficult for parents,[65] but withholding this information must be balanced against the parents right (*autonomy*) to knowledge. An important argument in favor of disclosure of VUS is the fact that this interpretation may change over time, and thus a VUS may be reclassified to pathogenic or benign if reanalysis is performed. Regular reanalysis may create an emotional burden on families and financial strain for the health-care system,[66-68] and it has been suggested that this should be decided in shared decision-making between parents and providers.[69]

Clinical Utility and Cost

The ethical principle of *justice* considers equitable access to health-care and medical resources. WES and WGS are costly tests and are still performed for prenatal diagnosis at a relatively small scale outside research settings. Fetal genome and exome sequencing is not reimbursed by all private health insurers or national health systems, who have to assure equitable distribution of limited resources.[66-68] The cost-effectiveness and clinical utility of WES or WGS for ongoing pregnancies have not yet been comprehensively evaluated, but such studies are underway.[69] Important considerations include not only the price of the test but also counseling, follow-up testing, data storage, and reinterpretation costs, which should be compared with the cost of an unknown diagnosis or an unsuccessful lengthy and expensive "diagnostic odyssey."

WHAT ARE CURRENT PROFESSIONAL GUIDELINES REGARDING PRENATAL NEXT-GENERATION SEQUENCING?

Few organizations have provided guidance on the use of WES and WGS for prenatal diagnosis, in part because large prospective trials on their use in ongoing pregnancies have not yet been completed. ACOG and ACMG state that the clinical utility of fetal WES and WGS in ongoing pregnancies has not yet been demonstrated and that it should therefore not yet be routinely used.[70,71] Recently, the International Society for Prenatal Diagnosis (ISPD), Society for Maternal-Fetal Medicine (SMFM), and the Perinatal Quality Foundation (PQF)[27] issued a joint position statement about fetal genome sequencing. Although this joint statement largely agrees with the ACOG/ACMG recommendations and highlights the need for more research on the benefits and limitations of WES/WGS, this statement did conclude that diagnostic prenatal genome-wide sequencing may be acceptable if done by teams of experts for certain specific indications where a single gene disorder is highly suspected and routine testing has yielded no genetic diagnosis.[27,71]

WHAT ARE THE CLINICAL CONSIDERATIONS AND RECOMMENDATIONS FOR PRENATAL USE OF NEXT-GENERATION SEQUENCING?

1. Genome-wide DNA sequencing is a new technology that improves the ability to find the genetic variants that cause single gene disorders. There are two approaches, the first and most commonly used clinically at the present time is WES, which focuses on the 1%–2% of the genome that codes for proteins and some noncoding RNAs. The second, lesser used alternative is WGS, which sequences the entire genome, including promoters and other regulatory regions. WGS is currently more expensive and not yet widely used for clinical diagnosis. Although it

can identify more potentially deleterious sequence variants, including those in noncoding regions, it is more difficult to prove that these are disease-causing and to interpret the very large quantity of data obtained. Low-coverage WGS can detect structural and numerical chromosomal abnormalities rearrangements, which are more difficult to find with WES.

2. WES has an incremental diagnostic yield of 25%–40% over standard testing in pediatric and adult populations, but its diagnostic yield when used for prenatal diagnosis is much more variable and ranges from 6% to more than 80% and varies by indication and patient selection, with higher detection rates for skeletal dysplasias, fetuses with multiple anomalies, and clinical presentations suggestive of autosomal recessive inheritance.

3. Although WES has promise for prenatal diagnosis, its indications, benefits and pitfalls, overall incremental diagnostic rate and clinical utility have not yet been established and will have to await the data from larger prospective studies that are currently ongoing and planned. Until then it is best done in a research protocol but could be offered clinically in rare circumstances when a single gene disorder is highly suspected and under guidance of experts in genetics who have experience with prenatal use of diagnostic genome-wide sequencing.

4. For prenatal diagnosis, time to results is critical, and WES is best performed in a trio-sequencing approach, in which parental DNA is sequenced along with the fetal DNA to expedite interpretation of the pathogenicity of sequence variants found in the fetal DNA.

5. With genome-wide genetic testing strategies, there is a chance for detecting incidental and secondary findings, VUSs, or of not obtaining a diagnosis. Other possible outcomes are discovery of nonpaternity, close parentage, and findings that are relevant to the health of family members. Parents should be counseled about the benefits of WES and these pitfalls and be informed on options they have for receiving certain types of results as part of the informed consent process.

6. Because WES is a new technology, data collection and sharing in a deidentified fashion will be important to monitor the clinical utility and advance the field, and this should be included in the informed consent for testing. Likewise, because knowledge about the pathogenic changes in the genome is rapidly evolving, regular sequence variant reinterpretation, in particular before or early in subsequent pregnancies will be important.

SUMMARY

Genome-wide sequencing, WES and WGS, is an evolving technology with great potential. Early data suggest that it will significantly increase our ability to prenatally identify the cause of genetic disorders and birth defects. More studies are needed to establish its true clinical utility and the balance of benefits of an increased diagnostic rate to pitfalls, such as risk for incidental and uncertain findings. Currently, the depth and coverage required to survey the entire exome or genome for single gene disorders through sequencing will continue to require fetal DNA obtained through an invasive procedure and a trio-sequencing approach to have timely results. Nevertheless, it is already technically possible to survey the fetal genome noninvasively, but both the cost and time needed to obtain single-nucleotide resolution results, currently preclude this from being applied clinically. However, as both technology and genomic knowledge increase, this may become a reality in the remote future.

REFERENCES

1. Van den Veyver IB. Recent advances in prenatal genetic screening and testing. *F1000Res*. 2016;5:2591.
2. Hillman SC, McMullan DJ, Hall G, et al. Use of prenatal chromosomal microarray: prospective cohort study and systematic review and meta-analysis. *Ultrasound Obstet Gynecol*. 2013;41:610–620.
3. Wapner RJ, Martin CL, Levy B, et al. Chromosomal microarray versus karyotyping for prenatal diagnosis. *N Engl J Med*. 2012;367:2175–2184.
4. Hillman SC, Willams D, Carss KJ, et al. Prenatal exome sequencing for fetuses with structural abnormalities: the next step. *Ultrasound Obstet Gynecol*. 2015;45:4–9.
5. Best S, Wou K, Vora N, et al. Promises, pitfalls and practicalities of prenatal whole exome sequencing. *Prenat Diagn*. 2017;38:10–19.
6. Baird PA, Anderson TW, Newcombe HB, Lowry RB. Genetic disorders in children and young adults: a population study. *Am J Hum Genet*. 1988;42:677–693.
7. Beaudet AL, Scriver CR, Sly WS, Valle D. Genetics, biochemistry, and molecular bases of variant human phenotypes. In: Valle D, Beaudet AL, Vogelstein B, et al., eds. *The Online Metabolic and Molecular Bases of Inherited Disease*. New York, NY: McGraw-Hill; 2014. http://ommbid.mhmedical.com.ezproxyhost.library.tmc.edu/content.aspx?bookid=971&sectionid=62632821.
8. Scriver CR, Neal JL, Saginur R, Clow A. The frequency of genetic disease and congenital malformation among patients in a pediatric hospital. *Can Med Assoc J*. 1973;108:1111–1115.
9. Bamshad MJ, Ng SB, Bigham AW, et al. Exome sequencing as a tool for Mendelian disease gene discovery. *Nat Rev Genet*. 2011;12:745–755.

10. Biesecker LG, Green RC. Diagnostic clinical genome and exome sequencing. *N Engl J Med.* 2014;371:1170.

11. Normand EA, Alaimo JT, Van den Veyver IB. Exome and genome sequencing in reproductive medicine. *Fertil Steril.* 2018;109:213–220.

12. Rehm HL, Bale SJ, Bayrak-Toydemir P, et al. ACMG clinical laboratory standards for next-generation sequencing. *Genet Med.* 2013;15:733–747.

13. Abou Tayoun AN, Spinner NB, Rehm HL, et al. Prenatal DNA sequencing: clinical, counseling, and diagnostic laboratory considerations. *Prenat Diagn.* 2018;38:26–32.

14. Genomes Project C, Auton A, Brooks LD, et al. A global reference for human genetic variation. *Nature.* 2015;526:68–74.

15. Gonzaga-Jauregui C, Lupski JR, Gibbs RA. Human genome sequencing in health and disease. *Annu Rev Med.* 2012;63:35–61.

16. Richards S, Aziz N, Bale S, et al. Standards and guidelines for the interpretation of sequence variants: a joint consensus recommendation of the American College of medical genetics and genomics and the association for molecular pathology. *Genet Med.* 2015;17:405–424.

17. Rehm HL, Berg JS, Brooks LD, et al. ClinGen–the clinical genome resource. *N Engl J Med.* 2015;372:2235–2242.

18. Xue Y, Ankala A, Wilcox WR, Hegde MR. Solving the molecular diagnostic testing conundrum for Mendelian disorders in the era of next-generation sequencing: single-gene, gene panel, or exome/genome sequencing. *Genet Med.* 2015;17:444–451.

19. Lek M, Karczewski KJ, Minikel EV, et al. Analysis of protein-coding genetic variation in 60,706 humans. *Nature.* 2016;536:285–291.

20. Landrum MJ, Lee JM, Benson M, et al. ClinVar: public archive of interpretations of clinically relevant variants. *Nucleic Acids Res.* 2016;44:D862–D868.

21. Stenson PD, Mort M, Ball EV, et al. The Human Gene Mutation Database: towards a comprehensive repository of inherited mutation data for medical research, genetic diagnosis and next-generation sequencing studies. *Hum Genet.* 2017;136:665–677.

22. Firth HV, Richards SM, Bevan AP, et al. DECIPHER: database of chromosomal imbalance and phenotype in humans using Ensembl resources. *Am J Hum Genet.* 2009;84:524–533.

23. Adzhubei IA, Schmidt S, Peshkin L, et al. A method and server for predicting damaging missense mutations. *Nat Methods.* 2010;7:248–249.

24. Kumar P, Henikoff S, Ng PC. Predicting the effects of coding non-synonymous variants on protein function using the SIFT algorithm. *Nat Protoc.* 2009;4:1073–1081.

25. Schwarz JM, Cooper DN, Schuelke M, Seelow D. MutationTaster2: mutation prediction for the deep-sequencing age. *Nat Methods.* 2014;11:361–362.

26. ACMG Board of Directors. Laboratory and clinical genomic data sharing is crucial to improving genetic health care: a position statement of the American College of Medical Genetics and Genomics. *Genet Med.* 2017;19:721–722.

27. International Society for Prenatal Diagnosis. Society for maternal-fetal medicine, perinatal quality Foundation. Joint position statement from the International Society for Prenatal Diagnosis (ISPD), the Society for Maternal Fetal Medicine (SMFM), and the Perinatal Quality Foundation (PQF) on the use of genome-wide sequencing for fetal diagnosis. *Prenat Diagn.* 2018;38:6–9.

28. Robinson PN, Mundlos S. The human phenotype ontology. *Clin Genet.* 2010;77:525–534.

29. Van den Veyver IB, Eng CM. Genome-wide sequencing for prenatal detection of fetal single-gene disorders. *Cold Spring Harb Perspect Med.* 2015:5.

30. Gao J, Wan C, Zhang H, et al. Anaconda: AN automated pipeline for somatic COpy Number variation Detection and Annotation from tumor exome sequencing data. *BMC Bioinformatics.* 2017;18:436.

31. Dong Z, Zhang J, Hu P, et al. Low-pass whole-genome sequencing in clinical cytogenetics: a validated approach. *Genet Med.* 2016;18:940–948.

32. Dong Z, Wang H, Chen H, et al. Identification of balanced chromosomal rearrangements previously unknown among participants in the 1000 Genomes Project: implications for interpretation of structural variation in genomes and the future of clinical cytogenetics. *Genet Med.* 2017.

33. Green RC, Berg JS, Grody WW, et al. ACMG recommendations for reporting of incidental findings in clinical exome and genome sequencing. *Genet Med.* 2013;15:565–574.

34. ACMG Board of Directors. ACMG policy statement: updated recommendations regarding analysis and reporting of secondary findings in clinical genome-scale sequencing. *Genet Med.* 2015;17:68–69.

35. Kalia SS, Adelman K, Bale SJ, et al. Recommendations for reporting of secondary findings in clinical exome and genome sequencing, 2016 update (ACMG SF v2.0): a policy statement of the American College of Medical Genetics and Genomics. *Genet Med.* 2017;19:249–255.

36. Meng L, Pammi M, Saronwala A, et al. Use of exome sequencing for infants in intensive care units: ascertainment of severe single-gene disorders and effect on medical management. *JAMA Pediatr.* 2017:e173438.

37. Yang Y, Muzny DM, Xia F, et al. Molecular findings among patients referred for clinical whole-exome sequencing. *Jama.* 2014;312:1870–1879.

38. Yang Y, Muzny DM, Reid JG, et al. Clinical whole-exome sequencing for the diagnosis of mendelian disorders. *N Engl J Med.* 2013;369:1502–1511.

39. Retterer K, Juusola J, Cho MT, et al. Clinical application of whole-exome sequencing across clinical indications. *Genet Med.* 2016;18:696–704.

40. Trujillano D, Bertoli-Avella AM, Kumar Kandaswamy K, et al. Clinical exome sequencing: results from 2819 samples reflecting 1000 families. *Eur J Hum Genet.* 2017;25:176–182.

41. Sawyer SL, Hartley T, Dyment DA, et al. Utility of whole-exome sequencing for those near the end of the diagnostic odyssey: time to address gaps in care. *Clin Genet.* 2016;89:275–284.

42. Srivastava S, Cohen JS, Vernon H, et al. Clinical whole exome sequencing in child neurology practice. *Ann Neurol*. 2014;76:473–483.

43. Stark Z, Tan TY, Chong B, et al. A prospective evaluation of whole-exome sequencing as a first-tier molecular test in infants with suspected monogenic disorders. *Genet Med*. 2016;18:1090–1096.

44. Talkowski ME, Ordulu Z, Pillalamarri V, et al. Clinical diagnosis by whole-genome sequencing of a prenatal sample. *N Engl J Med*. 2012;367:2226–2232.

45. Shamseldin HE, Swaid A, Alkuraya FS. Lifting the lid on unborn lethal Mendelian phenotypes through exome sequencing. *Genet Med*. 2013;15:307–309.

46. Filges I, Nosova E, Bruder E, et al. Exome sequencing identifies mutations in KIF14 as a novel cause of an autosomal recessive lethal fetal ciliopathy phenotype. *Clin Genet*. 2014;86:220–228.

47. Alamillo CL, Powis Z, Farwell K, et al. Exome sequencing positively identified relevant alterations in more than half of cases with an indication of prenatal ultrasound anomalies. *Prenat Diagn*. 2015;35:1073–1078.

48. Carss KJ, Hillman SC, Parthiban V, et al. Exome sequencing improves genetic diagnosis of structural fetal abnormalities revealed by ultrasound. *Hum Mol Genet*. 2014;23:3269–3277.

49. Drury S, Williams H, Trump N, et al. Exome sequencing for prenatal diagnosis of fetuses with sonographic abnormalities. *Prenat Diagn*. 2015;35:1010–1017.

50. Vora NL, Powell B, Brandt A, et al. Prenatal exome sequencing in anomalous fetuses: new opportunities and challenges. *Genet Med*. 2017;19:1207–1216.

51. Fu F, Li R, Li Y, et al. Whole exome sequencing as a diagnostic adjunct to clinical testing in a tertiary referral cohort of 3988 fetuses with structural abnormalities. *Ultrasound Obstet Gynecol*. 2017.

51a. Normand EA, Braxton A, Nassef S, et al., Clinical exome sequencing for fetuses with ultrasound abnormalities and a suspected Mendelian disorder. *Genome Med*. 2018;10:74. Epub 2018/09/30. https://doi.org/10.1186/s13073-018-0582-x.

52. Lei TY, Fu F, Li R, et al. Whole-exome sequencing for prenatal diagnosis of fetuses with congenital anomalies of the kidney and urinary tract. *Nephrol Dial Transplant*. 2017;32:1665–1675.

53. Chandler N, Best S, Hayward J, et al. Rapid prenatal diagnosis using targeted exome sequencing: a cohort study to assess feasibility and potential impact on prenatal counseling and pregnancy management. *Genet Med*. 2018.

54. Filges I, Friedman JM. Exome sequencing for gene discovery in lethal fetal disorders - harnessing the value of extreme phenotypes. *Prenat Diagn*. 2015;35:1005–1009.

55. Ellard S, Kivuva E, Turnpenny P, et al. An exome sequencing strategy to diagnose lethal autosomal recessive disorders. *Eur J Hum Genet*. 2015;23:401–404.

56. Stals KL, Wakeling M, Baptista J, et al. Diagnosis of lethal or prenatal-onset autosomal recessive disorders by parental exome sequencing. *Prenat Diagn*. 2018;38:33–43.

57. Westerfield L, Darilek S, Van den Veyver IB. Counseling challenges with variants of uncertain significance and incidental findings in prenatal genetic screening and diagnosis. *J Clin Med*. 2014;3:1018–1032.

58. Fonda Allen J, Stoll K, Bernhardt BA. Pre- and post-test genetic counseling for chromosomal and Mendelian disorders. *Semin Perinatol*. 2016;40:44–55.

59. Sobreira N, Schiettecatte F, Valle D, Hamosh A. GeneMatcher: a matching tool for connecting investigators with an interest in the same gene. *Hum Mutat*. 2015;36:928–930.

60. Horn R, Parker M. Opening Pandora's box?: ethical issues in prenatal whole genome and exome sequencing. *Prenat Diagn*. 2017.

61. Yurkiewicz IR, Korf BR, Lehmann LS. Prenatal whole-genome sequencing–is the quest to know a fetus's future ethical? *N Engl J Med*. 2014;370:195–197.

62. Burke W, Matheny Antommaria AH, Bennett R, et al. Recommendations for returning genomic incidental findings? We need to talk!. *Genet Med*. 2013;15:854–859.

63. Mand C, Gillam L, Duncan RE, Delatycki MB. "It was the missing piece": adolescent experiences of predictive genetic testing for adult-onset conditions. *Genet Med*. 2013;15:643–649.

64. Anderson JA, Hayeems RZ, Shuman C, et al. Predictive genetic testing for adult-onset disorders in minors: a critical analysis of the arguments for and against the 2013 ACMG guidelines. *Clin Genet*. 2015;87:301–310.

65. Bernhardt BA, Roche MI, Perry DL, et al. Experiences with obtaining informed consent for genomic sequencing. *Am J Med Genet*. 2015;167A:2635–2646.

66. Westerfield LE, Stover SR, Mathur VS, et al. Reproductive genetic counseling challenges associated with diagnostic exome sequencing in a large academic private reproductive genetic counseling practice. *Prenat Diagn*. 2015;35:1022–1029.

67. Chitty LS, Friedman JM, Langlois S. Current controversies in prenatal diagnosis 2: should a fetal exome be used in the assessment of a dysmorphic or malformed fetus? *Prenat Diagn*. 2016;36:15–19.

68. Quinlan-Jones E, Kilby MD, Greenfield S, et al. Prenatal whole exome sequencing: the views of clinicians, scientists, genetic counsellors and patient representatives. *Prenat Diagn*. 2016;36:935–941.

69. Westerfield LE, Braxton AA, Walkiewicz M. Prenatal diagnostic exome sequencing: a review. *Curr Gen Med Rep*. 2017.

70. ACOG Committee on Genetics and Society for Maternal-Fetal Medicine. Committee opinion no. 682: microarrays and next-generation sequencing technology: the use of advanced genetic diagnostic tools in Obstetrics and Gynecology. *Obstet Gynecol*. 2016;128:e262–e268.

71. ACMG Board of Directors. Points to consider in the clinical application of genomic sequencing. *Genet Med*. 2012;14:759–761.

CHAPTER 14

Prenatal Diagnostic Testing

MARY E. NORTON, MD

INTRODUCTION

Testing is available for an ever-increasing number of genetic disorders. Although prenatal testing originally focused primarily on Down syndrome, it is now possible to detect a broad range of genetic conditions. Prenatal diagnostic testing is most commonly performed on fetal tissue obtained with amniocentesis or chorionic villus sampling (CVS), although umbilical cord blood obtained through percutaneous sampling is occasionally used. In the early embryo, preimplantation genetic testing (PGT) is also used for genetic diagnosis in families at risk for specific genetic disorders (see Chapter 15). The focus of this chapter is on CVS and amniocentesis, as these are the techniques most commonly used for routine prenatal testing.

Prenatal genetic testing is focused on every woman's values and preferences, which vary greatly.[1] Before undergoing prenatal diagnostic testing, women should understand the benefits and limitations of such testing, the conditions that are being tested for, as well as the conditions that will not be detected, and the risks of the procedure. Prenatal genetic testing can provide reassurance when results are normal, identify disorders for which in utero treatment might be available, improve neonatal outcomes by assuring the best location for delivery and that appropriate pediatric specialists are available to care for affected infants, and can also provide the opportunity for pregnancy termination for women who choose that option.

Fetal genetic disorders that are amenable to prenatal genetic testing include those abnormalities in structure or function that are caused by variants in an individual's genes, in contrast to those caused primarily by environmental or other disruptive causes; these latter conditions may be best identified by imaging. These distinctions are not always clear, as a genetic predisposition may increase the susceptibility to environmental influences, and some genetic abnormalities may only become apparent under specific environmental conditions or circumstances. Some disorders may have an epigenetic basis; in other words, gene functions may be turned on or silenced by modifications that may depend on the parent of origin or other influences (see Chapter 2). With improvements in our ability to study genetics and genomics, it is increasingly appreciated that inheritance and genetics are complex and our understanding is still relatively limited. For this reason, prenatal diagnosis can be complicated, and it is not always possible to predict the outcome based on a prenatal genetic test. It is important that patients understand that prenatal diagnostic testing is possible for many, but not all, genetic disorders.

WHAT CONDITIONS CAN BE DIAGNOSED BY PRENATAL GENETIC TESTING?

In general, chromosomal abnormalities and single gene disorders can be identified by analysis of fetal tissue, and it is these categories of conditions that are most often the target of prenatal diagnostic testing. Chromosomal abnormalities are relatively common in pregnancy, and about 1/150 live births has a chromosomal abnormality that causes an abnormal phenotype.[2] About 5% of stillbirths and 5–7% of infant and childhood deaths result from chromosomal abnormalities,[3] and chromosomal abnormalities are commonly associated with structural fetal abnormalities.[4] Copy number variants (CNVs), which can be detected with chromosomal microarray analysis (CMA), are present in about 1–1.7% of structurally normal fetuses and about 6% of those with an abnormality detected by ultrasound.[5]

Chromosomal abnormalities include variations in chromosome number or structure. The most common abnormality of chromosome number found by prenatal testing is aneuploidy, which is the presence of an extra or missing chromosome or chromosomes. It is also possible to have one or more extra sets of chromosomes, as in triploidy or tetraploidy. Abnormalities in chromosome number can be mosaic, in which the abnormal number of chromosomes is not present in all cells (see Chapter 4).

In addition to abnormalities of chromosome number, there can also be aberrations in chromosome structure, such as deletions, duplications, translocations,

Perinatal Genetics. https://doi.org/10.1016/B978-0-323-53094-1.00014-X

and other rearrangements. In some cases, rearrangements are balanced, meaning the appropriate genomic content is present but rearranged, whereas in other cases, translocations or other rearrangements can result in extra or missing pieces of chromosomes. Balanced translocations most often are associated with a normal phenotype, although they can lead to recurrent miscarriage or an increased risk of abnormal offspring. Deletions and duplications can be quite large, and easily seen by a karyotype, or can be small microdeletions or duplications only detectable with chromosomal microarray analysis (CMA), fluorescence in situ hybridization (FISH), or other specialized methods (see Chapter 6) (Table 14.1).

Some genetic disorders, such as cystic fibrosis, hemophilia, and Tay–Sachs disease, are caused by variants in single genes. Diseases caused solely by abnormalities in a single gene are relatively uncommon. The phenotype of some single gene disorders can be impacted by modifying genes, or by combinations of additional genes, as well as by environmental influences and therefore not all individuals who inherit a genetic variant will have the exact same phenotype. Single gene disorders can be detected by prenatal diagnostic testing if the disorder has been diagnosed with certainty and the particular variant within the family has been identified.

The most common congenital anomalies are isolated birth defects, such as heart defects, neural tube defects, and facial clefts. These traits are determined by multiple genes and environmental factors rather than by single genes. Because there is a genetic component, they often recur more commonly within a family. However, because they are not caused by a single gene variant but rather a complex interplay of genetic and environmental factors, prenatal diagnostic genetic testing is not available using specific DNA methods; rather diagnosis is usually made by ultrasound or

TABLE 14.1
Tests Available for Prenatal Genetic Diagnosis

Test	Turnaround Time	Conditions Detected	Comments
Karyotype	7–14 d	Chromosomal abnormalities >5–10 Mb	Traditional method for diagnosis of chromosomal abnormalities
Fluorescence in situ hybridization (FISH)—Interphase	24–48 h	Rapid assessment of major aneuploidies (typically chromosomes 13,18,21,X,Y)	Less accurate with chorionic villus sampling versus amniocentesis
FISH—Metaphase	7–14 d	Microdeletions and duplications	Can be used to test for specific abnormalities when clinically suspected; CMA often preferable
Chromosomal microarray analysis (CMA)	3–5 d (direct); 10–14 d (cultured cells)	Copy number variants (CNVs) >50–200 kb	Whole genome screen for CNVs. Detects major chromosomal abnormalities except balanced rearrangements and some triploidies
Molecular DNA testing	3–14 d (faster with direct testing than when cultured cells are required)	Genetic variants previously demonstrated to be present in a family or suspected based on ultrasound or other findings	Usually a targeted test focusing on a specific disorder (or category of disorders) suspected to be present in a fetus based on ultrasound findings or family history
Gene panels	10–14 days	Sets of genes or gene regions that are associated with common features or phenotypes, such as skeletal dysplasia	Often not as comprehensive as targeted single gene testing
Whole exome sequencing	Several weeks to months	Sequencing of all or most of the protein-coding genes in a genome	Often difficult to interpret in prenatal cases

other imaging. In some cases, an apparently isolated structural anomaly is associated with a cytogenetic abnormality or CNV, therefore karyotyping and/or chromosomal microarray analysis is recommended when one or more structural abnormalities is identified by ultrasound (see Chapter 12).

Although most genes are encoded in the nuclear genome, the mitochondria each contain their own genome. Variants can also occur in the mitochondrial DNA, and a number of mitochondrial diseases are due to these disorders. Mitochondria are essential for aerobic respiration, and mitochondrial diseases commonly affect tissues with high-energy requirements, such as the central nervous system, heart, and muscle. Mitochondria are all maternally inherited, and prenatal diagnosis for mitochondrial diseases can be complex and clinical outcomes are difficult to predict, due to variation in the number of abnormal mitochondria and the association with predicted phenotype (see Chapter 2).

HOW IS PRENATAL DIAGNOSTIC TESTING PERFORMED?

Prenatal diagnostic testing refers to genetic testing done on fetal tissue obtained most commonly by amniocentesis or CVS. Less commonly, fetal blood is obtained through percutaneous umbilical blood sampling. Testing of early embryos can also be done in conjunction with in vitro fertilization in a procedure known as preimplantation genetic testing (PGT) (see Chapter 15). Finally, fetal cell-free DNA (cfDNA) or potentially nucleated fetal cells can be obtained from the maternal circulation and tested for genetic disorders. However, such techniques at present are considered screening methods and are discussed elsewhere in this book (see Chapter 9).

Cytogenetic or karyotype analysis requires viable cells that can be cultured; such cells can be obtained by CVS, amniocentesis, or fetal blood sampling. DNA for molecular testing (including chromosomal microarray analysis) can be obtained from any cell with a nucleus, regardless of viability, including blood lymphocytes, skin, hair, cheek cells or saliva, and paraffin tissue blocks. Cultured amniocytes, chorionic villi, and fetal blood are tissues that can be used for prenatal DNA testing of the fetus; if adequate tissue is obtained, DNA can be extracted without the need for culture. Other fetal tissue biopsy, such as biopsy of fetal skin, muscle, or liver, was done in the past for direct measurement of fetal enzyme activity or other physiologic parameters. Such biopsies have been largely replaced by molecular DNA methods that can directly detect the underlying genetic basis of many congenital disorders (see Table 14.1).

Amniocentesis
Genetic amniocentesis is usually performed between 15 and 20 weeks of gestation. Typically, a 22-gauge spinal needle is inserted into the amniotic sac under ultrasound guidance, and approximately 20 mL of amniotic fluid is withdrawn. It is common to avoid penetrating the placenta to decrease the chance of causing bleeding into the amniotic fluid, which can lead to difficulty in culturing cells and can also lead to false-positive amniotic fluid alpha-fetoprotein measurement. In addition, placental penetration can potentially lead to alloimmunization if there is maternal-fetal red cell incompatibility. However, transplacental amniocentesis does not appear to be associated with an increased risk of pregnancy loss.[6,7]

Chorionic Villus Sampling
CVS is typically performed between 10–13 weeks of gestation. Placental villi may be obtained through either a transcervical or transabdominal approach. With transcervical CVS, a specialized catheter is inserted through the cervical os and guided into the placenta under ultrasound guidance. The transabdominal procedure is more similar to amniocentesis, and a needle (typically 20-gauge) is inserted into the placenta under ultrasound guidance. Typically, 15–25 mg of chorionic villi are obtained.

Although there are limited data comparing transcervical and transabdominal CVS, there does not appear to be a significant difference in fetal loss rates between the two approaches.[8,9] The primary advantage of CVS over amniocentesis is that results are available earlier in pregnancy, which provides reassurance for parents when results are normal and, when results are abnormal, may allow for earlier and safer pregnancy termination. In addition, for patients in whom specialized direct DNA testing is to be performed, CVS samples are more cellular and provide larger amounts of DNA for direct analysis, allowing a more rapid turnaround time.

WHAT ARE THE RISKS OF DIFFERENT PRENATAL DIAGNOSIS PROCEDURES?
The procedure-related loss rate of midtrimester amniocentesis at 16–20 weeks' gestation has decreased over time, likely because of increasing experience, as well as improvements in imaging. Patients at less than

24 weeks' gestation have a background loss rate without an invasive procedure, and this needs to be accounted for in calculating the excess loss rate due to amniocentesis or other tests. A recent metaanalysis of miscarriage risk after amniocentesis, including more than 42,000 women who underwent a procedure and 138,000 women who did not, estimated the loss rate because of the procedure at approximately 0.11% (95% CI, –0.04 to 0.26) or 1 in 900.[10] In this large study, the miscarriage rate was not statistically different in patients who did, or did not, have a procedure (P = .14). These data were collected relatively recently, so represent contemporary statistics.[11–17] Importantly, these data were collected from high-volume, experienced centers and may not apply to small sites or low-volume providers.

Minor complications from amniocentesis, including transient vaginal spotting or amniotic fluid leakage, occur after approximately 1%–2% of procedures. The outcomes of amniotic membrane rupture after amniocentesis are far better than after spontaneous ruptured membranes; the perinatal survival rate after amniotic fluid leakage following midtrimester amniocentesis is greater than 90%.[18] Direct injury to the fetus during amniocentesis has been reported but is rare when amniocentesis is performed under continuous ultrasound guidance. Amniotic fluid cell culture failure occurs in 0.1% of samples. In numerous studies, it has been reported that pregnancy loss, and complications such as blood-contaminated specimens, leaking of amniotic fluid, and the need for more than one needle puncture are related to the experience of the operator, the use of small-gauge needles, and ultrasound guidance.[19–21]

As with amniocentesis, determination of procedure-related loss rates after CVS requires consideration of the background loss rate, which is substantially higher in the first trimester during the gestational age window when CVS is performed. As with amniocentesis, the loss rate from CVS has decreased over time.[7] The most recent metaanalysis, including 54,000 women who had CVS and 670,000 who had no procedure, reported a procedure related loss rate of 0.1%. Including only those studies that specifically included a control group, the procedure-related loss rate was 0.22% (95% CI, –0.71–1.16). As in the analysis of amniocentesis, the loss rate in those patients who had a CVS procedure was not higher than the background rate (P = .638).[10,15,16,22]

Once again, an important caveat is that these data are from experienced, high-volume centers and may not apply to lower volume, less experienced providers. In several studies, it has been shown that there is a significant learning curve associated with the performance of CVS.[23,24]

Although there have been reports of associations between CVS and limb reduction and oromandibular defects, the risk for these anomalies appears to be low and to correlate with procedures performed at <10 weeks' gestation.[25] In an analysis by the World Health Organization, an incidence of limb-reduction defects of 6 per 10,000 was reported in infants to women who had undergone CVS, which is not significantly different from the incidence in the general population.[26] An increased risk of hemangiomas in the newborn has also been reported after CVS, primarily after transcervical CVS, in some but not all studies.[27,28] Hemangiomas are generally benign and resolve without treatment in early childhood. Other complications after CVS include vaginal spotting or bleeding, which occurs in up to 32% of patients after transcervical CVS and at a lower rate after transabdominal CVS. The incidence of culture failure, amniotic fluid leakage, or infection after CVS is less than 0.5%.

Early amniocentesis has been reported between 11 and 13 weeks of gestation using a technique similar to midtrimester amniocentesis.[29–31] However, early amniocentesis has been found to result in significantly higher rates of pregnancy loss and other complications compared with midtrimester amniocentesis. In a multicenter randomized trial, the spontaneous pregnancy loss rate after early amniocentesis was 2.5%, compared with 0.7% with traditional amniocentesis.[32] In addition, the incidence of club foot was markedly increased, occurring in 1.4% after early amniocentesis compared with 0.1% (comparable with the background rate) after midtrimester amniocentesis. Membrane rupture was also more likely after early amniocentesis, and significantly more amniotic fluid culture failures occurred. For these reasons, amniocentesis at less than 14 weeks of gestation is no longer recommended and is rarely performed as CVS is considered a safer early option. Most data on the safety of amniocentesis are based on studies of procedures performed after 16 weeks' gestation, and the safety and complication rates of procedures undertaken between 14 and 16 weeks are less certain.

Chromosomal mosaicism, the presence of more than one cell line identified during cytogenetic analysis, occurs in approximately 0.25% of amniocentesis specimens and 1–2% of chorionic villus specimens. After mosaicism is found using CVS, amniocentesis typically is performed to assess whether mosaicism is present in amniocytes. In most cases, approximately 90%, the amniocentesis result is normal, and the mosaicism is assumed to be confined to the trophoblast.[33] Although such confined placental mosaicism (CPM) is unlikely to cause congenital abnormalities in the fetus, it may result in third trimester growth restriction.[34]

Clinical outcomes of fetal mosaicism depend on the specific mosaic cell line(s) and may range from normal to findings consistent with the abnormal chromosome result. Counseling after the finding of chromosomal mosaicism is complex, and referral for genetic counseling may be useful in these cases. In the past, cordocentesis was often performed for further evaluation; more recently, it has been recognized that this adds little to the prediction of outcome. Placental mosaicism can also lead to false-positive results from noninvasive prenatal testing, which is based on testing of DNA thought to arise from trophoblasts.

CPM can be associated with so-called trisomy rescue of an originally trisomic conception. When this occurs, the fetus may be disomic but have uniparental disomy (UPD), a condition in which both chromosomes were inherited from the same parent. Trisomy rescue and UPD can potentially involve any chromosome, but if imprinted genes are present on the particular chromosome involved, this may have consequences on the fetus. Therefore, testing for UPD is indicated as a follow-up to CPM detected by CVS when a chromosome containing known imprinted genes is involved (e.g., chromosomes 6, 7, 11, 14, 15, and 20). If the chromosome involved in the original trisomy does not contain imprinted genes, no phenotypic consequences for the fetus would be predicted (see Chapter 2).

Mosaicism can also be suggested when the fetal specimen contains maternal cell contamination. This can be minimized by discarding the first 1–2 mL of the amniocentesis specimen and by careful dissection of chorionic villi from maternal decidua.

HOW HAS THE VOLUME OF PRENATAL DIAGNOSIS PROCEDURES CHANGED OVER TIME?

Recent years have seen a marked decrease in the rate of prenatal invasive diagnostic procedures.[35] Much of this decrease is thought to be attributable to improvements in aneuploidy screening, initially with the introduction of first trimester serum screening and nuchal translucency ultrasound, and later with the development of cell-free DNA analysis.[36–40] In addition to improved screening, the trend toward more informed and shared patient decision-making also appears to be associated with lower rates of prenatal testing, including diagnostic testing.[41]

Although lowering the number of diagnostic procedures performed is clearly of benefit, it is important that patients choosing screening instead of diagnostic testing are aware of the trade-off in detection, as currently available screening tests do not detect the broad range of chromosomal abnormalities detectable with invasive diagnostic testing, especially if chromosomal microarray analysis is used.[5,42] The common aneuploidies detectable with current screening modalities are present in about 1 pregnancy in 500 in the midtrimester, whereas CMA detects a significant abnormality in 1 in 100; therefore screening techniques can identify just 20% of the chromosomal anomalies detectable by diagnostic testing with CMA.

The lower rates of diagnostic testing have also resulted in fewer procedures available for training and the maintenance of clinical competence for providers who perform amniocentesis and CVS.[43] Although a precise threshold number necessary for training or for maintenance of skills is not known, data indicate that the rates of miscarriage associated with amniocentesis and CVS procedures have both decreased over time with increasing experience.[9,11,44] As the rate of procedures at some institutions and in some practices has become very low, it is uncertain whether the very low rates of procedure-related complications and loss reported in large series are still appropriate to quote to patients when providing informed consent.

ARE PRENATAL DIAGNOSIS PROCEDURES SAFE FOR WOMEN WITH CHRONIC VIRAL INFECTIONS, SUCH AS HEPATITIS AND HUMAN IMMUNODEFICIENCY VIRUS?

Although data are somewhat limited, available data indicate that the risk of neonatal infection as a result of amniocentesis in women who are chronically infected with hepatitis B appears to be increased, with the rate of vertical transmission being dependent on viral load.[45] Older data had indicated that the rate of neonatal infection was no different than in women who did not have an amniocentesis, although in older series viral load data were not generally available. In addition, limited data suggest that women who are HbeAg positive have a higher risk of vertical transmission after amniocentesis.[46] There are far more limited data available regarding amniocentesis in women with hepatitis C, although the risk of transmission appears to be low.[47,48]

Amniocentesis in women infected with human immunodeficiency virus who are on combination antiretroviral therapy does not appear to significantly increase the risk of vertical transmission, particularly if the viral load is undetectable, but women should be counseled that limited data are available on this issue. For women not on combined antiretroviral therapy, the risk of vertical transmission is increased by performing amniocentesis.[49] When possible, combined antiretroviral therapy should be initiated, and the procedure postponed until the viral load is undetectable.

There are insufficient data in the literature to assess the risk of CVS in women with chronic viral infections. As with all women, both invasive and noninvasive testing and screening options should be discussed.

WHAT LABORATORY PROCEDURES ARE PERFORMED ON PRENATAL SAMPLES?

The laboratory testing performed to diagnose fetal genetic disorders varies with the indication for the test, as well as with gestational age and patient preferences. In general, chromosomal analysis with karyotyping and/or chromosomal microarray analysis is always performed, regardless of indication. Alpha-fetoprotein level is usually also measured in amniotic fluid samples to assess for neural tube defects, although the need for this has been questioned.[50]

Metaphase analysis of a karyotype obtained from cultured amniocytes or chorionic villus cells is the traditional method for chromosomal analysis; this approach is highly accurate for chromosomal abnormalities larger than 5–10 Mb. However, CMA provides assessment of the chromosomes at a higher resolution than traditional karyotype and can detect microdeletions and duplications in addition to aneuploidies. This technique can detect essentially all abnormalities detectable by karyotype, except for balanced translocations and some cases of triploidy. As with karyotype, some cases of low-level mosaicism may not be identified. CMA can be performed either directly on uncultured tissue or on cultured cells. The advantage of direct CMA analysis is a much faster turnaround time (3–5 days) when culture is not required and potential benefits if cells are not viable and therefore prone to culture failure.

When structural abnormalities are detected by prenatal ultrasound, CMA has been demonstrated to detect significant chromosomal abnormalities in approximately 6% of fetuses with a normal karyotype.[5,42] For this reason, it is recommended that CMA be offered to patients in whom a structural abnormality is detected by ultrasound.[51] CMA has also been found to detect a pathogenic, or likely pathogenic, CNV in about 1% of

patients with a normal ultrasound and a normal karyotype. This risk is high enough that it is recommended that CMA should be available to any patient choosing to undergo invasive diagnostic testing. Finally, in part because CMA does not require cell culture, it has been shown to be more effective in the evaluation of stillbirth.[52]

FISH can be performed on uncultured tissue collected via amniocentesis or CVS to provide a rapid assessment of the common aneuploidies. FISH can also be performed on metaphase cells, after cell culture, to assess for specific microdeletions or duplications. Measurement of enzyme activity or other biochemical or physiologic parameters is possible when indicated to determine the presence of biochemical and other disorders. Such testing, however, is less commonly used as DNA testing for specific variants is increasingly available and generally more accurate. In rare circumstances, testing of fetal blood or other tissues is the only option for prenatal diagnosis.

Some structural malformations, or patterns of malformations, are characteristic of specific genetic disorders. Increasingly, molecular DNA testing for single conditions are available and may be appropriate in some conditions. For other findings, such as a skeletal dysplasia, a panel of genes for common and similar conditions may be available to screen for several disorders at the same time. Postnatally, if a pattern of abnormalities and/or the family history strongly suggests a genetic condition, but does not point to a known disorder, whole genome or whole exome sequencing may be recommended. This is rarely pursued at present in a prenatal setting, in part because of the long turnaround time, which often requires several months for the sequencing and the subsequent analysis. However, it is very likely that genomic sequencing will be increasingly used in prenatal settings in the future.

WHAT ARE THE INDICATIONS FOR PRENATAL DIAGNOSTIC TESTING?

Both CVS and amniocentesis collect tissue that can be cultured, or from which DNA can be extracted, for genetic testing of the fetus. Therefore, the indications for these two procedures and the laboratory tests that can be performed are generally the same. The major differences in the procedures include the gestational age at which they are performed and the tissue that is sampled (placenta vs. amniotic fluid). Both ACOG and the Society for Maternal-Fetal Medicine have recommended that invasive diagnostic testing as well as screening for aneuploidy should be available to all women, regardless of maternal age or risk status. Aneuploidy testing should be discussed as early as possible in pregnancy so that first trimester options are available.

Women who have an increased risk of a fetal genetic disorder and who may therefore request prenatal diagnostic testing include those with:

- Advanced maternal age, as the rate of fetal trisomy increases with maternal age. In contrast, structural chromosomal abnormalities, including microdeletions and duplications, do not increase in frequency with maternal age.
- A previous fetus or child with a chromosomal abnormality, as this increases the risk of recurrence.[53,54]
- Structural anomalies identified by sonography, as these increase the likelihood of aneuploidy, CNVs such as microdeletions, or other genetic syndromes.[5,42,55,56]
- Parental balanced chromosomal rearrangements, such as translocations or inversions. The chance of having unbalanced offspring depends on the precise rearrangement, and varies from essentially 0% to as high as 30%.[3]
- Parental aneuploidy or aneuploidy mosaicism, as this may increase the risk of aneuploid offspring.
- Parents who are carriers of genetic disorders, such as Tay Sachs disease or cystic fibrosis, as well as individuals who are affected by autosomal dominant disorders, such as neurofibromatosis.

WHAT ARE THE DIFFERENCES IN PRENATAL DIAGNOSTIC TESTING IN MULTIPLE GESTATIONS?

Data regarding the risk of aneuploidy as well as the risks of diagnostic testing are more limited in multiple gestations compared with singletons. In women with twins, formulas have been used to estimate the risk of aneuploidy based on maternal age and, when known, chorionicity as a proxy for zygosity.[57,58] Recent data suggest that such models may not be accurate and likely overestimate the risk of aneuploidy. Recent studies have estimated that the risk of Down syndrome per fetus from multiple pregnancies is only about half of that from singletons.[59,60]

Limited data exist concerning fetal loss in women with a twin gestation when amniocentesis or CVS is performed. According to some series, the fetal loss rate is approximately 3.5% when amniocentesis is performed in women with multiple gestations; this was not higher than the background loss rate for twins in the second trimester in one series with a control group.[61,62] Other more recent studies have estimated the attributable loss rate of amniocentesis in twins at about 2%.[63,64] There are no data concerning loss rates after amniocentesis in women with high-order multiple gestations. Similar information for twin gestations from small, nonrandomized series exists for CVS.[62,65] In one recent systematic review, the procedure-related loss rate for both CVS and amniocentesis in twin pregnancies was estimated at 1%. With CVS, there exists the additional potential for cross-contamination, or inadvertent sampling of both fetuses; this risk has been estimated at about 1%.[66]

With monochorionic (and therefore monozygotic) twin gestations, the karyotype is almost always concordant, and patients may opt for having testing performed on only one fetus. In this situation, it is important to consider the accuracy of ultrasound assessment of chorionicity, which is most accurate if ultrasonography is performed at or before 14 weeks of gestation. The positive predictive value of monochorionicity is 97.8% at this gestation age but decreases to 88% after 14 weeks.[67,68] Overall, chorionicity can be determined correctly in 94%–95% of cases. In addition, in rare circumstances, monochorionic twins can be discordant for chromosomal abnormalities; the rate of such discordance is unknown.

Counseling for multiple gestations should include a discussion of the options for pregnancy management if only one fetus is found to be affected. Such options include termination of the entire pregnancy, selective second trimester termination of the affected fetus, and continuing the pregnancy.

WHAT ARE THE IMPORTANT COMPONENTS OF PRE- AND POSTTEST PRENATAL GENETIC TESTING?

Pretest counseling should include a discussion of the risks and benefits of invasive diagnostic testing compared with screening; how many women will have a positive result with screening (screen-positive rate) and, of those, how many will have a true positive result (positive predictive value); the detection rate of aneuploidies other than Down syndrome; and the type and prognosis of chromosomal abnormalities likely to be missed by maternal serum and/or cell-free DNA screening. The differences between screening and diagnostic testing should be discussed with all women. A woman's decision as to whether to have screening, an amniocentesis or CVS is based on many factors, including the chance that the fetus will have a chromosomal abnormality, the risk of pregnancy loss from an invasive procedure, and the consequences of having an affected child. Studies that have evaluated women's preferences have shown that women weigh these potential outcomes very differently. The decision to perform invasive testing should take into account these preferences and should not be based solely on age. Ideally, all options should be offered to all women, after informed consent. Concerns that offering all test options to all women may lead to an increased rate of procedures and procedure-related losses are unfounded, as studies have demonstrated that the offer of all testing options after informed consent actually decreases the rate of invasive diagnostic testing, while at the same time providing patients options more aligned with their values and preferences.[41,69]

Ideally, patients should be provided general information about the disorders potentially detectable with any genetic test before making a decision as to whether to undergo the specific testing being offered. Although prenatal testing has historically focused largely on Down syndrome, the range of clinically significant disorders that can now be detected has greatly expanded far beyond this one condition. When the diagnosis of a chromosomal abnormality or another genetic disorder in the fetus is made, the patient should receive detailed information, to the extent the disorder or finding has been previously reported, about the natural history of the specific condition. With most fetal genetic or structural abnormalities, referral to specialists with expertise in the specific disorder is indicated, as patient decision-making requires accurate and detailed counseling by providers with expertise. For many CNVs identified by chromosomal microarray analysis, interpretation requires consultation with a genetic counselor or geneticist with expertise in prenatal genetic diagnosis. In some cases, national or other advocacy groups can provide information to help the patient make an informed decision.

The option of pregnancy termination should be discussed when a genetic disorder or major structural abnormality is detected prenatally. Patients may benefit from additional testing, including ultrasonography or fetal echocardiography and referral to appropriate obstetric and pediatric specialists or neonatologists to discuss pregnancy and neonatal management issues. Referral to parent support groups, counselors, social workers, or clergy may provide additional information and support.

Prenatal diagnosis is not performed solely for assistance in the decision of pregnancy termination, as such testing provides useful information for the physician and the patient. Nondirective counseling before prenatal diagnostic testing should not suggest that a patient commit to pregnancy termination if the result is abnormal. Rather, counseling should be nondirective, informative, and respectful of any decision desired by the patient. If a diagnosis of a genetic abnormality is made, counseling should include family education and preparedness, referral to a tertiary care center for the newborn if appropriate, adoption, pregnancy termination, or perinatal hospice, and comfort care for a delivery of a child with a diagnosis or fetal presentation incompatible with life. If it is determined that the fetus has a chromosomal abnormality, the physicians and family can plan ahead and develop a management plan for the remainder of the pregnancy, labor, and delivery.[70]

REFERENCES

1. Kuppermann M, Nease RF, Learman LA, et al. Procedure-related miscarriages and Down syndrome-affected births: implications for prenatal testing based on women's preferences. *Obstet Gynecol.* 2000;96(4):511–516.
2. https://www.marchofdimes.org/baby/chromosomal-conditions.aspx; accessed November 3, 2018.
3. Gardner RJ, Sutherland GR. *Chromosome Abnormalities and Genetic Counseling.* 3rd ed. New York (NY): Oxford University Press; 2004.
4. Nyberg DA, Crane JP. Chromosome abnormalities. In: Nyberg DA, Mahony BS, Pretorius DH, eds. *Diagnostic Ultrasound of Fetal Anomalies: Text and Atlas.* Chicago (IL): Year Book Medical; 1990:676–724.
5. Wapner RJ, Martin CL, Levy B, et al. Chromosomal microarray versus karyotyping for prenatal diagnosis. *N Engl J Med.* 2012;367:2175–2178.
6. Bombard AT, Powers JF, Carter S, Schwartz A, Nitowsky HM. Procedure-related fetal losses in transplacental versus nontransplacental genetic amniocentesis. *Am J Obstet Gynecol.* 1995;172:868–872.
7. Giorlandino C, Mobili L, Bilancioni E, et al. Transplacental amniocentesis: is it really a higher-risk procedure? *Prenat Diagn.* 1994;14:803–806.
8. Alfirevic Z, Sundberg K, Brigham S. Amniocentesis and chorionic villus sampling for prenatal diagnosis. *Cochrane Database Syst Rev.* 2003;(3):CD003252.

9. Jackson LG, Zachary JM, Fowler SE, et al. A randomized comparison of transcervical and transabdominal chorionic-villus sampling. The U.S. National Institute of child health and human development chorionic-villus sampling and amniocentesis study group. *N Engl J Med*. 1992;327:594–598.

10. Akolekar R, Beta J, Picciarelli G, Ogilvie C, D'Antonio F. Procedure-related risk of miscarriage following amniocentesis and chorionic villus sampling: a systematic review and meta-analysis. *Ultrasound Obstet Gynecol*. 2015; 45(1):16–26.

11. Caughey AB, Hopkins LM, Norton ME. Chorionic villus sampling compared with amniocentesis and the difference in the rate of pregnancy loss. *Obstet Gynecol*. 2006;108:612–616.

12. Eddleman KA, Malone FD, Sullivan L, et al. Pregnancy loss rates after midtrimester amniocentesis. *Obstet Gynecol*. 2006;108:1067–1072.

13. Mazza V, Pati M, Bertucci E, et al. Age-specific risk of fetal loss post second trimester amniocentesis: analysis of 5,043 cases. *Prenat Diagn*. 2007;27:180–183.

14. Muller F, Thibaud D, Poloce F, et al. Risk of amniocentesis in women screened positive for Down syndrome with second trimester maternal serum markers. *Prenat Diagn*. 2002;22:1036–1039.

15. Odibo AO, Gray DL, Dicke JM, Stamilio DM, Macones GA, Crane JP. Revisiting the fetal loss rate after second-trimester genetic amniocentesis: a single center's 16-year experience. *Obstet Gynecol*. 2008;111:589–595.

16. Odibo AO, Dicke JM, Gray DL, et al. Evaluating the rate and risk factors for fetal loss after chorionic villus sampling. *Obstet Gynecol*. 2008;112:813–819.

17. Tabor A, Vestergaard CH, Lidegaard O. Fetal loss rate after chorionic villus sampling and amniocentesis: an 11-year national registry study. *Ultrasound Obstet Gynecol*. 2009; 34:19–24.

18. Borgida AF, Mills AA, Feldman DM, Rodis JF, Egan JF. Outcome of pregnancies complicated by ruptured membranes after genetic amniocentesis. *Am J Obstet Gynecol*. 2000;183:937–939.

19. Mennuti MT, DiGaetano A, McDonnell A, Cohen AW, Liston RM. Fetal-maternal bleeding associated with genetic amniocentesis: real-time versus static ultrasound. *Obstet Gynecol*. 1983;62:26–30.

20. Romero R, Jeanty P, Reece EA, et al. Sonographically monitored amniocentesis to decrease intraoperative complications. *Obstet Gynecol*. 1985;65:426–430.

21. Leschot NJ, Verjaal M, Treffers PE. Risks of midtrimester amniocentesis; assessment in 3,000 pregnancies. *Br J Obstet Gynaecol*. 1985;92(8):804–807.

22. Lau KT, Leung YT, Fung YT, Chan LW, Sahota DS, Leung NT. Outcome of 1,355 consecutive transabdominal chorionic villus samplings in 1,351 patients. *Chin Med J*. 2005;118:1675–1681.

23. Silver RK, MacGregor SN, Sholl JS, Hobart ED, Waldee JK. An evaluation of the chorionic villus sampling learning curve. *Am J Obstet Gynecol*. 1990;163:917–922.

24. Wijnberger LD, van der Schouw YT, Christiaens GC. Learning in medicine: chorionic villus sampling. *Prenat Diagn*. 2000;20:241–246.

25. Kuliev A, Jackson L, Froster U, et al. Chorionic villus sampling safety. Report of World health Organization/EURO meeting in association with the seventh International conference on early prenatal diagnosis of genetic diseases, Tel-Aviv, Israel, May 21, 1994. *Am J Obstet Gynecol*. 1996;174: 807–811.

26. Botto LD, Olney RS, Mastroiacovo P, et al. Chorionic villus sampling and transverse digital deficiencies: evidence for anatomic and gestational-age specificity of the digital deficiencies in two studies. *Am J Med Genet*. 1996;62: 173–178.

27. Bauland CG, Smit JM, Bartelink LR, Zondervan HA, Spauwen PH. Hemangioma in the newborn: increased incidence after chorionic villus sampling. *Prenat Diagn*. 2010;30(10):913–917.

28. Bauland CG, Smit JM, Scheffers SM, et al. Similar risk for hemangiomas after amniocentesis and transabdominal chorionic villus sampling. *J Obstet Gynaecol Res*. 2012;38(2):371–375.

29. Johnson JM, Wilson RD, Winsor EJ, Singer J, Dansereau J, Kalousek DK. The early amniocentesis study: a randomized clinical trial of early amniocentesis versus midtrimester amniocentesis. *Fetal Diagn Ther*. 1996;11: 85–93.

30. Nicolaides K, Brizot Mde L, Patel F, Snijders R. Comparison of chorionic villus sampling and amniocentesis for fetal karyotyping at 10–13 weeks' gestation. *Lancet*. 1994;344:435–439. [published erratum appears in: Lancet 1994;344:830].

31. Sundberg K, Bang J, Smidt-Jensen S, et al. Randomised study of risk of fetal loss related to early amniocentesis versus chorionic villus sampling. *Lancet*. 1997;350: 697–703.

32. Canadian Early and Mid-trimester Amniocentesis Trial (CEMAT) Group. Randomised trial to assess safety and fetal outcome of early and midtrimester amniocentesis. *Lancet*. 1998;351:242–247.

33. Goldberg JD, Wohlferd MM. Incidence and outcome of chromosomal mosaicism found at the time of chorionic villus sampling. *Am J Obstet Gynecol*. 1997;176(6):1349–1352.

34. Baffero GM, Somigliana E, Crovetto F, et al. Confined placental mosaicism at chorionic villous sampling: risk factors and pregnancy outcome. *Prenat Diagn*. 2012;32(11):1102–1108.

35. Warsof SL, Larion S, Abuhamad AZ. Overview of the impact of noninvasive prenatal testing on diagnostic procedures. *Prenat Diagn*. 2015;35(10):972–979.

36. Norton ME, Brar H, Weiss J. Non-Invasive Chromosomal Evaluation (NICE) Study: results of a multicenter prospective cohort study for detection of fetal trisomy 21 and trisomy 18. *Am J Obstet Gynecol*. 2012;207(2):137.e1–8.

37. Beamon CJ, Hardisty EE, Harris SC, Vora NL. A single center's experience with noninvasive prenatal testing. *Genet Med.* 2014;16(9):681–687.

38. Chetty S, Garabedian MJ, Norton ME. Uptake of noninvasive prenatal testing (NIPT) in women following positive aneuploidy screening. *Prenat Diagn.* 2013;33(6):542–546.

39. Tiller GE, Kershberg HB, Goff J, Coffeen C, Liao W, Sehnert AJ. Women's views and the impact of noninvasive prenatal testing on procedures in a managed care setting. *Prenat Diagn.* 2014. https://doi.org/10.1002/pd.4495. [Epub ahead of print].

40. Wax JR, Cartin A, Chard R, Lucas FL, Pinette MG. Noninvasive prenatal testing: impact on genetic counseling, invasive prenatal diagnosis, and trisomy 21 detection. *J Clin Ultrasound.* 2015;43(1):1–6.

41. Kuppermann M, Pena S, Bishop JT, et al. Effect of enhanced information, values clarification, and removal of financial barriers on use of prenatal genetic testing: a randomized clinical trial. *J Am Med Assoc.* 2014;312(12):1210–1217.

42. de Wit MC, Srebniak MI, Govaerts LC, Van Opstal D, Galjaard RJ, Go AT. Additional value of prenatal genomic array testing in fetuses with isolated structural ultrasound abnormalities and a normal karyotype: a systematic review of the literature. *Ultrasound Obstet Gynecol.* 2014;43(2):139–146.

43. Rose NC, LaGrave D, Hafen B, Jackson M. The impact of utilization of early aneuploidy screening on amniocenteses available for training in obstetrics and fetal medicine. *Prenat Diagn.* 2013;233:242–244.

44. Rhoads GG, Jackson LG, Schlesselman SE, et al. The safety and efficacy of chorionic villus sampling for early prenatal diagnosis of cytogenetic abnormalities. *N Engl J Med.* 1989;320:609–617.

45. Yi W, Pan CQ, Hao J, et al. Risk of vertical transmission of hepatitis B after amniocentesis in HBs antigen-positive mothers. *J Hepatol.* 2014;60(3):523–529.

46. Ko TM, Tseng LH, Chang MH, et al. Amniocentesis in mothers who are hepatitis B virus carriers does not expose the infant to an increased risk of hepatitis B virus infection. *Arch Gynecol Obstet.* 1994;255:25–30.

47. Delamare C, Carbonne B, Heim N, et al. Detection of hepatitis C virus RNA (HCV RNA) in amniotic fluid: a prospective study. *J Hepatol.* 1999;31(3):416–420.

48. Prasad MR, Honegger JR. Hepatitis C virus in pregnancy. *Am J Perinatol.* 2013;30(2):149–159.

49. Simões M, Marques C, Gonçalves A, et al. Amniocentesis in HIV pregnant women: 16 years of experience. *Infect Dis Obstet Gynecol.* 2013;2013:914272.

50. Flick A, Krakow D, Martirosian A, Silverman N, Platt LD. Routine measurement of amniotic fluid alpha-fetoprotein and acetylcholinesterase: the need for a reevaluation. *Am J Obstet Gynecol.* 2014;211(2). 139.e1–6.

51. American College of Obstetricians and Gynecologists Committee on Genetics. Committee Opinion No. 581: the use of chromosomal microarray analysis in prenatal diagnosis. *Obstet Gynecol.* 2013;122(6):1374–1377.

52. Reddy UM, Page GP, Saade GR, et al. NICHD Stillbirth Collaborative Research Network. Karyotype versus microarray testing for genetic abnormalities after stillbirth. *N Engl J Med.* 2012;367(23):2185–2193.

53. Uehara S, Yaegashi N, Maeda T, et al. Risk of recurrence of fetal chromosomal aberrations: analysis of trisomy 21, trisomy 18, trisomy 13, and 45,X in 1,076 Japanese mothers. *J Obstet Gynaecol Res.* 1999;25(6):373–379.

54. Warburton D, Dallaire L, Thangavelu M, Ross L, Levin B, Kline J. Trisomy recurrence: a reconsideration based on North American data. *Am J Hum Genet.* 2004;75:376–385.

55. Williamson RA, Weiner CP, Patil S, Benda J, Varner MW, Abu-Yousef MM. Abnormal pregnancy sonogram: selective indication for fetal karyotype. *Obstet Gynecol.* 1987;69:15–20.

56. Wladimiroff JW, Sachs ES, Reuss A, Stewart PA, Pijpers L, Niermeijer MF. Prenatal diagnosis of chromosome abnormalities in the presence of fetal structural defects. *Am J Med Genet.* 1988;29:289–291.

57. Meyers C, Adam R, Dungan J, Prenger V. Aneuploidy in twin gestations: when is maternal age advanced? *Obstet Gynecol.* 1997;89:248–251.

58. Rodis JF, Egan JF, Craffey A, Ciarleglio L, Greenstein RM, Scorza WE. Calculated risk of chromosomal abnormalities in twin gestations. *Obstet Gynecol.* 1990;76:1037–1041.

59. Boyle B, Morris JK, McConkey R, et al. Prevalence and risk of Down syndrome in monozygotic and dizygotic multiple pregnancies in Europe: implications for prenatal screening. *BJOG.* 2014;121(7):809–819.

60. Sparks TN, Norton ME, Flessel M, Goldman S, Currier RJ. Observed rate of down syndrome in twin pregnancies. *Obstet Gynecol.* 2016;128(5):1127–1133.

61. Librach CL, Doran TA, Benzie RJ, Jones JM. Genetic amniocentesis in seventy twin pregnancies. *Am J Obstet Gynecol.* 1984;148:585–591.

62. Wapner RJ, Johnson A, Davis G, Urban A, Morgan P, Jackson L. Prenatal diagnosis in twin gestations: a comparison between second-trimester amniocentesis and first trimester chorionic villus sampling. *Obstet Gynecol.* 1993; 82:49–56.

63. Cahill AG, Macones GA, Stamilio DM, Dicke JM, Crane JP, Odibo AO. Pregnancy loss rate after mid-trimester amniocentesis in twin pregnancies. *Am J Obstet Gynecol.* 2009;200(3):257.e1–e6.

64. Millaire M, Bujold E, Morency AM, Gauthier RJ. Mid-trimester genetic amniocentesis in twin pregnancy and the risk of fetal loss. *J Obstet Gynaecol Can.* 2006;28(6): 512–518.

65. van den Berg C, Braat AP, Van Opstal D, et al. Amniocentesis or chorionic villus sampling in multiple gestations? Experience with 500 cases. *Prenat Diagn.* 1999;19: 234–244.

66. Agarwal K, Alfirevic Z. Pregnancy loss after chorionic villus sampling and genetic amniocentesis in twin pregnancies: a systematic review. *Ultrasound Obstet Gynecol.* 2012;40(2):128–134.

67. Blumenfeld YJ, Momirova V, Rouse DJ, et al. Eunice Kennedy shriver national Institute of child health and human development maternal-fetal medicine units network. Accuracy of sonographic chorionicity classification in twin gestations. *J Ultrasound Med.* 2014;33(12):2187–2192.
68. Lee YM, Cleary-Goldman J, Thaker HM, Simpson LL. Antenatal sonographic prediction of twin chorionicity. *Am J Obstet Gynecol.* 2006;195:863–867.
69. Norton ME, Nakagawa S, Norem C, Gregorich SE, Kuppermann M. Effects of changes in prenatal aneuploidy screening policies in an integrated health care system. *Obstet Gynecol.* 2013;121(2 Pt 1):265–271.
70. Clark SL, DeVore GR. Prenatal diagnosis for couples who would not consider abortion. *Obstet Gynecol.* 1989; 73(6):1035–1037.

CHAPTER 15

Preimplantation Genetic Testing

SVETLANA A. YATSENKO, MD • ALEKSANDAR RAJKOVIC, MD, PHD

ABBREVIATIONS

aCGH Array comparative genomic hybridization
AF Amniotic fluid
CRISPR Clustered regularly interspaced short palindromic repeat
CVS Chorionic villus sampling
FISH Fluorescence in situ hybridization
HDR Homology directed repair
ICM Inner cell mass
ICSI Intracytoplasmic sperm injection
mtDNA Mitochondrial DNA
nDNA Nuclear DNA
NGS Next-generation sequencing
NHEJ Nonhomologous end joining
cfDNA cell-free DNA
PCR Polymerase chain reaction

PGD Preimplantation genetic diagnosis
PGS Preimplantation genetic screening
PGT Preimplantation genetic testing
PGT-A Preimplantation genetic testing for aneuploidies
PGT-M Preimplantation genetic testing for monogenic/single-gene defects
PGT-SR Preimplantation genetic testing for chromosomal structural rearrangements
qPCR Quantitative polymerase chain reaction
SNP Single nucleotide polymorphism
STR Short tandem repeat
TE Trophectoderm
UPD Uniparental disomy
WGA Whole-genome amplification

INTRODUCTION

Over the past two decades, in vitro fertilization has become routine clinical practice. Technological advances in genetics and DNA amplification now allow preimplantation diagnosis (PGD in the past, now known as preimplantation genetic testing for monogenic/single-gene defects [PGT-M]) to be performed by testing a few cells of a developing preimplantation (usually day 5 or day 6) blastocyst embryo. This technique was developed initially to benefit couples at high risk of producing an embryo with a known genetic disorder. Preimplantation testing allows for selection of unaffected embryos for implantation and avoids the emotional stress of termination of an affected pregnancy. Most of these diagnoses are for heritable Mendelian disorders.[1]

Because first-trimester and earlier miscarriages are known to have aneuploidy rates in excess of 40%,[2] screening preimplantation embryos for aneuploidies was proposed to potentially improve implantation rates and take-home pregnancy rates.[3,4] Preimplantation aneuploidy testing (PGS in the past, now known

as preimplantation genetic testing for aneuploidies [PGT-A]) was specifically applied to improve singleton embryo transfer pregnancy rates and therefore reduce twinning and higher-order pregnancy rates, to improve outcomes for patients with recurrent miscarriages, and to improve pregnancy rates for women of advanced maternal age. Randomized controlled trials to support many of these indications are lacking, although there is significant support for testing among experts.[1]

Preimplantation genetic testing (PGT) is advancing rapidly and will continue to benefit from new genomic technologies. Coupled with preconception carrier screening of parents, whole-genome sequencing of embryo genomes can theoretically diagnose most heritable and de novo Mendelian disorders. Noninvasive approaches to embryo genotyping show promise and will likely make PGT more widespread. Genome editing technologies are raising tantalizing possibilities of correcting pathogenic variants in affected embryos and fears that such technologies will be used to "enhance" embryos for certain traits. Moreover, PGT raises many ethical questions before conception including whether

Perinatal Genetics. https://doi.org/10.1016/B978-0-323-53094-1.00015-1

to test for adult onset disorders; whether to use for sex selection outside of medical indications; and whether to transfer embryos with identified pathogenic variants because of family wishes. It is important to keep in mind that any form of genetic testing of the embryo or parents should involve genetic counseling and careful documentation of such counseling by the healthcare provider. Vigorous research in the area of preimplantation genetic testing needs to continue to further understand the fundamentals of embryo development and benefits/clinical utility of genomic testing.

WHAT ARE THE RATES OF ANEUPLOIDY AT DIFFERENT STAGES OF EMBRYO DEVELOPMENT?

Incorrect number of chromosomes (aneuploidy) is the most common contributor to miscarriage and congenital birth defects in humans. Aneuploidy can occur in dividing cells as the result of chromosome

missegregation during meiosis or mitosis, leading to gametes with an extra or missing chromosome. Chromosome nondisjunction during meiosis of the oocytes is the cause of most trisomic/monosomic embryos, and the risk of aneuploidy increases with maternal age. Chromosome gains and losses happen during spermatogenesis; however, male surveillance mechanisms are thought to eliminate aneuploid sperm at higher efficiency than eggs. After oocyte fertilization, the resulting zygote, a single diploid cell, undergoes rapid mitotic cell divisions to develop into an 8-cell blastomere at day 3 postfertilization and into a 100- to 200-cell blastocyst at days 5–6 (Fig. 15.1A). Human embryos at the early stages (days 1–3) of development are susceptible to unequal distributions of chromosomes or chromosome misallocation between the daughter cells (Fig. 15.1B). Therefore, an elevated level of chromosomal anomalies is commonly present at the day 3 embryo biopsy (Fig. 15.2A). A systematic review of data from a large cohort study[5] showed that ~35% of embryos in

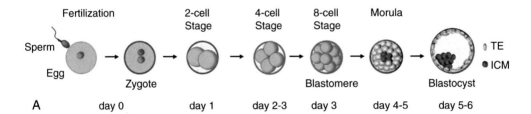

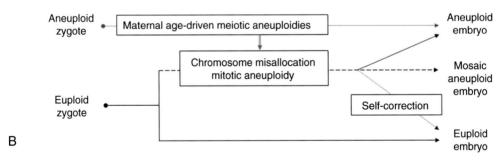

FIG. 15.1 Stages of human embryo development. **(A)**. Approximately 30 h after fertilization, the first division will produce a 2-cell embryo. Further embryo cleavages will occur every 10–12 h, producing a 4-cell embryo on day 2 and 8-cell embryo on day 3. On day 5 or 6, the human embryo is called blastocyst and contains inner cell mass (ICM) that will give rise to the fetus and the trophectoderm (TE) that will give rise to the placenta. **(B)** Origin of aneuploidy in human embryos. The majority (90%) of aneuploidy detected in embryos is due to maternal meiotic errors, 1%–2% is due to affected spermatozoa, and the remaining 8%–9% is due to a chromosome nondisjunction during early postzygotic mitotic cell divisions. Euploid zygotes may become aneuploid because of a chromosome missegregation during the day one to three mitotic divisions (mitotic aneuploidy). Chromosome misallocation affecting individual cells during embryo cleavage is a common event that may ultimately produce an aneuploid embryo or mosaic embryo. Self-correction of aneuploidy may give rise to a normal euploid embryo. Some aneuploid embryos may also experience postzygotic mitotic errors resulting in mosaicism.

day 3 biopsies are euploid, whereas ~65% of embryos are aneuploid or contain both normal and abnormal cells (mosaic aneuploid embryos). The rate of mitotic aneuploidy (aneuploidy that arises postfertilization, also termed postzygotic) is relatively similar among women of all age groups, suggesting that the occurrence of aneuploidy by postzygotic mitotic errors is not influenced by maternal age and equally affects maternal and paternal chromosomes. Furthermore, individual couples with compromised response to repair double-stranded DNA breaks that occur during meiosis and mitosis may experience extremely high rates of aneuploidy and chromosomal rearrangements.

Importantly, comparison between the chromosome status of embryos on day 3 and day 5 demonstrates that ~20–30% of aneuploid embryos that developed to the blastocyst stage undergo self-correction. Thus, the rate of euploid embryos at day 5 is higher than the proportion of chromosomally normal embryos at day 3 (Fig. 15.2B). Postzygotic aneuploidy resulting from zygotic chromosome loss, chromosome gain, or mitotic nondisjunction is a common defect in human embryos, and the process of embryo self-correction via apoptosis and death of aneuploid cells or growth advantage for proliferation of chromosomally normal cells requires further investigation.

WHAT IS THE DIFFERENCE BETWEEN INNER CELL MASS AND TROPHECTODERM?

The fertilized egg is totipotential, capable of differentiation into any cell type. After asymmetric division, a few cells positioned inside the embryo remain pluripotent and will give rise to the inner cell mass (ICM), whereas the rest differentiates into trophectoderm (TE). The ICM will become the fetus, whereas trophectoderm

(TE) will give rise to the placenta and umbilical cord (Fig. 15.1A). This differentiation into ICM versus TE occurs circa the 16-cell stage (day 4–5). The ICM can develop into any specialized cell in the human body. At the blastocyst stage, most of the aneuploidies appear to be meiotic in origin and present in both ICM and TE cells. Mitotic errors during the first cleavage divisions result in mosaicism for aneuploid cells and random distribution of abnormal cells within a developing embryo, which can cause discrepant findings between ICM and TE in ~3.3% of blastocysts.[6] The frequency of mitotic aneuploidies in human preimplantation embryos can be deduced from the frequency of mosaic embryos. Mosaic embryos may implant at a lower success rate, but more investigation is necessary to determine its clinical utility.

WHAT ARE THE DIFFERENT EMBRYONIC STAGES AT WHICH DIAGNOSTICS APPLY?

Testing can be performed on a biopsy obtained from either a polar body, blastomere at the cleavage stage (day 3 after fertilization), or trophectoderm at the blastocyst stage (day 5 or 6 after fertilization). The earliest approach was based on polar body removal, and the genetic status of the oocyte was inferred from the results of the polar body assay. In some countries, religious influences have led to sanctity of life laws that forbid embryo biopsy, and polar body biopsy remains the only option. Polar body biopsy disadvantages include that it only provides information about the maternal contribution to the embryo and autosomal recessive disorders can only partially be diagnosed. Polar body biopsy also carries increased risk of diagnostic error because of the degradation of the genetic material or effects of recombination. The second assay to be developed was blastomere biopsy performed on embryo day 3.

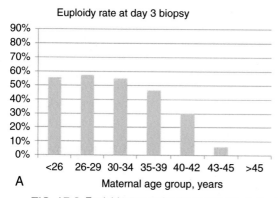
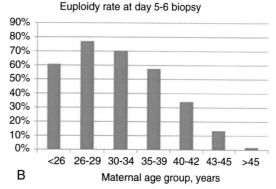

FIG. 15.2 Euploidy rate at the day 3 and day 5 developmental stages. **(A)** Percent of embryos at the day 3 stage that are euploid by women's age groups. **(B)** Rate of euploid embryos at the day 5/6 development. The rate of aneuploidy, as determined by analysis for all 24 chromosomes, is higher at day 3 (blastomere stage).

Initially, one or two cells were biopsied and evaluated by a fluorescence in situ hybridization (FISH) technique for aneuploidy involving a limited set of chromosomes commonly associated with first-trimester miscarriages. The FISH approach was abandoned because of a high rate of chromosomal mosaicism on day 3, the limited number (one or two) of cells available for analysis, and a large randomized trial[3,4] that showed no benefit to using FISH for selected chromosomes (18, 21, 13, X, Y, 1, 16, and 17). In this trial, testing using FISH significantly reduced the rates of ongoing pregnancies and live births after IVF in women of advanced maternal age. Misdiagnosis is also more common in blastomere biopsy because of the technical limitations of DNA amplification from a single cell by PCR. Erroneous amplification of sperm DNA from the zona pellucida, and/or allele dropout of one of the parental alleles during amplification, may lead to false-negative results. Current molecular technologies using single nucleotide polymorphisms and short tandem repeats to identify informative markers from both parents can eliminate the risk of misdiagnosis because of contamination with extraneous DNA or because of allele dropout (one of the two alleles is not amplified). Nonetheless, blastomere biopsy has lost its appeal mainly because of the low number of cells that are available for analysis. At the present time, testing at the blastocyst stage (days 5–6) is most popular because of a greater number of cells available for analysis (4–10), accurate and reliable evaluation for meiotic and mitotic nondisjunction errors, and little known negative impact on embryo viability.[7]

WHAT IS THE DIFFERENCE BETWEEN PGD AND PGS?

In the past, PGD referred to a targeted analysis of variants in the embryo, at risk of inheriting a Mendelian disorder, such as cystic fibrosis, from the parents. PGS referred to screening for aneuploidies to improve implantation and take-home baby rates. Recently, the terms preimplantation genetic diagnosis (PGD) and preimplantation genetic screening (PGS) have been replaced by preimplantation genetic testing (PGT) and descriptive suffixes.[8] PGT-A refers to analysis for aneuploidies and replaces the term PGS; PGT-M replaces the term PGD and refers to testing for monogenic/single gene defects, whereas PGT-SR refers to testing for chromosomal structural rearrangements. Couples undergoing in vitro fertilization (IVF) may select specific PGT options based on the primary referral reason(s) (Table 15.1).

TABLE 15.1
General approaches to preimplantation genetic testing, IVF treatment, and prenatal follow-up testing.

Primary referral reason	PGT-A Aneuploidy	PGT-M Monogenic Disease*	PGT-SR Structural Rearrangements	Prenatal testing
Advanced maternal age, IVF for nongenetic reasons	+			cfDNA, CVS, amniocentesis
Repeated pregnancy losses	+			cfDNA, CVS, amniocentesis
Donor egg/sperm	+			cfDNA, CVS, amniocentesis
Infertility, repeated IVF failure, embryonic arrest	+			cfDNA, CVS, amniocentesis
Family history of X-linked disorder, male lethal condition of unknown etiology	+			cfDNA, CVS, amniocentesis
Gender identification/selection	+			cfDNA, CVS, amniocentesis
Known alteration in a single gene (carriers of autosomal dominant or autosomal recessive condition)	+	+		CVS, amniocentesis
Known alteration in a single X-linked gene	+	+		CVS, amniocentesis
Family history of a gene defect for a late-onset autosomal dominant disorder	+	+		CVS, amniocentesis

TABLE 15.1

General approaches to preimplantation genetic testing, IVF treatment, and prenatal follow-up testing—cont'd

Primary referral reason	PGT-A Aneuploidy	PGT-M Monogenic Disease*	PGT-SR Structural Rearrangements	Prenatal testing
Mitochondrial disorder due to a known alteration in a gene encoded by nuclear genome	+	+		Amniocentesis
Mitochondrial disorder due to an alteration in mitochondrial genome^	+			Amniocentesis
HLA-matched donor	+	+		CVS, amniocentesis
Parent with a chromosome rearrangement				
• Robertsonian translocation	+			CVS, amniocentesis, UPD
• Other chromosome translocation	+		+	CVS, amniocentesis
• Inversion	+		+	CVS, amniocentesis
• Deletion	+		+	CVS, amniocentesis
• Duplication	+		+	CVS, amniocentesis
• Other structural rearrangement	+		+	CVS, amniocentesis

cfDNA, cell free DNA screening; *CVS*, chorionic villus sampling; *UPD*, uniparental disomy testing.
*ICSI is preferred to minimize the risk of contamination from sperm DNA.
^Nuclear transfer or mitochondria replacement therapy may prevent the transmission of mtDNA variants.

PGT-A is used to evaluate embryos for numerical chromosomal alterations such as trisomy and monosomy and to select chromosomally balanced embryos for transfer. The incidence of aneuploidy is high in IVF-produced embryos and significantly increases with advanced maternal age. Therefore, aneuploidy testing of blastocyst stage embryos for all 24 chromosomes has been advocated to improve implantation and delivery rates.[1] At present, however, there is insufficient evidence to recommend the routine use of blastocyst biopsy with aneuploidy testing in all infertile patients.

PGT-M is a test performed on embryos to identify their status for known genetic defect(s), such as pathogenic variants in the CFTR (cystic fibrosis) gene, when these are carried by the parent(s). The aim of PGT-M is to provide a reproductive option to parents with a risk of offspring with inherited disorders to select embryo(s) for pregnancy that are free of a genetic disease.

PGT-SR is a test to identify genomic imbalances that arise from parental structural chromosomal rearrangements such as translocations, inversions, deletions, and duplications affecting a part of chromosome. Carriers of structural chromosome rearrangements are at high risk to produce gametes with extra and missing DNA segments of rearranged chromosomes (segmental aneuploidies). Several technologies used for aneuploidy analysis can also detect segmental aneuploidy. In some patients with structural chromosome rearrangements, gametes are expected to contain imbalances for large DNA segments such as whole-chromosome aneuploidy in carriers of Robertsonian translocations. Consultation with laboratory personnel is recommended before biopsy to determine techniques and the optimal PGT-SR protocol to identify products of patient-specific chromosomal rearrangement.

WHAT ARE THE CURRENT TECHNOLOGIES UTILIZED TO ACHIEVE PREIMPLANTATION GENETIC TESTING?

To date, genetic testing of preimplantation embryos has moved from polar body and blastomere biopsy toward the use of trophectoderm biopsy from the 5- to 6-day blastocysts as the standard of clinical practice. DNA obtained from 4 to 10 cells from a blastocyst is amplified using commercially available whole-genome amplification (WGA) kits. The amplified DNA can be tested for aneuploidy using available PGT-A molecular techniques, such as quantitative polymerase chain reaction (qPCR), array comparative genome hybridization (aCGH), single nucleotide polymorphism (SNP) microarray, or next-generation sequencing (NGS). These methods enable accurate identification of aneuploidy for 24 chromosomes (22 autosomes and the X and Y sex chromosomes). aCGH and NGS techniques can identify mosaic whole-chromosome aneuploidy[9–11] and detect nonmosaic gains and losses of chromosomal segments as small as 5–10 Mb in size.[12,13] The ability and sensitivity to detect segmental imbalances are greatly influenced by the type of WGA method,[14] platform utilized, data analysis algorithm, and customized bioinformatics approaches.[15] For embryos derived from parents with structural chromosome rearrangements, the use of microarray or NGS assays that can simultaneously test for both aneuploidy and segmental chromosome imbalances is beneficial. FISH analysis or qPCR using region-specific probes can also be performed on the biopsied cells when PGT-SR is indicated. The more challenging task is to distinguish embryos that carry the same balanced translocation as the parent from those that have a normal karyotype. Balanced translocations are associated with a higher risk of infertility and miscarriage, and many patients would prefer to avoid transmitting their balanced translocation to their offspring. Recent reports indicate that this can be done utilizing SNP array technology.[16]

PGT-M involves WGA followed by targeted analysis of the DNA sequences to detect pathogenic variants. Currently, the most common PGT-M methods utilize direct sequencing or allele-specific genotyping approaches. Direct sequencing of PCR products for the known parental pathogenic variants often requires custom primer design and validation. Analysis of short tandem repeats (STRs) or SNP-based genotyping via SNP microarray or PCR-based methods to assay SNPs (TaqMan) is used to examine for informative SNPs near the disease locus and can help diminish the chance of allelic dropout.

WHAT ARE THE ADVANTAGES AND RISKS OF PGT-A?

Preimplantation genetic testing requires IVF, embryo biopsy, and genetic analysis. These procedures are associated with a low risk of accidental damage to the embryo during biopsy, unsuccessful biopsy, failure of DNA amplification, and false-positive and false-negative results (Fig. 15.3). Genetic testing may reveal that there are no suitable embryos for a transfer, and additional IVF cycles may be required. Embryos that undergo biopsy do not appear to have increased risk for miscarriage or birth defects; however, the long-term health consequences to offspring, if any, are currently unknown.

Careful counseling of couples regarding the pros and cons of PGT-A is very important. It is also critical to understand the limitations of PGT-A and to communicate these limitations to couples considering this procedure. PGT-A may be considered to be a screening test as the detection rate is not 100%. Screening is limited to whole-chromosome gain or loss and will not detect subchromosomal deletions/duplications. PGT-A also does not test for triploidy (three sets of all chromosomes) or genetic conditions caused by single-gene variants (such as cystic fibrosis). The negative and positive predictive values for microarray PGT-A are ~98% and ~95%, respectively, and the false-negative rate is lower than 2% (Fig. 15.3). Every couple, regardless of their ethnic background and family history, has a 3%–5% risk for birth defects with each pregnancy, and even if the result of PGT-A is normal, the baby could still have one or more birth defects or intellectual disability from causes not detected by testing approaches. PGT-A does not replace prenatal testing such as chorionic villus sampling (CVS) or amniocentesis. Standard prenatal screening or testing should still be made available to patients undergoing IVF, including patients who had PGT-A. Women who do not wish to undergo diagnostic procedures because of their associated risk of loss can be offered the usual aneuploidy screening tests such as traditional first-trimester serum screening, cell-free DNA, and detailed ultrasound examination with all the caveats associated with such screening.[17]

DOES CURRENT CLINICAL EVIDENCE SUPPORT THE EFFICACY OF PGT-A?

Aneuploidy is recognized as the most common genetic abnormality resulting in embryonic demise, pregnancy loss, and congenital birth defects. At the preimplantation stage, ~50% of the IVF-derived embryos have chromosomal abnormalities that are incompatible with implantation or normal fetal development. As maternal age increases, the rate of aneuploidy in human oocytes escalates dramatically. Patients seeking IVF treatment are also commonly of an advanced age, which significantly reduces their chances for a live birth.

The aim of PGT-A is to select euploid embryos to theoretically increase successful pregnancy rates and reduce miscarriage rates. In the past, FISH analysis on a single-cell blastomere was used to assess aneuploidy for chromosomes 13, 15, 16, 18, 21, 22, X, and Y, which are the most common abnormalities found in products of conception. This approach failed to show a beneficial effect of PGT-A on the implantation and live birth rate after IVF.[3,4,18]

In recent years, application of PGT-A shifted to analysis of all 24 chromosomes and the ability to test multiple cells from blastocyst stage embryos. Implantation of embryos determined to be euploid by the new methodology has resulted in an increased live

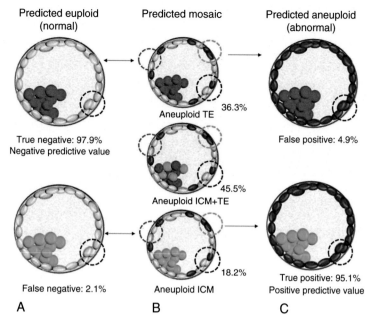

Predicted euploid (normal) Predicted mosaic Predicted aneuploid (abnormal)

Aneuploid TE 36.3%

True negative: 97.9%
Negative predictive value

False positive: 4.9%

Aneuploid ICM+TE 45.5%

False negative: 2.1% Aneuploid ICM 18.2%

True positive: 95.1%
Positive predictive value

A B C

FIG. 15.3 Outcomes of preimplantation genetic screening using TE biopsy. After successful PGS, embryos are predicted to be **(A)** euploid (~43%), **(C)** aneuploid (~32%), or **(B)** mosaic (~22%).[9] Other defects such as triploidy and nonmosaic segmental chromosomal copy number alterations are discovered in ~3% of samples. Possible sites of TE biopsy during preimplantation genetic testing are outlined by dashed circles. Euploid (normal) cells in TE and ICM are depicted by pink and red colored cells; aneuploid (abnormal) cells in TE and ICM are depicted by *dark blue* and *light blue* colored cells, respectively. *Black dashed circles* show TE content composed of euploid, aneuploid, or a euploid-aneuploid cell mixture that undergoes genetic testing to predict embryo karyotype. Among blastocysts predicted to be euploid **(A)**, negative predictive value is ~97.9%. Discordant TE and ICM cell lineages (false negative) are found in ~2.1% of embryos. Aneuploid embryos are true aneuploid (positive predictive value) in ~95.1% of cases and have euploid ICM (false-positive) content in ~4.9% of samples **(C)**. In mosaic embryos **(B)**, the result of TE biopsy is not predictive of ICM contents. Studies utilizing analysis from multiple TE and ICM biopsies from the same embryo have been performed on a very limited number of mosaic blastocysts. Out of 11 embryos, mosaicism in both TE and ICM was found in 5 embryos (45.5%), aneuploidy confined to TE was detected in 4 embryos (36.3%), and 2 embryos (18.1%) showed aneuploid ICM. Red and blue dashed circles exemplify situation when TE biopsy predominately contains euploid or aneuploid cells, and embryonic mosaicism is missed. As a result, some embryos will be misdiagnosed as euploid and if transferred may result in miscarriage or an affected fetus. *ICM*, inner cell mass; *TE*, trophectoderm.

birth delivery rate in women older than 37 years and a markedly decreased miscarriage rate.[19-21] PGT-A performed on a large cohort of patients showed that all 23 autosomes and sex chromosomes can be affected with trisomy and monosomy,[22] explaining high rate of miscarriages and implantation failures in earlier studies using targeted chromosome testing by FISH. The current clinical evidence shows that aneuploidy testing at the blastocyst stage provides the most accurate and consistent results, leading to improved IVF outcomes[23,24]; however, there are not enough data to recommend PGT-A as an universal approach to all IVF patients.[1] Additional studies are underway to

determine outcomes, evidence-based value of PGT-A, relative advantages and disadvantages, and specific recommendations for its use for patients of a certain age or a clinical indication.

WHAT IS A MOSAIC EMBRYO? SHOULD MOSAIC EMBRYOS BE IMPLANTED?

The presence of cells with both normal and abnormal chromosome complements in the embryo is defined as mosaicism. Embryonic mosaicism is a natural condition that exists at the early stages of embryo development. Up to 60% of IVF-derived embryos have at least one aneuploid cell at the 8-cell stage.[25] The proportion of abnormal cells in a mosaic embryo depends on the timing of when the chromosomal nondisjunction occurred. Missegregation of chromosomes at the 2-cell stage will result in a greater percentage of affected cells than mitotic errors at the 8-cell or 16-cell stages. Nearly 50% of mosaic embryos undergo self-correction; thus, abnormal cells are eliminated and embryos appear to be euploid at the blastocyst stage.[26] The rate of mosaic blastocysts has been estimated to be 5%–30%, depending on the detection technique, sensitivity of the analysis method, and clinic-specific reporting policies. Based on the proportion of aneuploid cells, mosaic embryos can be categorized as low-, middle-, and high-grade mosaics. Importantly, a low-grade mosaicism is difficult to distinguish from a technical artefact caused by an uneven representation of individual chromosomes after whole-genome amplification. Reanalysis of multiple TE and ICM biopsies initially diagnosed as mosaic blastocysts confirmed mosaicism in 48%–58% of embryos,[27,28] while the remaining embryos were in fact euploid. Therefore, the false-positive rate of an embryonic mosaicism is ~47%. On the other hand, detection of mosaicism is prejudiced by the content of TE biopsy. In mosaic embryos, a 4- to 10-cell TE sample may be composed of predominantly normal or abnormal cells depending on the biopsy location (Fig. 15.3B), precluding the detection of mosaicism. In fact, reanalysis by NGS assay of amplified DNA from euploid embryos showed mosaicism in ~30% of embryos that ended in spontaneous abortion.[27]

Embryos with true mosaicism can be classified into three categories: those that contain aneuploid cells confined to TE, aneuploidy affecting the ICM, or embryos with mosaicism in both TE and ICM cells (Fig. 15.3B). Overall concordance between TE and ICM has been demonstrated to be ~98% (negative predictive value) for fully euploid (Fig. 15.3A) and ~95% (positive predictive value) for fully aneuploid blastocysts (Fig. 15.3C); however, little is known about concordance between TE and ICM in mosaic embryos.[6]

In contrast to euploid embryos, mosaic embryos have a higher chance of carrying genetic abnormalities, including aneuploidy and uniparental disomy, leading to an increased risk of pregnancy loss as well as a liveborn child affected by chromosomal abnormalities and imprinting disorders. There are a few cases reported of the transfer of mosaic embryos resulting in live births, but the overall incidence of such events is unknown.[28] The impact of mosaicism on implantation, fetal development, and pregnancy outcome is not known and is likely underestimated. A broader range of genetic alterations, including whole-chromosome aneuploidy,

microdeletions/microduplications, and point mutations, have been observed in the mosaic state. Mosaic trisomy for chromosomes 2, 4, 5, 7, 8, 9, 12, 13, 14, 15, 16, 17, 18, 20, 21, 22, and X, as well as monosomy for chromosomes 7, 14, 15, 16, 18, 20, 21, 22, and X, have been reported in live births. Individuals with mosaic alterations may present with recognizable genetic diseases, developmental defects, neurodevelopmental conditions, and tissue-specific functional deficiencies that lead to disorders such as leukemia, reproductive problems, or an apparently normal phenotype. There is also an increased risk that mosaic individuals will transmit the aneuploidy to the offspring in a nonmosaic state. To date, there are no guidelines regarding the transfer of mosaic embryos. For couples with only mosaic embryos available for transfer, genetic counseling is encouraged to discuss several aspects influencing the decision-making process, such as the type of chromosomal alteration, the affected chromosome(s), copy number state (trisomy or monosomy), degree of mosaicism, detection method and the risk of false-positive results, benefits and limitations of prenatal testing, and potential clinical outcomes.

WHAT ARE THE REQUIREMENTS FOR PGT-M?

PGT-M has been used to detect more than 400 genetic conditions (https://www.hfea.gov.uk/pgd-conditions/) and is available for almost any genetic condition in specialized laboratories. PGT-M is now commonly available for disorders tested on routine and expanded carrier screening panels, genes implicated in inherited cancer predisposition syndromes, and adult-onset neuromuscular disorders.

The ability to offer PGT-M is dependent not only on the gene itself but also on the ability to implement a reliable test based on the patient-unique DNA alteration, available technologies, and their sensitivity in detection of a specific alteration type. PGT-M is a complex procedure that requires coordination between geneticists, embryologists, and infertility specialists. Couples undergoing PGT-M should have genetic counseling to provide detailed explanation of the risk of having an affected child, the impact of the disease, the benefits and limitations of prenatal diagnosis, and available options for preimplantation testing. PGT-M is suitable only for couples where one or both parents are affected or carry a disease-causing variant(s) identified by prior genetic analysis. The precise molecular diagnosis of the pathogenic variant(s) in the affected child and/or parents is a prerequisite for PGT-M testing. Parental DNA samples and/or affected family member must be available for

PGT-M for validation of the testing protocol for the specific gene variant of interest before an IVF cycle.

Intracytoplasmic sperm injection (ICSI) has been recommended for IVF cycles that will undergo PGT-M testing to minimize the risk of contamination from sperm DNA, although some studies have demonstrated negligible contamination by sperm cells after insemination methods in IVF cycles.[29] The simultaneous amplification of multiple polymorphic markers and comparison with the available parental samples is necessary to rule out DNA amplification failure of both alleles or a single allele (known as allele dropout).

WHAT ARE THE BENEFITS OF PARENTAL PRECONCEPTION GENETIC SCREENING AND HOW DOES IT AFFECT PREIMPLANTATION TESTING OF EMBRYOS?

On average, humans carry one to two variants per person that can cause severe genetic disorders or prenatal death if both copies of the same gene are defective.[30] About 0.2% of couples carry alterations in the same autosomal recessive gene.[31] Each couple that is a carrier for the same recessive disease will have a 25% risk of an affected fetus in each pregnancy. Parental preconception carrier screening is recommended to determine the couple's risk for a future pregnancy to be affected with severe recessive diseases.[32–34]

Ethnic-based, pan-ethnic, and expanded carrier screening tests include the analysis for pathogenic variants in genes associated with autosomal recessive and X-linked inherited disorders (see Chapter 7). The aim of preconception genetic testing is to determine parental carrier status and whether parents are at risk of conceiving a child with a genetic disorder. Termination of an affected pregnancy may be unacceptable or emotionally stressful for some couples; thus, preimplantation genetic testing may be the best option to avoid the birth of a child with a genetic disorder. Alternatively, parents may choose to use a gamete donor who has tested negative for the genetic condition that the couple carries.

SHOULD FOLLOW-UP PRENATAL TESTING AND SCREENING BE OFFERED FOR WOMEN WHO HAVE HAD PREIMPLANTATION GENETIC TESTING?

Although preimplantation genetic testing helps in the selection of healthy embryos, the risk of genetic disorders is not eliminated. Prenatal testing is recommended to all couples undergoing PGT-A, PGT-M, or PGT-SR (Table 15.1). Prenatal testing includes both screening tests (cell-free DNA and maternal serum screening) and diagnostic tests (chorionic villus sampling [CVS] and amniocentesis). Cell-free DNA screening, derived from placenta, also known as noninvasive prenatal screening (NIPS), can be performed as early as 10 weeks of gestation. Cell-free DNA is a screening method for detection of the most common trisomies (chromosomes 13, 18, 21), and sex chromosome aneuploidies. Aneuploidy for other chromosomes, mosaicism, chromosomal structural rearrangements, and DNA sequence variants in single genes are not available or reliable with cell-free DNA screening and require diagnostic testing on cells or tissues derived from the fetoplacental unit by karyotype, chromosomal microarray or sequencing.

In addition, testing for uniparental disomy (UPD) is recommended if the implanted embryo was reported to be mosaic, trisomic, or monosomic for a potentially imprinted chromosome (6, 7, 11, 14, 15, 16, or 20). Amniocentesis and UPD testing are also recommended in pregnancies when one of the parents carries a structural rearrangement involving imprinted chromosomes, such as balanced translocations involving chromosome 7 or Robertsonian translocations involving chromosome 14 or 15.[35]

Because of a chance of PGT-M DNA variant misdiagnosis in ~2% of cases due to DNA amplification inefficiencies or technical problems,[36,37] CVS or amniocentesis should be considered to confirm PGT findings. For any patient who has had PGT, diagnostic testing should be offered when a structural abnormality is found on fetal ultrasound to test for other genetic causes of birth defects regardless of a normal PGT result.

WHAT IS GENOME EDITING?

Genome editing refers to a collection of biomedical techniques that can be used to modify genomes. Researchers have been able to modify genomes of many organisms and some mammals for decades. Most of these modifications involved deleting or replacing large portions of the gene, but recent scientific breakthroughs allow introduction and correction of single nucleotide variants. The most popular technique is commonly known as CRISPR-Cas9 (short for clustered regularly interspaced short palindromic repeats and CRISPR-associated protein 9) genome editing. This method has gained enormous popularity in biomedical research because of the ease of introducing nucleotide variants. CRISPR-Cas9 is naturally used by bacteria to defend themselves from viral infections.[38,39] CRISPR-Cas9 has been used to genetically modify mammalian embryos (mice, rats) and nonhuman primate embryos. Scientific research shows that harmful variants can be repaired in human embryos[40,41]; however, genome editing of human embryos has several potential drawbacks. These include DNA modifications in regions that were not targeted, and the prevalence of such "off-target" modifications is unknown in human embryos. Moreover, CRISPR-Cas9 genome editing in mice causes mosaicism in a significant proportion of animals. This also occurs in human embryos although recent studies suggest a potential work-around by the coinjection of sperm and CRISPR–Cas9 components into metaphase II (MII) oocytes.[40] The ease of genome editing by CRISPR-Cas9 has led to fears that such technology could lead to a brave new world of genetic engineering and has led to widespread condemnation and a ban on such research in the United States.[42] However, most scientists and bioethicists agree that research involving human embryos is necessary to answer fundamental questions related to human biology[43] and should continue without implantation of such embryos. The genome editing of embryos is currently experimental[44] and not available for clinical use.

WHAT IS MITOCHONDRIAL DNA TRANSFER (THREE-PARENT IVF) AND WHAT ARE THE INDICATIONS FOR ITS USE?

Mitochondria, the cellular organelles located in the cytoplasm of all eukaryotic cells, contain their own mitochondrial DNA (mtDNA) and play a critical role in the generation of metabolic energy. In contrast to nuclear DNA (nDNA), which is inherited from both parents, mitochondrial DNA is transmitted from the mother to her offspring. Each human oocyte contains from 100,000 to 600,000 mitochondria, which are essential for oocyte maturation, fertilization, and embryonic development.[45] Changes in mtDNA or nDNA genes that encode mitochondrial proteins can lead to dysfunction of the mitochondria, causing a wide spectrum of severe mitochondrial disorders and diseases such as Leigh syndrome or mitochondrial myopathy, encephalopathy, lactic acidosis, and strokelike symptoms (MELAS), and can be associated with chronic progressive failure of multiple organ systems and early death. Variability in the proportion of normal and mutant copies of mtDNA (heteroplasmy) among different tissues may influence the resulting clinical phenotype, age of onset, and disease severity.

Parents harboring pathogenic variants for mitochondrial disorders in nuclear genes have an option to utilize PGT-M (Table 15.1). Preimplantation genetic testing for women with alterations in the mitochondrial genome itself is complicated by heteroplasmy and the inability to accurately determine the proportion of defective mtDNA in embryo biopsy samples.

A technique termed mitochondrial replacement therapy (MRT), also known as nuclear transfer or mitochondrial donation, has been recently developed to reduce the risk of transmission of defective mtDNA from a woman to her biological children.[46,47] Utilizing this IVF technology, DNA from three individuals, the maternal nuclear DNA, the donor's mitochondrial DNA, and the paternal genome, are combined together to produce a diploid zygote (Fig. 15.4). Even though MRT is an approved treatment option for selected patients in the United Kingdom,[48] the effectiveness and long-term outcome for children born using this experimental technique is not known.[49] The technique is not perfect, as a small number of maternal mutant mitochondria may be carried over during the sampling of maternal nuclear DNA, transferred into the donor egg, and distributed unequally between the various fetal tissues to cause potential pathology.[50] This procedure is currently banned in the United States because of concern for the effects of donor mitochondria on a "child's experiences of identity, kinship, or ancestry" and fear of introducing heritable genetic modifications to future offspring. Because all mtDNAs are inherited from the mother, MRT producing male offspring would not constitute heritable genetic modification because the modifications would not be passed down. A National Academy of Sciences study recommended that it is ethically permissible to conduct MRT clinical investigations. A recommendation has been made to allow mitochondrial replacement therapy for males first, as males will not be able to transmit the mitochondria to the next generation.[51]

COULD A PHYSICIAN REFUSE TO PROPAGATE HARMFUL TRAITS TO OFFSPRING?

Although rare, patients may request for the transfer of an embryo carrying a known disease causing pathogenic variant. For example, some individuals who themselves are affected with conditions such as hearing loss or achondroplasia may wish to raise children with a similar phenotype. Extensive and highly individualized counseling in such situations is important, as for any PGT procedure, and should involve discussion about the condition, the full spectrum of the phenotype including expressivity and penetrance, as well as potential lethality, and the emotional, physical, and financial effects that such conditions may have on the family unit. If the provider is not willing to assist the patients with their requests, patients should be given the option to seek help elsewhere. Overwhelming numbers of individuals with genetic conditions are born to couples without infertility, and therefore individuals

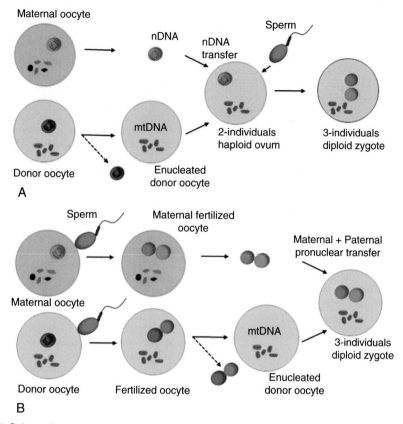

FIG. 15.4 Schematic representation of nuclear transfer techniques. **(A)** In a spindle transfer, the maternal spindle and chromosomes at metaphase stage of the second meiotic division (MII) are removed from an oocyte and inserted into enucleated MII donor egg. The spindle transfer results in an ovum containing maternal nuclear genome and the donor's healthy mitochondria, which is subsequently fertilized. **(B)** In a pronuclear transfer, both maternal and donor's eggs are fertilized. Maternal and paternal pronuclei are inserted into an enucleated donor's zygote comprising the donor's mitochondria, forming a diploid zygote.

who seek assisted reproductive services should potentially have the same choices. Nonetheless, in circumstances in which a child is highly likely to be born with a condition that is associated with severe handicap and suffering, the physician can refuse to transfer such embryos. Healthcare providers should consider many aspects of the decision-making, including the patient's reproductive autonomy, the welfare of resulting offspring, physician's autonomy and professional ethics, and the impact on the patient's family and society. The American Society for Reproductive Medicine encourages fertility clinics to establish written policies outlining unacceptable procedures, make them available to the patients before a treatment cycle, and coordinate referrals to genetic counseling or other professionals for a consultation about the parental reproductive risks and benefits.[52]

IS THERE AN INCREASED RISK OF BIRTH DEFECTS ASSOCIATED WITH ASSISTED REPRODUCTIVE TECHNOLOGY?

ART is associated with a small increase in birth defects. A meta-analysis comparing 92,671 babies conceived with ART with 3,870,760 naturally conceived children reported a somewhat higher risk of birth defects among infants conceived with ART (RR1.32; 95% CI: 1.24–1.42). The risk was increased when the analysis was limited to major birth defects (RR1.42, 95% CI: 1.29–1.56).[53] Studies have been performed to attempt to identify whether the observed increase in birth defects is attributable to the associated manipulation of the oocyte and the embryo, the underlying cause of infertility, or other specific characteristics, health risks, and behaviors in individuals undergoing ART. A large Australian study[54] of more than 300,000 births including 6163 ART pregnancies reported an increased risk of birth defects in pregnancies achieved with any type of ART (adjusted OR 1.28; 95% CI: 1.16–1.41) and a higher risk of birth defects associated with the use of intracytoplasmic sperm injection (ICSI) (adjusted OR 1.57; 95% CI: 1.30–1.90). A history of infertility, either with or without assisted conception, was also significantly associated with birth defects.[55]

A specific pattern of birth defects or disorders that can potentially be detected with targeted screening has not been identified.[55] ART has been associated with epigenetic alterations, involving methylation and imprinting disorders such as Beckwith-Wiedemann and Prader-Willi syndromes.[56] Epigenetic changes are heritable changes that do not involve alterations in the DNA sequence (see Chapter 2). A 2016 ACOG Committee Opinion states that "it seems judicious to make patients aware of the low level risk of birth defects and to offer ultrasonographic surveillance for structural abnormalities in these pregnancies." ACOG acknowledges that although some professional organizations recommend fetal echocardiography, the incremental yield following a reassuring targeted ultrasound is unclear and needs to be balanced against available resources.[56]

REFERENCES

1. Practice Committees of the American Society for Reproductive Medicine and the Society for Assisted Reproductive Technology. The use of preimplantation genetic testing for aneuploidy (PGT-A): a committee opinion. *Fertil Steril.* 2018;109(3):429–436.
2. Hassold T, Chen N, Funkhouser J, et al. A cytogenetic study of 1000 spontaneous abortions. *Ann Hum Genet.* 1980;44:151–178.
3. Mastenbroek S, Twisk M, van der Veen F, et al. Preimplantation genetic screening: a systematic review and meta-analysis of RCTs. *Hum Reprod Update.* 2011;17:454–466.
4. Rubio C, Bellver J, Rodrigo L, et al. Preimplantation genetic screening using fluorescence in situ hybridization in patients with repetitive implantation failure and advanced maternal age: two randomized trials. *Fertil Steril.* 2013;99:1400–1407.
5. Demko ZP, Simon AL, McCoy RC, et al. Effects of maternal age on euploidy rates in a large cohort of embryos analyzed with 24-chromosome single-nucleotide polymorphism-based preimplantation genetic screening. *Fertil Steril.* 2016;105:1307–1313.
6. Capalbo A, Rienzi L. Mosaicism between trophectoderm and inner cell mass. *Fertil Steril.* 2017;107:1098–1106.
7. Scott Jr RT, Upham KM, Forman EJ, et al. Cleavage-stage biopsy significantly impairs human embryonic implantation potential while blastocyst biopsy does not: a randomized and paired clinical trial. *Fertil Steril.* 2013;100:624–630.
8. Zegers-Hochschild F, Adamson GD, Dyer S, et al. The international glossary on infertility and fertility care, 2017. *Hum Reprod.* 2017;32:1786–1801.
9. Munné S, Blazek J, Large M, et al. Detailed investigation into the cytogenetic constitution and pregnancy outcome of replacing mosaic blastocysts detected with the use of high-resolution next-generation sequencing. *Fertil Steril.* 2017;108:62–71.
10. Munné S, Wells D. Detection of mosaicism at blastocyst stage with the use of high-resolution next-generation sequencing. *Fertil Steril.* 2017;107:1085–1091.
11. Harton GL, Cinnioglu C, Fiorentino F. Current experience concerning mosaic embryos diagnosed during preimplantation genetic screening. *Fertil Steril.* 2017;107:1113–1119.
12. Fiorentino F, Bono S, Biricik A, et al. Application of next-generation sequencing technology for comprehensive aneuploidy screening of blastocysts in clinical preimplantation genetic screening cycles. *Hum Reprod.* 2014;29:2802–2813.
13. Rodrigo L, Mateu E, Mercader A, et al. New tools for embryo selection: comprehensive chromosome screening by array comparative genomic hybridization. *BioMed Res Int.* 2014;2014:517125.
14. Treff NR, Zimmerman RS. Advances in preimplantation genetic testing for monogenic disease and aneuploidy. *Annu Rev Genomics Hum Genet.* 2017;18:189–200.
15. Treff NR, Franasiak JM. Detection of segmental aneuploidy and mosaicism in the human preimplantation embryo: technical considerations and limitations. *Fertil Steril.* 2017;107:27–31.
16. Treff NR, Thompson K, Rafizadeh M, et al. SNP array-based analyses of unbalanced embryos as a reference to distinguish between balanced translocation carrier and normal blastocysts. *J Assist Reprod Genet.* 2016;33:1115–1119.
17. Heron M. Deaths: leading causes for 2014. *Natl Vital Stat Rep.* 2016;65:1–96.
18. Northrop LE, Treff NR, Levy B, et al. SNP microarray-based 24 chromosome aneuploidy screening demonstrates that cleavage-stage FISH poorly predicts aneuploidy in embryos that develop to morphologically normal blastocysts. *Mol Hum Reprod.* 2010;16:590–600.
19. Dahdouh EM, Balayla J, García-Velasco JA. Comprehensive chromosome screening improves embryo selection: a meta-analysis. *Fertil Steril.* 2015;104:1503–1512.
20. Rubio C, Bellver J, Rodrigo L, et al. In vitro fertilization with preimplantation genetic diagnosis for aneuploidies in advanced maternal age: a randomized, controlled study. *Fertil Steril.* 2017;107:1122–1129.
21. Ubaldi FM, Cimadomo D, Capalbo A, et al. Preimplantation genetic diagnosis for aneuploidy testing in women older than 44 years: a multicenter experience. *Fertil Steril.* 2017;107:1173–1180.
22. Babariya D, Fragouli E, Alfarawati S, et al. The incidence and origin of segmental aneuploidy in human oocytes and preimplantation embryos. *Hum Reprod.* 2017;8:1–12.
23. Chang J, Boulet SL, Jeng G, et al. Outcomes of in vitro fertilization with preimplantation genetic diagnosis: an analysis of the United States Assisted Reproductive Technology Surveillance Data, 2011-2012. *Fertil Steril.* 2016;105:394–400.

24. Munné S, Cohen J. Advanced maternal age patients benefit from preimplantation genetic diagnosis of aneuploidy. *Fertil Steril.* 2017;107(5):1145–1146. https://doi.org/10.1016/j.fertnstert.2017.03.015. Epub 2017 Apr 6. PubMed PMID: 28390694.

25. Munné S, Chen S, Colls P, et al. Maternal age, morphology, development and chromosome abnormalities in over 6000 cleavage-stage embryos. *Reprod Biomed Online.* 2007;14(5):628–634.

26. Bazrgar M, Gourabi H, Valojerdi MR, et al. Self-correction of chromosomal abnormalities in human preimplantation embryos and embryonic stem cells. *Stem Cells Dev.* 2013;22(17):2449–2456.

27. Maxwell SM, Colls P, Hodes-Wertz B, et al. Why do euploid embryos miscarry? A case-control study comparing the rate of aneuploidy within presumed euploid embryos that resulted in miscarriage or live birth using next-generation sequencing. *Fertil Steril.* 2016;106(6). 1414–1419.e5.

28. Greco E, Minasi MG, Fiorentino F. Healthy babies after intrauterine transfer of mosaic aneuploid blastocysts. *N Engl J Med.* 2015;373(21):2089–2090.

29. Feldman B, Aizer A, Brengauz M, et al. Pre-implantation genetic diagnosis-should we use ICSI for all? *J Assist Reprod Genet.* 2017;34:1179–1183.

30. Gao Z, Waggoner D, Stephens M, Ober C, Przeworski M. An estimate of the average number of recessive lethal mutations carried by humans. *Genetics.* 2015;199(4):1243–1254.

31. Azimi M, Schmaus K, Greger V, Neitzel D, Rochelle R, Dinh T. Carrier screening by next-generation sequencing: health benefits and cost effectiveness. *Mol Genet Genomic Med.* 2016;4(3):292–302.

32. Franasiak JM, Olcha M, Bergh PA, et al. Expanded carrier screening in an infertile population: how often is clinical decision making affected? *Genet Med.* 2016;18(11):1097–1101.

33. Committee opinion no. 690 summary: carrier screening in the age of genomic medicine. *Obstet Gynecol.* 2017;129(3):595–596.

34. Committee opinion no. 691. Carrier screening for genetic conditions. American College of Obstetricians and Gynecologists. *Obstet Gynecol.* 2017;129:e41–55.

35. Liehr T. Cytogenetic contribution to uniparental disomy (UPD). *Mol Cytogenet.* 2010;29(3):8.

36. Grati FR, Malvestiti F, Ferreira JC, et al. Fetoplacental mosaicism: potential implications for false-positive and false-negative noninvasive prenatal screening results. *Genet Med.* 2014;16(8):620–624.

37. Dreesen J, Destouni A, Kourlaba G, et al. Evaluation of PCR-based preimplantation genetic diagnosis applied to monogenic diseases: a collaborative ESHRE PGD consortium study. *Eur J Hum Genet.* 2014;22(8):1012–1018.

38. Hsu PD, Lander ES, Zhang F. Development and applications of CRISPR-Cas9 for genome engineering. *Cell.* 2014;157:1262–1278.

39. Komor AC, Badran AH, Liu DR. CRISPR-based technologies for the manipulation of eukaryotic genomes. *Cell.* 2017;168(1–2):20–36.

40. Ma H, Marti-Gutierrez N, Park SW, et al. Correction of a pathogenic gene mutation in human embryos. *Nature.* 2017;548(7668):413–419.

41. Liang P, Ding C, Sun H, et al. Correction of β-thalassemia mutant by base editor in human embryos. *Protein Cell.* 2017;8(11):811–822.

42. Baltimore D, Berg P, Botchan M, et al. A prudent path forward for genomic engineering and germline gene modification. *Science.* 2015;348(6230):36–38.

43. Fogarty NME, McCarthy A, Snijders KE, et al. Genome editing reveals a role for OCT4 in human embryogenesis. *Nature.* 2017;550(7674):67–73.

44. Ormond KE, Mortlock DP, Scholes DT, et al. Human germline genome editing. *Am J Hum Genet.* 2017;101(2):167–176.

45. Liu Y, Han M, Li X, et al. Age-related changes in the mitochondria of human mural granulosa cells. *Hum Reprod.* 2017;32(12):2465–2473.

46. Craven L, Tuppen HA, Greggains GD, et al. Pronuclear transfer in human embryos to prevent transmission of mitochondrial DNA disease. *Nature.* 2010;465(7294):82–85.

47. Tachibana M, Amato P, Sparman M, et al. Towards germline gene therapy of inherited mitochondrial diseases. *Nature.* 2013;493(7434):627–631.

48. Herbert M, Turnbull D. Mitochondrial donation clearing the final regulatory hurdle in the United Kingdom. *N Engl J Med.* 2017;376(2):171–173.

49. Zhang J, Liu H, Luo S, et al. Live birth derived from oocyte spindle transfer to prevent mitochondrial disease. *Reprod Biomed Online.* 2017;34(4):361–368.

50. Treff NR, Campos J, Tao X, et al. Blastocyst preimplantation genetic diagnosis (PGD) of a mitochondrial DNA disorder. *Fertil Steril.* 2012;98:1236–1240.

51. Committee on the Ethical and Social Policy Considerations of Novel Techniques for Prevention of Maternal Transmission of Mitochondrial DNA Diseases, Board on Health Sciences Policy, Institute of Medicine, National Academies of Sciences, Engineering, and Medicine. In: Claiborne A, English R, Kahn J, eds. *Mitochondrial Replacement Techniques: Ethical, Social, and Policy Considerations.* Washington (DC): National Academies Press (US); 2016.

52. Ethics Committee of the American Society for Reproductive Medicine, Ethics Committee of the American Society for Reproductive Medicine. Transferring embryos with genetic anomalies detected in preimplantation testing: an ethics committee opinion. *Fertil Steril.* 2017;107(5):1130–1135. Electronic address: ASRM@asrm.org.

53. Hansen M, Kurinczuk JJ, Milne E, de Klerk N, Bower C. Assisted reproductive technology and birth defects: a systematic review and meta-analysis. *Hum Reprod Update.* 2013;19:330–353.

54. Hansen M, Kurinczuk JJ, de Klerk N, Burton P, Bower C. Assisted reproductive technology and major birth defects in western Australia. *Obstet Gynecol.* 2012;120:852–863.

55. Davies MJ, Moore VM, Willson KJ, et al. Reproductive technologies and the risk of birth defects. *N Engl J Med.* 2012;366:1803–1813.

56. Perinatal risks associated with reproductive technology. Committee opinion no. 671. American College of Obstetricians and Gynecologists. *Obstet Gynecol.* 2016;128:e61–e68.

CHAPTER 16

Fetal Treatment of Genetic Disorders

QUOC-HUNG L. NGUYEN, MD • RUSSELL G. WITT, MD • TIPPI C. MACKENZIE, MD

IN UTERO STEM CELL TRANSPLANTATION

In utero hematopoietic stem cell transplantation (IUHCT) is a promising approach to treat congenital genetic disorders. IUHCT offers multiple therapeutic advantages over postnatal bone marrow transplantation due in part to the fetal immune system's ability to support transplanted donor cells and develop donor-specific tolerance.[1,2] The immunologic immaturity of the developing fetus allows antigens that are introduced early in development to not elicit an immune response. Fetal stem cell therapy provides access to hematopoietic stem cell niches at an important time in development when stem cells are migrating to their destined tissues and offers the ability to treat a disease before birth.[3,4]

WHAT IS THE RATIONALE FOR IN UTERO STEM CELL TRANSPLANTATION, AND WHAT BARRIERS DO REMAIN IN THE DEVELOPMENT OF THIS THERAPY?

Rationale, Experimental Work, and Barriers to Success

Conceptualization of hematopoietic stem cell transplantation dates back to 1945 when Owen found that dizygotic cattle twins shared placental circulation.[5] Later, Billingham et al. demonstrated that early fetal exposure to antigens allowed for tolerance to the exposed antigen, meaning that postnatal treatment was better tolerated.[6] These investigators isolated cells from various organs in one strain of mice, and these were then injected into fetuses of a different strain. After birth, these mice were able to tolerate skin grafts from mice of the transplanted strain. This early study set the groundwork for future research exploring the fetal environment as an avenue for tolerance to foreign antigens.

IUHCT was later performed in anemic mice with a mutation in the c-kit gene, which is responsible for the differentiation, proliferation, and survival of hematopoietic stem cells.[7,8] Using a transplacental injection of hematopoietic stem cells, it was shown that stem cells from either fetal livers or adult bone marrow were able to correct the anemia. Mice that were more anemic supported the engraftment of stem cells, whereas mice that were not anemic did not engraft. Further studies demonstrated that engraftment of stem cells after IUHCT could be achieved in mice that had no stem cells[9] or mice with severe combined immunodeficiency (SCID), in which a genetic defect prevents the proper maturation of T and B cells.[10] Mice that were deficient in stem cells demonstrated donor-derived multilineage engraftment, whereas SCID-transplanted mice were only able to produce donor-derived lymphocytes. These were the first studies to show that IUHCT could lead to successful engraftment if the host was deficient in that particular lineage of cell, whereas host cell competition limited the effectiveness of IUHCT and explained why IUHCT in immunocompetent hosts had not led to successful engraftment.

Studies of stem cell engraftment after IUHCT in animals without inherent defects in their hematopoiesis showed engraftment below clinically relevant levels including mice,[11-14] dogs,[15,16] goats,[17,18] and primates.[19,20] Further research has improved techniques for delivery of transplanted cells. Intrahepatic and intravascular cell delivery allows greater numbers of hematopoietic stem cells to be transplanted and results in increases in overall chimerism.[21] Reaching levels of 1%–2% engraftment result in donor-specific tolerance of donor cells. Mice that reach these levels of chimerism have been found to be able to accept donor skin grafts and do not show immunoreactivity to donor antigens.[14,22,23]

Even in the fetal environment, an immune response can still limit donor cell engraftment. In fetal mice, although the fetal immune system matures later than in humans, the main culprit for rejection of transplanted cells has been shown to be the maternal immune system. A barrier to engraftment are maternal T cells that cross the placenta.[24] In human fetuses, in which there is earlier maturation of the immune system, it has been demonstrated that the trafficking of maternal antigens to the fetus makes fetal T cells less reactive to the

Perinatal Genetics. https://doi.org/10.1016/B978-0-323-53094-1.00016-3

mother.[25] Thus, transplantation of maternal stem cells into fetuses should overcome the maternal immune response to the transplantation, particularly because the human fetus should have T cells specific for these maternal antigens.

Studies of In Utero Stem Cell Transplantation in Large Animal Models

One of the major early successes with IUHCT was in the sheep model. Using an intraperitoneal injection of fetal stem cells, allogeneic engraftment could be shown in 75% of recipients with engraftment as high as 30%.[1] The sheep continued to have chimerism 9 months after transplantation and never developed evidence of graft-versus-host disease. This early success leads to a great deal of enthusiasm; however, initial clinical application of IUHCT failed for numerous diseases.[26]

Studies in the pig model were more encouraging, and it was demonstrated that IUHCT recipients were able to develop donor-specific tolerance and to tolerate donor-matched kidney transplants without immunosuppression.[27,28] In studies of a canine model of leukocyte adhesion deficiency (CLAD), dogs underwent IUHCT via an intraperitoneal injection, which resulted in low levels of engraftment in two dogs and improvement in the disease phenotype. The dogs were then able to undergo a booster transplant to improve their chimerism to clinically relevant levels.[29] Around this time, discoveries made in the murine model of IUHCT were used to further improve donor cell engraftment, specifically the use of maternal cells.[24] Dogs were then treated with maternally derived donor stem cells via intracardiac injection.[30] Chimerism was significantly improved with the new approach, and 21 of 24 dogs had engraftment greater than 1% with an average of 11%. This verified that the barriers found in the mouse model were limiting in the large animal models as well.

Early Clinical Experience in Humans

There has been little clinical success in IUHCT in humans due in large part to the unforeseen barriers to engraftment that were only identified after the early trials. At this time, 26 cases of IUHCT have been attempted in human fetuses for a variety of diseases with only bare lymphocyte syndrome[31] and X-linked SCID,[32,33] demonstrating clinically relevant engraftment and disease amelioration.[2] It appears that in all successful cases, engraftment occurred due to the lack of host immune cell competition. Despite limited success, numerous lessons were learned from these early experiences and multiple improvements have been made based in part on the identified barriers found in animal studies. Fetal

access has improved significantly. Ultrasound guidance allows for safe access to the umbilical vein and allows for a more efficient intravascular delivery of hematopoietic stem cells. In addition, it is now recognized that a protocol based on transplantation of a high dose of maternal-derived stem cells, injected intravascularly, has the best chance of allowing engraftment. Even if clinically significant levels are not achieved, a low level of chimerism could allow a postnatal "booster" transplantation with minimal conditioning.[34] This approach has been used in mouse models of thalassemia and sickle cell disease.[35]

WHAT DISEASES ARE AMENABLE TO IN UTERO STEM CELL THERAPY?

Hemoglobinopathies

Hemoglobinopathies are a group of clinical disorders caused by genetic defects that cause either an abnormal structure of hemoglobin or insufficient production.[36] IUHCT can potentially correct or lessen the disease burden of any disease that results from defective hematopoiesis, including hemoglobinopathies.[31,37,38] Hemoglobinopathies are ideal targets for IUHCT by virtue of their overall prevalence in the general population and their deficiency arising from within the hematopoietic stem cell population.[37,39] Postnatal allogeneic stem cell transplantation for sickle cell disease has been demonstrated as curative for patients with symptomatic sickle cell disease[40] and thalassemia.[41] The most prevalent clinically severe hemoglobinopathy is sickle cell anemia. Its clinical manifestations and disease burden vary greatly from individual to individual.[42] The disease is characterized by vasoocclusive crises that require prolonged hospitalization. The overall cost of sickle cell disease in the United States was estimated at $460,151 per person[43] and this disorder afflicts approximately 100,000 Americans.[44] There have been several advances that have improved and prolonged the lives of patients with sickle cell disease[45,46]; however, hematopoietic stem cell transplantation remains the only curative treatment. Unfortunately, postnatal stem cell transplantation carries a lifetime risk of graft-versus-host disease and requires myeloablative preconditioning. Although clinical experience with high chimerism levels is sparse, in the preclinical and few clinical cases, graft-versus-host disease is rarely observed when the amount of mature T cells is controlled for.[47]

Thalassemias are also common; gene frequencies are estimated to range from 2.5% to 15% in the tropics and subtropics.[48,49] α-Thalassemia major manifests with severe anemia in utero, including hydrops fetalis and fetal demise.[50] If left untreated, α-thalassemia major (ATM) is lethal, but fetal therapy with in utero transfusions can be lifesaving for these fetuses, and fetuses who are treated with in utero transfusions can survive with reasonable neurologic outcomes.[51] This disease represents an ideal target for in utero therapy because it is fatal in utero without treatment. Because the fetus already needs to receive an invasive procedure in utero to survive, the HSC transplantation can be performed at the same time as the transfusions.

Lysosomal Storage Disorders

Lysosomal storage disorders are a group of diseases that result from a genetic deficiency in an enzyme required for the normal metabolic functions of the lysosome. Lysosomes are therefore unable to break down their complex substrates, which then accumulate within the cells leading to cellular dysfunction.[52] Consequences of the disease include intellectual disability, skeletal dysplasias, pulmonary insufficiency, and, in severe cases, hydrops fetalis and in utero fetal demise. Patients with certain lysosomal storage disorders can be treated after birth with enzyme replacement therapy (ERT). The deficient enzyme is transfused and taken up by various cells, decreasing the extent of cellular damage. This approach is limited, however, and ERT does not appear to cross the blood-brain barrier and does not significantly improve the central nervous system deterioration.[53] Additionally, the deficient enzyme is seen as foreign by the patient's immune system. Postnatal therapy is limited by the development of antibodies against the exogenous enzyme, which leads to decreased effectiveness of the enzyme and allergic responses.[54] As a result, immunosuppression is required for continued enzyme therapy.[55]

To improve outcomes in patients with lysosomal storage disorders, stem cell transplantation has been performed in multiple lysosomal storage disorders including Hurler disease, Batten disease, metachromatic leukodystrophy, Krabbe disease, and I-cell disease.[56] Clinical results have varied based on the disease, which stem cells were transplanted, age at transplantation, and chimerism levels, but overall clinical results have been promising.[57-61] In Hurler disease specifically, improvements were noted in survival, cognitive development, preservation of hearing, corneal clouding, and respiratory support requirements.[62] Earlier age at transplantation and posttransplant enzyme levels were predictive of outcome improvement.

In utero hematopoietic stem cell transplantation coupled with in utero enzyme replacement therapy could greatly improve outcomes for this group of patients for multiple reasons. First, many affected fetuses die before birth or before enzyme replacement therapy can be initiated. Second, fetal accumulation of toxic metabolic by-products leads to numerous developmental insults before the possible initiation of enzyme replacement. Neurologic outcomes may be improved with earlier therapy, particularly during fetal development, either by providing the enzyme before formation of the blood brain barrier or by early receptor-mediated transport. Third, fetal exposure to the exogenous enzyme may induce tolerance, which would make postnatal therapy more efficacious.

Osteogenesis Imperfecta

Osteogenesis imperfecta (OI) is a genetic connective tissue disorder that is caused by defects in the proper synthesis of type I collagen.[63] The disease is characterized by fragile bones among multiple other ailments, and there are multiple forms with significant variability in clinical presentation, from perinatal death to a normal life span.[64] Current medical therapies seek to improve bone strength, although efficacy is limited and, in the most severe form, is available too late to improve survival. In utero therapy has been focused on the use of mesenchymal stem cells because of their nonimmunogenic nature and ability to engraft and form bone.[65] In utero therapy with mesenchymal stem cells for OI is particularly appealing because it takes advantage of the chemotactic properties of MSCs that guide them to sites of injury (intrauterine fractures are common) and the small fetal size (30–100 g at 14–16 weeks' gestation) allows for lower stem cell dosing and greater potential proliferation throughout gestation.

In utero stem cell transplantation for OI has been performed previously. In 2003, Westgren et al. performed in utero stem cell transplantation at a gestational age of 29 weeks.[66] They found engraftment of 5% and no intrauterine fractures. In 2005, another transplantation was performed at 32 weeks' gestation with 7% chimerism. At 2 years of age, the patient had suffered three fractures.[67]

WHAT CURRENT TRIALS ARE UNDERWAY FOR IUHCT?

In 2014, the International Fetal Transplantation and Immunology Society was established to determine the most effective and ethical ways to conduct clinical trials.[68,69] The group released a consensus statement that stated that IUHCT is a viable strategy to treat congenital disorders, that the intravascular route may be the delivery method of choice for stem cell transplantation, that transplantation should utilize maternally derived donor cells and that suggested that an international registry be developed to facilitate the sharing of results.[68,69] This society has been instrumental in the coordination and planning of ongoing clinical trials.

Our group is currently conducting a phase 1 clinical trial using CD34+-selected maternal HSCs in fetuses with α-thalassemia major to explore the safety and feasibility in this setting.[70] In an attempt to circumvent the known barriers to successful engraftment, we are using high dose, maternally derived hematopoietic stem cells and transfusing them between 18 and 25 weeks because of limitations in umbilical vein access earlier in gestation.

There is also an ongoing trial for in utero mesenchymal stem cell transplantation for OI, the BOOSTB4 trial. It is a multicenter trial devised to evaluate the safety and efficacy of mesenchymal stem cell transplantation in severe forms of OI. The study includes three groups: prenatal and postnatal transplantation, postnatal transplantation, and historical and prospective controls.[71] These trials, although early, are exciting advances in the field of in utero therapy and are offering treatments for diseases with significant burden and limited options currently.

In Utero Gene Therapy

In utero gene therapy (IUGT) is another potential fetal molecular therapy for single-gene disorders with encouraging preclinical data. The general strategy for gene therapy involves packaging genetic sequences within inactivated viral vectors, which retain the ability to transduce genetic material to host cells. This takes advantage of existing viral infectious machinery but with the theoretical removal of treatment toxicity. As described in more detail below, some vectors have the ability to integrate into the host genome, allowing for transmission to daughter cell populations and long-term transgene expression. This section details the therapeutic advantages of using this treatment during the fetal period, outlines existing research with preclinical and postnatal clinical models, and describes some of the risks and potential adverse effects of this treatment modality.

WHAT ARE THE POTENTIAL ADVANTAGES OF IUGT OVER POSTNATAL APPROACHES?
Avoidance of Disease Onset

Prototypical diseases for in utero gene therapy are those that manifest early in life, including the thalassemias, hemophilia, and severe combined immunodeficiency (SCID). Many of these diseases result in severe and irreversible damage before birth. These diseases typically require lifelong treatment that is noncurative.

Correction in utero has the potential to improve the quality of life for the patient and family. The impact of genetic disease was assessed in a study out of the Case hospital system in Ohio; review of the hospital's records showed that 96% of children with chronic underlying disorders had a clear genetic etiology or susceptibility, with one-third of pediatric ICU admissions related to diseases with a genetic basis, such as cystic fibrosis and sickle cell disease.[72] Liver diseases such as urea cycle disorders typically present with severe neonatal manifestations in the first week of life; they can result in irreversible multiorgan damage and death.[73] In a study on patients with severe hemophilia, prophylactic treatment with clotting factors earlier in life resulted in lower incidence of arthropathies secondary to bleeding episodes later in life.[74]

Unique Immunologic Advantage

The fetal immune system provides several distinct advantages for gene therapy with respect to immune responses to the viral vector as well as the proteins encoded by the transgene. Fetuses have theoretically never encountered the common viral vectors for gene therapy; thus it is unlikely that preformed antibodies will exist against viral vectors. In adulthood, both innate and adaptive immune responses have been demonstrated in response to the administration of these vectors. Administering viral vectors in a fetal host before the formation of these antibodies could potentially avoid inflammatory reaction and associated vector neutralization.

Immune responses to the proteins encoded by the transgene can also limit the efficacy of postnatal therapy. Preclinical models have shown that adults are capable of developing an immune response that limits the effectiveness of viral transgene. In a study on rhesus macaques, different doses of human factor IX were given via first-generation adenoviral vector to determine whether sustained expression of the human coagulation factor could be achieved.[75] Human factor IX was detectable for several weeks but disappeared along with development of high titers of antifactor IX antibody. The relative immaturity of the fetal immune system could allow for immunologic tolerance and the avoidance of the above complications.

Many preclinical experiments have supported this idea of a tolerant fetal environment. Direct intraperitoneal injection of retroviral vector encoding β-galactosidase in fetal sheep led to development of postnatal tolerance to the protein product.[76] This was demonstrated by administering a postnatal booster of the protein and showing that the animals have a blunted ability to form an antibody response to the protein. A similar study in mice involved in utero yolk sac injection of adenoviral vector carrying human factor IX transgene.[77,78] Injection of the human protein in adult mice resulted in persistent expression of this protein as well as undetectable antifactor IX antibody levels, whereas control mice developed high antibody titers and associated loss of factor IX expression. This induction of tolerance facilitates postnatal repeat therapy as well, because both vector and vector transgene are introduced with in utero treatment.

These preclinical experiments have been expanded to nonhuman primates as well, where in utero treatment led to long-term expression of human factor IX, with evidence of tolerance induction.[79] AAV5 and 8 vectors were used to deliver human factor IX in late gestation with macaques, which led to liver tropism and stable expression for more than 6 years.[80] Challenge with postnatal AAV led to subclinical levels of anti-AAV antibody expression, indicating that tolerance had been induced with prenatal treatment. There was no evidence of toxicity from observed viral integration, nor was there evidence of germline transmission.

Crossing Blood-Brain Barrier

The blood-brain barrier provides a unique challenge in postnatal therapy—peripheral administration of drugs and therapies such as stem cell transplant or gene therapy generally does not cross this barrier. In utero gene therapy does show promise in the central nervous system—direct intraventricular injection of adenoviral vector carrying the missing enzyme in mucopolysaccharidosis VII (MPS7) resulted in widespread gene expression and amelioration of disease in early life.[81] Other studies have used postnatal full-body irradiation in mice to circumvent the blood-brain barrier, a toxic adjunctive procedure that would be avoided if in utero treatment can provide access to the brain before formation of that barrier. Several AAV vectors have been demonstrated to successfully cross the blood-brain barrier in the perinatal period in murine and nonhuman models.[82] Neonatal treatment in the mouse model with the AAV9 vector carrying the *SMN* gene has led to phenotypic rescue of spinal muscular atrophy. In the nonhuman primate model, both fetal and early neonatal treatments with AAV9 vector successfully transduced a wide range of systemic cells including neurons as well. Gaining access to the blood-brain barrier with in utero treatment, especially without toxic systemic treatments such as whole-body radiation, is another potential benefit to this approach.

Access to Stem Cell Populations

Similar to the rationales cited in fetal stem cell therapy, IUGT has the potential to access stem cell populations during a time when they exist in higher relative frequency to other cells. Usage of viral vectors that integrate into the host genome would allow for significant expansion of the viral transgene into daughter cells. An experiment using VSV-G pseudotype equine infectious anemia with a transgene for β-galactosidase in mice resulted in multiorgan gene expression that was uniquely found to be in clusters of cells. This suggested clonal expansions of originally transduced cells.[83] IUGT with lentiviral delivery of lacZ has resulted in transduction of muscle stem cells (satellite cells) in a murine muscular injury model.[84]

WHICH DISEASES HAVE DEMONSTRATED EFFICACY WITH POSTNATAL GENE THERAPY IN PRECLINICAL MODELS?

Hemophilia

There have been recent promising results in safety and efficacy of IUGT with preclinical models of hemophilia, suggesting that this may be a good candidate for initial IUGT clinical trials. Although the disease is no longer debilitating, it does relegate patients to a lifetime of frequent infusions, with alloantibody development reducing treatment efficacy.[85] With hemophilia A, the relatively large size of the factor VIII coding region has led to limited gene therapy applications, as vectors such as AAV have limited packaging capacity. A recent study overcame this obstacle, and six of seven patients had normal long-term factor VIII expression levels. No liver toxicity of neutralizing antibodies was developed, and although anti-AAV5 capsid antibodies were detected, no cellular immune responses were found.[86] These exciting phenotypic improvements after single doses, as well as the lack of significant adverse effects, indicate that hemophilia may be an ideal first target for IUGT. There were cases in these hemophilia studies where existing arthropathies secondary to recurrent bleeds could not be reversed despite successful long-term transgene expression—IUGT would address the disease before the development of such chronic sequelae.

In cases of severe human hemophilia B, another recent landmark study was published where a single injection of AAV-mediated hyperfunctional factor IX variant gene led to high levels of functional factor IX, along with decreased bleeding rates and factor infusion requirements.[87] Of the 10 patients treated, 8 patients did not require any further factor infusions over the follow-up period of over a year, and 9 patients had no further bleeding episodes after vector treatment. Although low titers of neutralizing antibody titers were detectable, the patients universally had lasting factor IX activity (35.5 ± 18.7% of the normal value) throughout the study period. The improvement in bleeding episodes and factor dependence in all patients provides further evidence that gene therapy had significant potential with this disease.

Lysosomal Storage Disorders

As described above, lysosomal storage disorders are good candidates for in utero treatment because phenotypic manifestations often occur before birth. Although early clinical studies with retrovirally transduced stem cells were unsuccessful, more recent efforts with AAV and retroviral-mediated vector in conjunction with liver-specific promoters have shown improved efficacy.[88] Retroviral vectors have been used in MPS7 to successfully transduce up to 20% of hepatocytes and have resulted in normal long-term expression of the missing B-glucuronidase.[89] These high expression levels were associated with phenotypic improvements in affected dogs. As the collective prevalence of lysosomal storage disease is common (1 in 9000), early diagnosis and treatment with gene therapy vectors has the potential to ameliorate storage accumulation before development of systemic symptoms.

Severe Combined Immunodeficiencies

Severe combined immunodeficiencies are attractive targets for IUGT because they are typically associated with a defective hematopoietic niche that confers a survival advantage to treated cells. In mice with absence of both B and T cells, bone marrow–derived stem cells successfully reconstituted functioning B and T cells.[90] This approach has been successful for multiple variants of SCID and has been extended into the clinical setting as well. X-linked SCID patients transplanted with autologous CD34+ stem cells that had been transduced with retroviral-mediated gamma chain cDNA resulted in immunologic reconstitution in 9 of 10 patients.[91] These resultant reconstituted T cells were demonstrated to function normally in response to immunologic challenges.

Hemoglobinopathies

Using a similar technique to that described above, gene-modified HSCs have shown efficacy in both preclinical and human β-thalassemia models. Initial mouse models using lentiviral vectors resulted in correction of anemia and red cell morphology.[92] The first human trial involved a β-thalassemia case where CD45+ cells were

transfected with lentiviral-delivered β-globin—this led to long-term transfusion independence attributed to the expansion of multiple HSC clones.[93] The study was extended to other patients with varying degrees of β-thalassemia severity, with correction of all but the most severe forms—this variant had partial correction with the treatment. As a result of these initial successes, multiple trials are now underway using postnatal gene therapy for both thalassemias and sickle cell anemias.

WHAT ARE THE RISKS OF IUGT?

Access to unique populations such as stem cells in the fetal environment allows for efficient and long-lasting transduction as discussed above, especially if the viral vector can successfully integrate into the host genome. These benefits do not come without risk, as genomic alterations can interfere with naturally growing organs, or the vectors themselves can theoretically have off-target effects on protein expression leading to unknown but potentially deleterious consequences. The latter effect has been described as "insertional mutagenesis." The delivered transgene can also potentially infiltrate germline cells, introducing the risk of transmission to future offspring. Finally, maternal risk must be taken into consideration as well—in fact, one study showed that AAV vector used for transduction of human factor IX in nonhuman primates led to transplacental transfer and subsequent transduction of multiple maternal tissues.[94] Although no adverse effects or germline transmission was found in the mothers, this study served as a reminder that maternal toxicity must be studied in future preclinical models. Regarding the potential for disruption of natural organ development, one study found that FGF-10 overexpression following localized IUGT in rat lungs led to development of cystic adenomatoid malformation-like lesions.

Insertional Mutagenesis

The risk of insertional mutagenesis was recognized when four cases of T-cell leukemia were found after treatment with retrovirus-transduced gamma chain gene.[79] These patients, who had been successfully transduced with phenotypic improvement, several years after treatment, were found to have leukemia. All cases were found to be secondary to insertional mutagenesis, where the viral vector had integrated near the LMO-2 gene (previously implicated in T-cell leukemia) and that high expression of the transgene was associated with concomitant overexpression of the oncogene.[95] Another study found leukemogenic potential in γ-retroviral vector used for treatment of Wiskott-Aldrich syndrome.[96] Whereas 9 of 10 patients had phenotypical correction after therapy, 7 patients developed acute leukemia secondary to viral vector insertion near several oncogenes. Unexpected chromosomal translocations also developed over time. A study in mice also found that nonprimate lentiviruses (equine infectious anemia virus) were capable of causing hepatocellular carcinoma, secondary to preferential insertion near oncogenes in the majority of cases.[97]

These studies highlight the risk of genomic integration, and further investigation on retroviruses has found that integration occurs in a nonrandom fashion. Vectors derived from HIV, avian sarcoma leukosis virus, and murine leukemia virus have preferential integration sites. These characteristics likely account for the high incidence of oncogenic mutagenesis in the above studies. Strategies to prevent mutagenesis include more directed targeting to both tissue and chromosome region, where insertion into noncoding regions could avoid off-target effect. Adding "insulating" elements around transgenes could prevent expression of nearby genes. Also, phage integrases have been used to direct the integration of transgenes to specific locations in the mouse genome, which could be used to avoid oncogenes.[98]

Germline Transmission

Another concern with gene therapy has been germline transduction and subsequent risk to future offspring. Primordial germ cells in humans are restricted to the gonads by 7 weeks of gestation; thus intravascular treatment with a genetic vector should not have access to this compartment.[99] Possible transduction of the germline is still a relevant concern, however, as in vitro models have shown that primordial germ cells are capable of being transduced by Moloney leukemia virus with subsequent passage of the transgene to daughter populations.[100] Concern was raised for this possibility when men undergoing AAV-mediated hemophilia treatment were found to have vector sequences in their semen.[101] A study in rams using in utero retroviral vector transfer showed via PCR that sperm cells were positive for provirus and via immunohistochemistry that multiple cell types within the testis had evidence of transduction.[86] Preclinical studies with sheep have shown that this therapy increases uterine blood flow and increases fetal growth.[102] The propensity for germline transduction was found to be strongly correlated with the gestational age of the fetus, with the conclusion that treatment should be avoided earlier in gestation, when germline cells are rapidly cycling, leading to levels of transduction up to 700-fold. Although this study revealed a preferential germline transduction in male

animals only, another study on lentiviral vectors in rhesus monkeys found that the female germline was exclusively affected.[103] In cases where transplacental passage of AAV vector was found in nonhuman primate, maternal oocytes were confirmed to be unaffected.[94]

WHAT CURRENT TRIALS AND FUTURE DIRECTIONS EXIST FOR IUGT?

All current and past research in prenatal gene therapy has existed in preclinical and in vitro models only. Although there are no plans in the near future for an in vivo study with this therapy, a European Consortium (EVERREST) has been developed, with a current clinical trial seeking to better characterize pregnancies affected by early-onset fetal growth restriction. Maternal and fetal tissue and imaging data will be collected to better understand the natural history of fetal growth restriction, as well as to identify predictors for cases with poorer outcomes. These findings will directly facilitate a clinical trial of in utero maternal gene therapy, studying the safety and efficacy of uterine artery VEGF injection.[104]

CONCLUSION

In this chapter, we have reviewed the rationales and preclinical models for both in utero stem cell transplantation and in utero gene therapy. The first clinical trials with in utero applications of these existing treatment modalities are now starting, which have the potential to start a new era in "personalized medicine" for many congenital disorders that were previously thought to be untreatable. The risks of treatment should be cautiously kept in mind, however, and application to clinical trials should only follow thorough assessment of both efficacy and potential adverse events in preclinical models.

REFERENCES

1. Flake AW, Harrison MR, Adzick NS, Zanjani ED. Transplantation of fetal hematopoietic stem cells in utero: the creation of hematopoietic chimeras. *Science.* 1986;233(4765):776–778.
2. Flake AW, Zanjani ED. In utero hematopoietic stem cell transplantation: ontogenic opportunities and biologic barriers. *Blood.* 1999;94(7):2179–2191.
3. Witt R, MacKenzie TC, Peranteau WH. Fetal stem cell and gene therapy. *Semin Fetal Neonatal Med.* 2017.
4. Nijagal A, Flake AW, MacKenzie TC. In utero hematopoietic cell transplantation for the treatment of congenital anomalies. *Clin Perinatol.* 2012;39(2):301–310.
5. Owen RD. Immunogenetic consequences of vascular anastomoses between bovine twins. *Science.* 1945;102(2651):400–401.

6. Billingham RE, Brent L, Medawar PB. Actively acquired tolerance of foreign cells. *Nature.* 1953;172(4379):603–606.

7. Fleischman RA, Mintz B. Prevention of genetic anemias in mice by microinjection of normal hematopoietic stem cells into the fetal placenta. *Proc Natl Acad Sci U S A.* 1979;76(11):5736–5740.

8. Fleischman RA, Mintz B. Development of adult bone marrow stem cells in H-2-compatible and -incompatible mouse fetuses. *J Exp Med.* 1984;159(3):731–745.

9. Blazar BR, Taylor PA, Vallera DA. Adult bone marrow-derived pluripotent hematopoietic stem cells are engraftable when transferred in utero into moderately anemic fetal recipients. *Blood.* 1995;85(3):833–841.

10. Blazar BR, Taylor PA, Vallera DA. In utero transfer of adult bone marrow cells into recipients with severe combined immunodeficiency disorder yields lymphoid progeny with T- and B-cell functional capabilities. *Blood.* 1995;86(11):4353–4366.

11. Carrier E, Lee TH, Busch MP, Cowan MJ. Induction of tolerance in nondefective mice after in utero transplantation of major histocompatibility complex-mismatched fetal hematopoietic stem cells. *Blood.* 1995;86(12):4681–4690.

12. Kim HB, Shaaban AF, Yang EY, Liechty KW, Flake AW. Microchimerism and tolerance after in utero bone marrow transplantation in mice. *J Surg Res.* 1998;77(1):1–5.

13. Howson-Jan K, Matloub YH, Vallera DA, Blazar BR. In utero engraftment of fully H-2-incompatible versus congenic adult bone marrow transferred into nonanemic or anemic murine fetal recipients. *Transplantation.* 1993;56(3):709–716.

14. Kim HB, Shaaban AF, Milner R, Fichter C, Flake AW. In utero bone marrow transplantation induces donor-specific tolerance by a combination of clonal deletion and clonal anergy. *J Pediatr Surg.* 1999;34(5):726–729; discussion 729–730.

15. Blakemore K, Hattenburg C, Stetten G, et al. In utero hematopoietic stem cell transplantation with haploidentical donor adult bone marrow in a canine model. *Am J Obstet Gynecol.* 2004;190(4):960–973.

16. Omori F, Lutzko C, Abrams-Ogg A, et al. Adoptive transfer of genetically modified human hematopoietic stem cells into preimmune canine fetuses. *Exp Hematol.* 1999;27(2):242–249.

17. Pearce RD, Kiehm D, Armstrong DT, et al. Induction of hemopoietic chimerism in the caprine fetus by intraperitoneal injection of fetal liver cells. *Experientia.* 1989;45(3):307–308.

18. Lovell KL, Kraemer SA, Leipprandt JR, et al. In utero hematopoietic stem cell transplantation: a caprine model for prenatal therapy in inherited metabolic diseases. *Fetal Diagn Ther.* 2001;16(1):13–17.

19. Harrison MR, Slotnick RN, Crombleholme TM, Golbus MS, Tarantal AF, Zanjani ED. In-utero transplantation of fetal liver haemopoietic stem cells in monkeys. *Lancet.* 1989;2(8677):1425–1427.

20. Shields LE, Gaur L, Delio P, et al. The use of CD 34(+) mobilized peripheral blood as a donor cell source does not improve chimerism after in utero hematopoietic stem cell transplantation in non-human primates. *J Med Primatol.* 2005;34(4):201–208.

21. Boelig MM, Kim AG, Stratigis JD, et al. The intravenous route of injection optimizes engraftment and survival in the murine model of in utero hematopoietic cell transplantation. *Biol Blood Marrow Transplant.* 2016;22(6):991–999.

22. Hayashi S, Isobe K, Emi N, et al. Inhibition of human complement-dependent cell lysis by bovine aortic endothelial cells transfected with membrane-bound complement-regulatory factor (DAF and HRF20) gene using a retroviral vector. *Eur Surg Res.* 1996;28(6):440–446.

23. Peranteau WH, Hayashi S, Hsieh M, Shaaban AF, Flake AW. High-level allogeneic chimerism achieved by prenatal tolerance induction and postnatal nonmyeloablative bone marrow transplantation. *Blood.* 2002;100(6):2225–2234.

24. Nijagal A, Wegorzewska M, Jarvis E, Le T, Tang Q, MacKenzie TC. Maternal T cells limit engraftment after in utero hematopoietic cell transplantation in mice. *J Clin Invest.* 2011;121(2):582–592.

25. Mold JE, Michaelsson J, Burt TD, et al. Maternal alloantigens promote the development of tolerogenic fetal regulatory T cells in utero. *Science.* 2008;322(5907):1562–1565.

26. De Santis M, De Luca C, Mappa I, et al. In-utero stem cell transplantation: clinical use and therapeutic potential. *Minerva Ginecol.* 2011;63(4):387–398.

27. Lee PW, Cina RA, Randolph MA, et al. In utero bone marrow transplantation induces kidney allograft tolerance across a full major histocompatibility complex barrier in swine. *Transplantation.* 2005;79(9):1084–1090.

28. Lee PW, Cina RA, Randolph MA, et al. Stable multilineage chimerism across full MHC barriers without graft-versus-host disease following in utero bone marrow transplantation in pigs. *Exp Hematol.* 2005;33(3):371–379.

29. Peranteau WH, Heaton TE, Gu YC, et al. Haploidentical in utero hematopoietic cell transplantation improves phenotype and can induce tolerance for postnatal same-donor transplants in the canine leukocyte adhesion deficiency model. *Biol Blood Marrow Transplant.* 2009;15(3):293–305.

30. Vrecenak JD, Pearson EG, Santore MT, et al. Stable long-term mixed chimerism achieved in a canine model of allogeneic in utero hematopoietic cell transplantation. *Blood.* 2014;124(12):1987–1995.

31. Touraine JL, Raudrant D, Royo C, et al. In-utero transplantation of stem cells in bare lymphocyte syndrome. *Lancet.* 1989;1(8651):1382.

32. Flake AW, Roncarolo MG, Puck JM, et al. Treatment of X-linked severe combined immunodeficiency by in utero transplantation of paternal bone marrow. *N Engl J Med.* 1996;335(24):1806–1810.

33. Wengler GS, Lanfranchi A, Frusca T, et al. In-utero transplantation of parental CD34 haematopoietic progenitor cells in a patient with X-linked severe combined immunodeficiency (SCIDXI). *Lancet.* 1996;348(9040):1484–1487.

34. Peranteau WH, Hayashi S, Abdulmalik O, et al. Correction of murine hemoglobinopathies by prenatal tolerance induction and postnatal nonmyeloablative allogeneic BM transplants. *Blood.* 2015;126(10):1245–1254.

35. Ashizuka S, Peranteau WH, Hayashi S, Flake AW. Busulfan-conditioned bone marrow transplantation results in high-level allogeneic chimerism in mice made tolerant by in utero hematopoietic cell transplantation. *Exp Hematol.* 2006;34(3):359–368.

36. Papanikolaou E, Anagnou NP. Major challenges for gene therapy of thalassemia and sickle cell disease. *Curr Gene Ther.* 2010;10(5):404–412.

37. Derderian SC, Jeanty C, Walters MC, Vichinsky E, MacKenzie TC. In utero hematopoietic cell transplantation for hemoglobinopathies. *Front Pharmacol.* 2014;5:278.

38. Vrecenak JD, Flake AW. In utero hematopoietic cell transplantation–recent progress and the potential for clinical application. *Cytotherapy.* 2013;15(5):525–535.

39. Michlitsch J, Azimi M, Hoppe C, et al. Newborn screening for hemoglobinopathies in California. *Pediatr Blood Cancer.* 2009;52(4):486–490.

40. Walters MC, Patience M, Leisenring W, et al. Bone marrow transplantation for sickle cell disease. *N Engl J Med.* 1996;335(6):369–376.

41. Lucarelli G, Galimberti M, Polchi P, et al. Bone marrow transplantation in patients with thalassemia. *N Engl J Med.* 1990;322(7):417–421.

42. Rees DC, Williams TN, Gladwin MT. Sickle-cell disease. *Lancet.* 2010;376(9757):2018–2031.

43. Kauf TL, Coates TD, Huazhi L, Mody-Patel N, Hartzema AG. The cost of health care for children and adults with sickle cell disease. *Am J Hematol.* 2009;84(6):323–327.

44. Singh R, Jordan R, Hanlon C. Economic impact of sickle cell hospitalization. *Blood.* 2014;124:5971.

45. Miller ST, Sleeper LA, Pegelow CH, et al. Prediction of adverse outcomes in children with sickle cell disease. *N Engl J Med.* 2000;342(2):83–89.

46. Wang WC, Ware RE, Miller ST, et al. Hydroxycarbamide in very young children with sickle-cell anaemia: a multicentre, randomised, controlled trial (BABY HUG). *Lancet.* 2011;377(9778):1663–1672.

47. Shields LE, Gaur LK, Gough M, Potter J, Sieverkropp A, Andrews RG. In utero hematopoietic stem cell transplantation in nonhuman primates: the role of T cells. *Stem Cells.* 2003;21(3):304–314.

48. Weatherall DJ. Phenotype-genotype relationships in monogenic disease: lessons from the thalassaemias. *Nat Rev Genet.* 2001;2(4):245–255.

49. Forget B, Cohen A. Thalassemia syndromes. *Hematology: Basic Principles and Practice.* 3. ; 2000.

50. Vichinsky EP. Alpha thalassemia major–new mutations, intrauterine management, and outcomes. *Hematology Am Soc Hematol Educ Program.* 2009;35–41.

51. Kreger EM, Singer ST, Witt RG, et al. Favorable outcomes after in utero transfusion in fetuses with alpha thalassemia major: a case series and review of the literature. *Prenat Diagn.* 2016;36(13):1242–1249.

52. Vellodi A. Lysosomal storage disorders. *Br J Haematol.* 2005;128(4):413–431.

53. Wynn RF, Wraith JE, Mercer J, et al. Improved metabolic correction in patients with lysosomal storage disease treated with hematopoietic stem cell transplant compared with enzyme replacement therapy. *J Pediatr.* 2009;154(4):609–611.

54. Sands MS, Vogler C, Torrey A, et al. Murine mucopolysaccharidosis type VII: long term therapeutic effects of enzyme replacement and enzyme replacement followed by bone marrow transplantation. *J Clin Invest.* 1997;99(7):1596–1605.

55. Salazar-Fontana LI, Desai DD, Khan TA, et al. Approaches to mitigate the unwanted immunogenicity of therapeutic proteins during drug development. *AAPS J.* 2017;19(2):377–385.

56. Siddiqi F, Wolfe JH. Stem cell therapy for the central nervous system in lysosomal storage diseases. *Hum Gene Ther.* 2016;27(10):749–757.

57. Boelens JJ, Aldenhoven M, Purtill D, et al. Outcomes of transplantation using various hematopoietic cell sources in children with hurler syndrome after myeloablative conditioning. *Blood.* 2013;121:3981–3987.

58. Peters C, Shapiro EG, Anderson J, et al. Hurler syndrome: II. Outcome of HLA-genotypically identical sibling and HLA-haploidentical related donor bone marrow transplantation in fifty-four children. The storage disease collaborative study group. *Blood.* 1998;91(7):2601–2608.

59. Solders M, Martin DA, Andersson C, et al. Hematopoietic SCT: a useful treatment for late metachromatic leukodystrophy. *Bone Marrow Transplant.* 2014;49(8):1046–1051.

60. Escolar ML, Poe MD, Provenzale JM, et al. Transplantation of umbilical-cord blood in babies with infantile krabbe's disease. *N Engl J Med.* 2005;352(20):2069–2081.

61. Krivit W, Shapiro EG, Peters C, et al. Hematopoietic stem-cell transplantation in globoid-cell leukodystrophy. *N Engl J Med.* 1998;338(16):1119–1126.

62. Aldenhoven M, Wynn RF, Orchard PJ, et al. Long-term outcome of hurler syndrome patients after hematopoietic cell transplantation: an international multicenter study. *Blood.* 2015;125(13):2164–2172.

63. Amin MT, Shazly SA. In utero stem cell transplantation for radical treatment of osteogenesis imperfecta: perspectives and controversies. *Am J Perinatol.* 2014;31(10):829–836.

64. Huber MA. Osteogenesis imperfecta. *Oral Surg Oral Med Oral Pathol Oral Radiol Endod.* 2007;103(3):314–320.

65. Horwitz EM, Prockop DJ, Fitzpatrick LA, et al. Transplantability and therapeutic effects of bone marrow-derived mesenchymal cells in children with osteogenesis imperfecta. *Nat Med.* 1999;5(3):309–313.

66. Westgren L, Anneren G, Axelsson O, Evald U, LeBlanc K, Ringden O. Donor chimerism across full allogenic barriers achieved by in utero transplantation of fetal mesenchymal stem cells in a case of osteogenesis imperfecta. *Am J Obstet Gynecol.* 2003;189(6):S215.

67. Le Blanc K, Götherström C, Ringdén O, et al. Fetal mesenchymal stem-cell engraftment in bone after in utero transplantation in a patient with severe osteogenesis imperfecta. *Transplantation.* 2005;79(11):1607–1614.

68. MacKenzie TC, David AL, Flake AW, Almeida-Porada G. Consensus statement from the first international conference for in utero stem cell transplantation and gene therapy. *Front Pharmacol.* 2015;6:15.

69. IFeTIS. International Fetal Transplantation and Immunology Society. 2016; https://www.fetaltherapies.org/.

70. TC M. *In Utero Hematopoietic Stem Cell Transplantation for Alpha-thalassemia Major (ATM)*; 2017. https://clinicaltrials.gov/ct2/show/NCT02986698.

71. Chitty L, David A, Gottschalk I, et al. EP21. 04: BOOSTB4: a clinical study to determine safety and efficacy of pre- and/or postnatal stem cell transplantation for treatment of osteogenesis imperfecta. *Ultrasound Obstet Gynecol.* 2016;48(S1):356.

72. McCandless SE, Brunger JW, Cassidy SB. The burden of genetic disease on inpatient care in a children's hospital. *Am J Hum Genet.* 2004;74(1):121–127.

73. Helman G, Pacheco-Colon I, Gropman AL. The urea cycle disorders. *Semin Neurol.* 2014;34(3):341–349.

74. Fischer K, van der Bom JG, Mauser-Bunschoten EP, et al. The effects of postponing prophylactic treatment on long-term outcome in patients with severe hemophilia. *Blood.* 2002;99(7):2337–2341.

75. Lozier JN, Metzger ME, Donahue RE, Morgan RA. Adenovirus-mediated expression of human coagulation factor IX in the rhesus macaque is associated with dose-limiting toxicity. *Blood.* 1999;94(12):3968–3975.

76. Tran ND, Porada CD, Almeida-Porada G, Glimp HA, Anderson WF, Zanjani ED. Induction of stable prenatal tolerance to beta-galactosidase by in utero gene transfer into preimmune sheep fetuses. *Blood.* 2001;97(11):3417–3423.

77. Waddington SN, Buckley SM, Nivsarkar M, et al. In utero gene transfer of human factor IX to fetal mice can induce postnatal tolerance of the exogenous clotting factor. *Blood.* 2003;101(4):1359–1366.

78. Sabatino DE, Mackenzie TC, Peranteau W, et al. Persistent expression of hF.IX after tolerance induction by in utero or neonatal administration of AAV-1-F.IX in hemophilia B mice. *Mol Ther.* 2007;15(9):1677–1685.

79. Hacein-Bey-Abina S, von Kalle C, Schmidt M, et al. A serious adverse event after successful gene therapy for X-linked severe combined immunodeficiency. *N Engl J Med.* 2003;348(3):255–256.

80. Mattar CNZ, Gil-Farina I, Rosales C, et al. In utero transfer of adeno-associated viral vectors produces long-term factor IX levels in a cynomolgus macaque model. *Mol Ther.* 2017;25(8):1843–1853.

81. Shen JS, Meng XL, Maeda H, Ohashi T, Eto Y. Widespread gene transduction to the central nervous system by adenovirus in utero: implication for prenatal gene therapy to brain involvement of lysosomal storage disease. *J Gene Med.* 2004;6(11):1206–1215.

82. Karda R, Buckley SM, Mattar CN, et al. Perinatal systemic gene delivery using adeno-associated viral vectors. *Front Mol Neurosci.* 2014;7:89.

83. Waddington SN, Mitrophanous KA, Ellard FM, et al. Long-term transgene expression by administration of a lentivirus-based vector to the fetal circulation of immunocompetent mice. *Gene Ther.* 2003;10(15):1234–1240.

84. MacKenzie TC, Kobinger GP, Louboutin JP, et al. Transduction of satellite cells after prenatal intramuscular administration of lentiviral vectors. *J Gene Med.* 2005;7(1):50–58.

85. van den Berg HM. A cure for hemophilia within reach. *N Engl J Med.* 2017;377(26):2592–2593.

86. Rangarajan S, Walsh L, Lester W, et al. AAV5-Factor VIII gene transfer in severe hemophilia A. *N Engl J Med.* 2017;377(26):2519–2530.

87. George LA, Sullivan SK, Giermasz A, et al. Hemophilia B gene therapy with a high-specific-activity factor IX variant. *N Engl J Med.* 2017;377(23):2215–2227.

88. Cheng SH, Smith AE. Gene therapy progress and prospects: gene therapy of lysosomal storage disorders. *Gene Ther.* 2003;10(16):1275–1281.

89. Ponder KP, Melniczek JR, Xu L, et al. Therapeutic neonatal hepatic gene therapy in mucopolysaccharidosis VII dogs. *Proc Natl Acad Sci U S A.* 2002;99(20):13102–13107.

90. Yates F, Malassis-Seris M, Stockholm D, et al. Gene therapy of RAG-2-/- mice: sustained correction of the immunodeficiency. *Blood.* 2002;100(12):3942–3949.

91. Hacein-Bey-Abina S, Le Deist F, Carlier F, et al. Sustained correction of X-linked severe combined immunodeficiency by ex vivo gene therapy. *N Engl J Med.* 2002;346(16):1185–1193.

92. May C, Rivella S, Callegari J, et al. Therapeutic haemoglobin synthesis in beta-thalassaemic mice expressing lentivirus-encoded human beta-globin. *Nature.* 2000;406(6791):82–86.

93. Malik P. Gene therapy for hemoglobinopathies: tremendous successes and remaining caveats. *Mol Ther.* 2016;24(4):668–670.

94. Mattar CN, Nathwani AC, Waddington SN, et al. Stable human FIX expression after 0.9G intrauterine gene transfer of self-complementary adeno-associated viral vector 5 and 8 in macaques. *Mol Ther.* 2011;19(11):1950–1960.

95. Staal FJ, Pike-Overzet K, Ng YY, van Dongen JJ. Sola dosis facit venenum. Leukemia in gene therapy trials: a question of vectors, inserts and dosage? *Leukemia.* 2008;22(10):1849–1852.

96. Braun CJ, Boztug K, Paruzynski A, et al. Gene therapy for Wiskott-Aldrich syndrome–long-term efficacy and genotoxicity. *Sci Transl Med.* 2014;6(227):227ra233.

97. Nowrouzi A, Cheung WT, Li T, et al. The fetal mouse is a sensitive genotoxicity model that exposes lentiviral-associated mutagenesis resulting in liver oncogenesis. *Mol Ther.* 2013;21(2):324–337.

98. Hollis RP, Stoll SM, Sclimenti CR, Lin J, Chen-Tsai Y, Calos MP. Phage integrases for the construction and manipulation of transgenic mammals. *Reprod Biol Endocrinol.* 2003;1:79.

99. David AL, Peebles D. Gene therapy for the fetus: is there a future? *Best Pract Res Clin Obstet Gynaecol.* 2008;22(1):203–218.

100. Jaenisch R. Germ line integration and mendelian transmission of the exogenous moloney leukemia virus. *Proc Natl Acad Sci U S A.* 1976;73(4):1260–1264.

101. Kelley K, Verma I, Pierce GF. Gene therapy: reality or myth for the global bleeding disorders community? *Haemophilia.* 2002;8(3):261–267.

102. Carr DJ, Wallace JM, Aitken RP, et al. Uteroplacental adenovirus vascular endothelial growth factor gene therapy increases fetal growth velocity in growth-restricted sheep pregnancies. *Hum Gene Ther.* 2014;25(4):375–384.

103. Lee CC, Jimenez DF, Kohn DB, Tarantal AF. Fetal gene transfer using lentiviral vectors and the potential for germ cell transduction in rhesus monkeys (*Macaca mulatta*). *Hum Gene Ther.* 2005;16(4):417–425.

104. Spencer R, Ambler G, Brodszki J, et al. EVERREST prospective study: a 6-year prospective study to define the clinical and biological characteristics of pregnancies affected by severe early onset fetal growth restriction. *BMC Pregnancy Childbirth.* 2017;17(1):43.

Index

A

Achondroplasia, 8, 106, 107f
Alleles, 2–3
Allelic heterogeneity, 3–4
α-Thalassemia major (ATM), 176–177
American Board of Genetic Counseling (ABGC), 22
American College of Obstetricians and Gynecologists (ACOG), 68
Amniocentesis, 151
  amniotic fluid leakage, 152
  chromosomal mosaicism, 152
  fetal imaging, 137
  genetic, 151
  human immunodeficiency virus infection, 153
  indications, 137, 154–155
  midtrimester, 151–152
  miscarriage risk after, 151–152
  multiple gestations, 155
  procedure-related loss rate, 151–152
  transplacental, 151
Aneuploidy
  anaphase lag, 32
  cell-free DNA (cfDNA) screening. (See Cell-free DNA (cfDNA)) screening
  in children, 30
  chromosome 45,X, 34–35
  consequences, 30
  early pregnancy loss, 31–32
  first trimester ultrasound markers
    ductus venosus blood flow, 80
    nasal bone sonography, 79–80
    NT and cystic hygroma, 78–79
    tricuspid regurgitation (TR), 80
  in late pregnancy loss, 31
  monosomy syndromes, 30
  mosaicism, 35, 155
  multiple gestations, 80–81
  in newborn infants, 30–31, 31t
  nondisjunction, 32
  nonmosaic, 30
  polyploidy, 34
  recurrent pregnancy loss, 35
  serum screening
    chromosomal abnormalities, 75–76, 76t
    detection rates and false positives, 77t
    first-trimester screening, 76–77
    history, 75

Aneuploidy (Continued)
    hypersensitive disorders, 81
    integrated screening, 77
    quadruple screen, 77
    screen-positive, 80
    sequential screening, 77
    stepwise sequential screen, 77–78
    trisomies, 30
Angelman syndrome, 15
Anticipation, 7
Array comparative genomic hybridization (aCGH) arrays, 126–127, 126f, 165–166
Assisted reproductive technology (ART), 15
  birth defects, 171–172
  epigenetic alterations, 172
Autosomal dominant inheritance
  allele penetrance and expressivity, 3–4
  biallelic (two copies) fashion, 3–4
  codominant gene expression, 4
  transmission, 3–4
  syndrome, 108
Autosomal recessive inheritance, 4, 5f
Azoospermia, 47

B

Balanced paracentric inversions, 41
Balanced structural chromosome rearrangements, 39
Beckwith–Wiedemann syndrome (BWS), 15, 54, 112–113
Beneficence, 144–145
Benign variant, 63
Bifid hallux, 108
Birth defects, 9, 17f
  structural, 16, 17t
BOOSTB4 trial, 178

C

Cell-free DNA (cfDNA) screening, 75
  advantages and disadvantages, 87
  false-positive
    confined placental mosaicism, 89
    maternal aneuploidy, 89
    maternal malignancy, 89–90
    organ transplantation, 90
    sample mix-up/human error, 90
    vanishing twin, 89
  fetal aneuploidy, 86, 86t, 90
  fetal anomalies, 118

Cell-free DNA (cfDNA) screening (Continued)
  first trimester ultrasound, 92
  low fetal fraction, 90–91
  low–molecular-weight heparin, 90
  massive parallel sequencing, 86
  microarray-based technology, 86
  microdeletions and microduplications, 130–131
  in multiple gestations, 91–92
  nuchal translucency (NT), 77
  obesity, 90
  performance characteristics, 86t
  placental cfDNA, 85
  posttest counseling, 91
  pretest counseling, 91
    microdeletion detection, 88
    RhD determination, 89
    single gene disorders, 88–89
  sex chromosome aneuploidies, 86–87
  single-nucleotide polymorphism-based approach, 86
  targeted sequencing, 86
  whole genome sequencing approach, 86
Certified Genetic Counselor (CGC), 22
CHARGE syndrome, ultrasound, 113
Chorionic villus sampling (CVS), 151
  chromosomal mosaicism, 152
  chronic viral infections, 153
  direct DNA testing, 151
  fetal anomalies detection, 117
  FISH, 154
  indications, 137, 154–155
  limb-reduction defects, 152
  multiple gestations, 155
  procedure-related loss rates, 152
  transabdominal procedure, 151
  transcervical, 149, 151
  vaginal spotting or bleeding, 152
Choroid plexus cyst, 96, 97f
Chromodomain helicase DNA-binding protein-7 (CHD7) gene, 113
Chromosomal microarray analysis (CMA), 15–16, 28, 39
  array comparative genomic hybridization (aCGH) arrays, 126–128, 126f
  benefits, 118
  computer algorithms, 125–126
  copy number variants (CNVs), 125

Note: Page numbers followed by "f" indicate figures, "t" indicate tables.

Chromosomal microarray analysis
  (CMA) (*Continued*)
  counseling challenges, 134
  cytogenetic etiology, 125
  fetal anomalies, 117–118
  fetal anomalies detection, 117–118
  fluorescence in situ hybridization,
    133
  genetic abnormalities, 133
  genetic material gains and loss
    detection, 117
  guidelines, pregnancy, 132
  incremental diagnostic yield, 137
  informed consent, 134
  vs. karyotype, 128–130
  limitations, 118
  maternal cell contamination testing,
    133
  microdeletion and duplication
    syndromes, 129t
  normal karyotypes, 118
  parental blood karyotype, 133
  pathogenic CNV drops, 133
  resources, 135
  results disclosure, 135
  results report
    language, 132f
    mosaicism, 132
    pathogenic result, 131
    region of homozygosity, 132
    VUS, 132
  single-nucleotide polymorphism
    (SNP) arrays, 127–128
  "targeted" CMA *vs.* "whole genome"
    CMA, 128
  vs. targeted gene testing, 130
  whole exome and whole genome
    sequencing (WES/WGS), 130
Chromosome abnormalities, 17f. *See
  also* Aneuploidy
Chromosome banding, 27
Chromosome-specific sequencing, 86
Clustered regularly interspaced short
  palindromic repeats-Ca9 (CRISPR-
  cas9), 59–60, 169–170
Codominant gene, 4
Codons, 1–2
Comparative genomic hybridization
  (CGH), 9–10
Complete blood count (CBC), 68
Complete penetrance, 3–4
Complex chromosome rearrangements
  (CCRs), 46–47
Compound heterozygotes, 4
Confined placental mosaicism (CPM),
  17–18, 85, 89, 153
Congenital anomalies of the kidneys
  and urinary tract (CAKUT), 142–143
Congenital heart malformations, 16
Consanguinity couples, genetic risk
  assessment, 24–25
Contiguous gene deletion syndromes, 6

Conventional karyotype analysis, 9–10
Copy number variants, 17f
Cri-du-chat syndrome, 30
Crown-rump length (CRL), 78
Cystic hygroma, 79
Cytogenetics
  autosomes, 27
  centromere, 27
  chromosomal microarray analysis
    (CMA), 28
  chromosome banding, 27
  chromosome testing, 27
  diploid chromosome, 27
  direct chromosome analysis, 29
  FISH testing, 27–28
  male G-banded karyotype, 27, 28f
  mitochondrial DNA, 27
  mitotic division, 28
  nuclear DNA, 27
  standard laboratory reports, 29–30
  tissue biopsies, 28
  tissue culture methods, 28–29

D
Deformations, 16
22q11.2 deletion syndrome, 88
De novo structural chromosome
  rearrangements, 39–40
Digenic inheritance, 9
DiGeorge syndrome, 88, 107–108
DNA
  alleles, 2–3
  codon, 1–2
  exons, 1–2
  length, 1
  methylation and histone acetylation,
    2
  mutations, 3
  regulatory elements and coding
    regions, 1–2
  regulatory polymorphisms, 3
  single nucleotide polymorphisms
    (SNPs), 3
DNA fingerprinting, 51f
Down syndrome
  chromosomal abnormalities, 75
  pathogenic CNVs, 125
  ultrasound, 108–109
Duchenne muscular dystrophy
  (DMD), 18

E
Echogenic bowel
  antenatal finding, 99
  congenital infection, 98–99
  cystic fibrosis, 98
  fetal CMV infection, 99
  gastrointestinal pathology, 99
  idiopathic, 98
  isolated, 98
  transducer frequency, 98
  trisomy 21, 98

Echogenic intracardiac focus (EIFs),
  96, 96f
Ectrodactyly-ectodermal dysplasia-
  clefting (EEC) syndrome, 108
Embryo development
  blastomere biopsy, 163–164
  chromosome misallocation,
    162–163
  chromosome nondisjunction,
    162–163
  euploid embryos, 163
  fluorescence in situ hybridization
    (FISH) technique, 163–164
  inner cell mass *vs.* trophectoderm,
    163
  mitotic aneuploidy, 162–163
  polar body biopsy, 163–164
  postzygotic aneuploidy, 163
  stages, 162f
Embryonic mosaicism, 167–168
Enoxaparin therapy, 90
Enzyme replacement therapy (ERT),
  177
Epigenetic modification, 7
Epigenomics, 51
Expanded carrier screening
  (ECS), 65
Expressivity, 64

F
Facial clefts, 108
Family history, 22
Fetal anomalies
  fetal echocardiography, 115–116
  magnetic resonance imaging (MRI),
    115
  prenatal genetic testing
    cell-free DNA, 118
    chorionic villus sampling (CVS),
      117
    chromosomal microarray analysis
      (CMA), 117–118
    fluorescent in situ hybridization,
      117
    karyotype abnormalities, 117
    pre- and posttest counseling,
      117
    targeted gene sequencing, 118
    twin gestations, 117
    whole-exome sequencing, 118
  twin gestations, 116
  ultrasound
    detection rates, 105
    late first-trimester scan,
      105–106
    pattern recognition (*See* Pattern
      recognition, ultrasound)
    second-trimester anatomic survey,
      106
    standard and anatomic scan,
      105
    third-trimester scans, 106

Fetal growth restriction (FGR), 97–98
Fluorescence in situ hybridization (FISH), 9–10
 chromosomal microarray (CMA), 133
 fetal anomalies detection, 117
Fragile X mental retardation 1 (FMR1) gene, 11
Fragile X syndrome
 CGG repeats, 11–12, 12f
 clinical characteristics, 11
 fragile X mental retardation 1 (FMR1) gene, 11
 premutation carrier, 12, 11–12
 prevalence, 11
Frameshift mutation, 3, 50–51

G

G-banded chromosome analysis, 39
G-banding, 27
Gene editing, 59–60
GeneMatcher, 144
Gene structure and organization
 chromosomes, 1
 DNA
  codon, 1–2
  length, 1
  methylation and histone acetylation, 2
  regulatory elements and coding regions, 1–2
  exons, 1–2
  introns, 2
  noncoding regulatory regions, 2
  protein-coding gene, 2f
Genetic anticipation, 11
Genetic carrier screening, 4
Genetic counseling
 consanguinity couples, 24–25
 definition, 21
 disclosure of genetic test results, 24
 genetic counselors, 21–22
 genetic information, 21
 indications, 21
 patient education, 25
 pre- and posttest counseling
  aneuploidy screening, 23–24
  carrier screening, 22–23
 referrals, 22
Genetic counselors, 21–22
Genetic inheritance
 autosomal dominant inheritance, 3–4
 autosomal recessive conditions, 4, 5f
 Mendelian genetics, 3
 sex-linked inheritance, 4–5
Genetics
 individual genes changes, 1
 principles, 1
Gene writing, 60
Genome editing, 169–170
Genomic disorders
 contiguous gene deletion syndromes, 6

Genomic disorders (Continued)
 digenic inheritance, 9
 DiGeorge syndrome, 5–6
 epigenetic modification, 7
 germline and somatic mosaicism, 8
 hereditary unstable DNA, 7
 imprinting, 7
 mitochondrial inheritance, 8, 8f
 multifactorial inheritance, 9
 nonallelic homologous recombination, 5–6
 screening and diagnostic tests, 9–10
 terminal deletions and duplications, 6
Genomic hybridization techniques, 1
Genomic imprinting disorders
 Angelman syndrome, 15, 15t
 Beckwith-Wiedemann syndrome, 15
 Prader-Willi syndrome, 14, 15t
 Russell-Silver syndrome, 15
Genomics, 1
Genotyping, 63–64, 66
Germline mosaicism, 8, 18
Gonadal mosaicism, 8

H

Health Insurance Portability and Accountability Act (HIPAA) regulations, 22–23
Hemoglobin electrophoresis, 69
Hemoglobinopathies
 in utero gene therapy (IUGT), 180
 in utero hematopoietic stem cell transplantation (IUHCT), 176–177
Hemophilia, 179–180
Hereditary unstable DNA, 7
Hereditary unstable DNA repeat disorders
 fragile X syndrome
  CGG repeats, 11–12, 12f
  clinical characteristics, 11
  fragile X mental retardation 1 (FMR1) gene, 11
  premutation carrier, 11–12
  prevalence, 11
 genetic anticipation, 11
 Huntington disease, 13
 myotonic dystrophy, 12–13
 trinucleotide repeat disorders, 12t
Heteroplasmy, 8
Heterozygous carrier, 4
Homologous Robertsonian translocation, 44–45
Homozygous mutation, 4
Human chorionic gonadotropin (hCG), 75
Human Genome Project–Write (HG-W) initiative, 60

Human Phenotype Ontology (HPO), 140
Huntington disease, 13
Hurler disease, 177
Hypoplastic left heart, 9

I

Imprinting, 7
Imprinting defects
 Angelman syndrome, 15, 15t
 Beckwith-Wiedemann syndrome, 15
 Prader-Willi syndrome, 14, 15t
 Russell-Silver syndrome, 15
Incomplete penetrance, 3–4
Informed consent process, 22
Inner cell mass (ICM), 163
Intracytoplasmic sperm injection (ICSI), 169, 171–172
In utero gene therapy (IUGT)
 access to stem cell populations, 179
 avoidance of disease onset, 178
 blood-brain barrier, 179
 current trials and future aspects, 181
 germline transmission, 181
 hemoglobinopathies, 180
 hemophilia, 179–180
 hemophilia B, 179–180
 immunologic advantage, 178–179
 insertional mutagenesis risk, 180–181
 lysosomal storage disorders, 180
 severe combined immunodeficiencies, 180
In utero hematopoietic stem cell transplantation (IUHCT)
 advantages, 175
 anemic mice, 175
 canine model, 176
 chimerism, 176
 conceptualization, 175
 current trials, 177–178
 early clinical experience in humans, 176
 hemoglobinopathies, 176–177
 immune response, 175–176
 in large animal models, 176
 lysosomal storage disorders, 177
 osteogenesis imperfecta (OI), 177
 pig model, 176
 SCID-transplanted mice, 175
 stem cell engraftment, 175
 in utero gene therapy (IUGT), 178
Isochromosomes, 40–41, 41f

J

"Junk" DNA, 2

K

Karyotyping, 125

L

Leukocyte adhesion deficiency (CLAD), 176
Licensure, 22
Likely benign variant, 63
Likely pathogenic variant, 63
Long contiguous stretch of homozygosity (LCSH), 127–128
Low–molecular-weight heparin, 90
Lysosomal storage disorders
  in utero gene therapy (IUGT), 180
  in utero hematopoietic stem cell transplantation, 177

M

Macroglossia, 112–113, 112f
Male G-banded karyotype, 27
Marker chromosomes, 47
"Massively parallel sequencing", 137–138
Maternal aneuploidy, 89
Maternal cell contamination testing, 133
Maternal serum alpha-fetoprotein (MSAFP), 75
Matrilineal inheritance, 16–17
Microarray-based technology, 86
Microdeletion and duplication syndromes, 129t
Miller–Dieker syndrome, 134
Missense mutation, 3
Mitochondrial DNA, 27
Mitochondrial DNA transfer, 170
Mitochondrial inheritance, 8, 8f, 16–17, 18t
Mitochondrial replacement therapy (MRT), 170
Molecular cytogenetic testing, 9–10
Molecular genetics
  cystic fibrosis (CF), 49
  DNA fingerprinting, 51f
  DNA sequence, 49
  DNA sequence variability, 49
  epigenomics, 51
  frameshift mutations, 50–51
  gene editing, 59–60, 60f
  gene sequencing, 53–54
  genetic mutation, 51
  gene writing, 60
  genomics, 49
  genotyping
    altered length of DNA segments, 51
    carrier detection, 52
    ethnic and racial populations, 52
    genetic carrier testing, 52
    prenatal genetic testing, 52
    Tay-Sachs disease, 52
  introns and exon, 50–51, 51f
  molecular tools, 49
  next-generation sequencing (See Next-generation sequencing)
  "nonsense" mutation, 50–51

Molecular genetics (Continued)
  PCR technique, 54–57, 57f–58f
  point mutation, 50–51
  preimplantation tests, 60
  prenatal genetics
    parental samples, 59
    tissues used, 59
    ultrasound anomaly, 58–59
  protein function changes, 49–50
  single gene disorders, 49, 50f
  Southern blot method, 54–56
Moloney leukemia virus, 181
Monochorionic twins, 116
Monosomy X, 110
Mosaic embryo, 167–168
Mosaicism
  chromosomal, 152
  chromosomal microarray (CMA), 132
  clinical features, 35
  confined placental mosaicism (CPM), 17–18
  counseling, 36
  germline mosaicism, 18
  imprinting disorder, 37
  low-level
    aneuploid pregnancy, 35–36
    trisomy, nondisjunction, 36
  placental, 152–153
  sex chromosome abnormalities, 35
  somatic mosaicism, 18
Mucopolysaccharidosis VII (MPS7), 179
Multifactorial inheritance, 9
  characteristics, 16t
  family and twin studies, 15
  neuropsychiatric disorders, 15–16
Multiplex ligation-dependent probe amplification (MLPA), 54–56
Mutation, 63
MutationTaster2, 139
Myotonic dystrophy (DM)
  myotonic dystrophy 1, 12–13
  myotonic dystrophy 2 (DM2), 13

N

"Negative" carrier screen, 22–23
Next-generation sequencing (NGS), 10, 63, 137
  clinical considerations and recommendations, 145–146
  genetic carrier screening, 53
  incidental and secondary findings, 141–142, 142t
  prenatal genetic carrier screening
    cost analysis, 70
    enzymatic screening, 69
    expanded carrier screening, 69–70, 72–73
    hemoglobin electrophoresis, 69
    pathogenic variants, 69
    Tay-Sachs screening, 69
  professional guidelines, 145

Next-generation sequencing (NGS) (Continued)
  single genes, 53
  variants detectable with, 141t
  whole exome sequencing (WES)
    bioinformatic interpretation, 53
    data-mining strategies, 53
    DNA sequence variants identification, 53
    exons, 53
    guidelines for, 54
    limitations, 54
    pretest counseling, 54
  whole genome sequencing (WGS), 54
Nonallelic homologous recombination, 5–6
Nonchromosomal congenital anomalies, twin gestations, 116
Noninvasive prenatal screening (NIPS), 85
Nonmaleficence, 144–145
Non-mendelian genetics
  hereditary unstable DNA repeats (See Hereditary unstable DNA repeat disorders)
  imprinting defects, 14–15, 14t
  mitochondrial disorder, 16–17
  mosaicism, 17–18
  multifactorial inheritance, 15–16
  structural birth defects, 16
  uniparental disomy (UPD), 13–14
Nonsense mutation, 3
Noonan syndrome (NS), 111–112, 130
Nuchal translucency (NT), 75
  cell-free DNA (cfDNA) screening, 77–78
  chromosomal abnormalities, 78
  crown-rump length (CRL), 78
  cystic hygroma, 79
  first-trimester screening, 76–77
  late first-trimester ultrasound, 105–106
  trisomy 18, 77
  trisomy 21, 78
Nuclear DNA, 27
Nuclear transfer techniques, 171f

O

Obesity, cell-free DNA (cfDNA) screening, 90
Oligospermia, 47
Omphalocele, 112
Oro-facial-digital syndrome, 108
Osteogenesis imperfecta (OI), in utero hematopoietic stem cell transplantation (IUHCT), 177

P

Pan-ethnic screening, 64
Paracentric inversions, 41, 42f
Parental aneuploidy, 155

Parental balanced chromosomal rearrangements, 155
Patau syndrome, 109, 109f
Pathogenic variant, 63
Pattern recognition, ultrasound
 Beckwith-Wiedemann syndrome, 112–113
 CHARGE syndrome, 113
 clefts palate without a disrupted lip, 107–108
 DiGeorge syndrome, 107–108
 facial clefts, 107–108
 monosomy X (Turner syndrome), 110
 Noonan syndrome (NS), 111–112
 Smith-Lemli-Opitz syndrome, 114
 triploidy, 110–111
 trisomy 13 (Patau syndrome), 109
 trisomy 18 (Edwards syndrome), 109
 trisomy 21, 108–109
 VACTERL sequence, 114–115
Penetrance, 3–4, 64
"Perception of uncertainties around genomic screening" (PUGS), 72
Pericentric inversions
 balanced, 41–43
 chromosome 9, 43
 inversion loop formation, 41–43
 trisomy and monosomy, 41–43
Perinatal medicine, 1
Placental mosaicism, 152–153
Point mutation, 50–51
Polymorphisms
 regulatory, 3
 single nucleotide polymorphisms, 3
PolyPhen 2, 139
Polysyndactyly, 108
Postzygotic aneuploidy, 163
Postzygotic mutation, 8
Prader-Willi syndrome, 14
Precision medicine, 1
Pregnancy-associated plasma protein A (PAPP-A), 75
Preimplantation diagnosis (PGD), 161
Preimplantation genetic testing (PGT)
 array comparative genome hybridization (aCGH), 165–166
 embryo genotyping, 161–162
 embryo transfer, harmful traits, 170–171
 follow-up prenatal testing, 169
 genome editing technologies, 161–162
 mitochondrial DNA transfer, 170
 mosaic embryo, 167–168
 parental preconception genetic screening, 169
 preconception carrier screening, 161–162
 vs. preimplantation genetic screening (PGS), 164, 164t–165t

Preimplantation genetic testing (PGT) (Continued)
 quantitative polymerase chain reaction (qPCR), 165–166
 whole-genome amplification (WGA) kits, 165–166
Preimplantation genetic testing for aneuploidies (PGT-A)
 advantages and risks, 166, 167f
 aneuploidy testing of blastocyst, 165
 efficacy, 166–167
Preimplantation genetic testing for chromosomal structural rearrangements (PGT-SR), 165
Preimplantation genetic testing for monogenic/single-gene defects (PGT-M)
 genetic defect(s), 165
 requirements for, 168–169
 whole-genome amplification (WGA) kits, 166
Preimplantation tests, 60
Premutation carrier, 11–12
Prenatal genetic carrier screening
 appropriateness, 67–68
 carrier frequency, 63
 congenital cardiac defects, 67
 decision-making, 67
 domains of uncertainty, 72
 expanded carrier screening, 65
 genotyping, 66
 goal of, 66–67
 human genome structure, 65–66
 ideal pan-ethnic panel, 68–69
 negative predictive value (NPV), 64
 next-generation sequencing (NGS)
  cost analysis, 70
  enzymatic screening, 69
  expanded carrier screening, 69–70, 72–73
  hemoglobin electrophoresis, 69
  pathogenic variants, 69
  Tay-Sachs screening, 69
 "perception of uncertainties around genomic screening" (PUGS), 72
 vs. primary or secondary prevention screening, 64
 principles, 64–65
 professional organizations for, 68
 Sanger sequencing, 66
 variants selection, 70–71
Prenatal genetic testing (PGT)
 amniocentesis See Amniocentesis
 benefits and limitations, 149
 cell-free DNA (cfDNA) screening
  counseling, 91
  microdeletion detection, 88
  RhD determination, 89
  single gene disorders, 88–89
 chorionic villus sampling (CVS)
  (See Chorionic villus sampling (CVS))

Prenatal genetic testing (PGT) (Continued)
 chromosomal abnormalities
  balanced translocations, 149–150
  chromosome number, 149–150
  copy number variants (CNVs), 149
  structural fetal abnormalities, 149
 cytogenetic or karyotype analysis, 151
 fetal genetic disorder, 149
 indications, 154–155
 laboratory procedures, 154
 metaphase analysis of karyotype, 154
 mitochondrial diseases, 151
 in multiple gestations, 155
 pre- and posttest, 155–156
 single gene disorders, 150–151
 skill training and maintenance, 153
 tests available, 150t
Prenatal genome sequencing
 clinical experience, 142–143
 interpretation considerations, 140
 pretest and posttest counseling
  disclosure and posttest counseling, 144
  genetic counseling, 143, 144t
  informed consent, 143
  pretest education, 143–144
  trio sequencing, 143
 technical considerations for, 139
Prenatal pretest counseling, 23t
Primary prevention, 63
Protein-coding gene, 2f
Punnet square, 5f
Pyloric stenosis, 9

Q
22q11.2 deletion syndrome, 107–108
Qualitative traits, 9
Quantitative polymerase chain reaction (qPCR), 165–166

R
Regulatory polymorphisms, 3
Residual risk, 63
Ring chromosomes, 40, 40f
Robertsonian translocation
 acrocentric chromosome fusion, 43
 balanced carrier, 43
 Down syndrome, 44
 homologous, 44–45
 reproductive risks, 43–44
Robertsonian translocations, 43
Rubik cube model, 65, 65f
Russell-Silver syndrome, 15

S
Sanger sequencing, 66
Schizophrenia, 15
Secondary prevention, 63

Severe combined immunodeficiency (SCID)
   in utero gene therapy (IUGT), 180
   in utero hematopoietic stem cell transplantation, 175
Sex chromosome aneuploidies, 86–87
Sex-linked inheritance
   X chromosome gene, 4
   X-linked dominant inheritance, 4–5, 6f
   X-linked recessive inheritance, 4–5, 6f
Shortened long bones, 100
Sickle cell disease, in utero stem cell therapy, 176
Silent mutation, 3
Single-gene defects, 17f, 88–89, 137
Single nucleotide polymorphisms (SNPs), 3
Single umbilical artery (SMA)
   fetal growth restriction (FGR), 97–98
   incidence, 97
Small extra structural abnormal (ESAC), 47
Smith-Lemli-Opitz syndrome (SLOS), 16, 114
Society for Maternal-Fetal Medicine (SMFM), 80–81, 125
Somatic mosaicism, 8, 18
Sorting Intolerant from Tolerant (SIFT), 139
Southern blot method, 54–56
Spinal muscular atrophy (SMA), 54–56
Splice site mutation, 3
Structural birth defects, 16, 17t
Structural chromosome
   rearrangements
   assessment, 39
   balanced inversion, 39
   balanced translocation, 43
   complex chromosome rearrangements (CCRs), 46–47
   de novo, 39–40
   G-banded chromosome analysis, 39
   isochromosomes, 40–41, 41f
   marker chromosomes, 47
   paracentric inversions, 41, 42f
   parental chromosome tests, 47
   pericentric inversions, 41–43
   reciprocal translocations
      in meiosis, 46
      reproductive risks, 45–46
      3:1 segregation, 46
   recurrent pregnancy loss, 47–48
   ring chromosomes, 40, 40f
   Robertsonian translocation
      acrocentric chromosome fusion, 43
      balanced carrier, 43
      Down syndrome, 44
      homologous, 44–45
      reproductive risks, 43–44

Structural chromosome rearrangements (*Continued*)
   terminal deletions, 40
   unbalanced rearrangements, 39
Supernumerary marker chromosomes, 47

T

"Targeted" chromosomal microarray (CMA), 128
Targeted gene sequencing, 118
Tay-Sachs screening, 69
Teratogens, 17f
Terminal deletions of chromosomes, 40
Tessier cleft, 108
Tetraploidy, 34
Thalassemia, in utero stem cell therapy, 176–177
Threshold traits, 9
Trinucleotide repeats, 7
Triploidy, 34, 110–111, 110f
Trisomy 13, 109, 109f
Trisomy 16, 27
Trisomy 18 (Edwards syndrome), 108f, 109
Trisomy 21, 44, 78, 137
   low-level mosaicism, 36
   ultrasound, 108–109
   and urinary tract dilation (UTD), 100
Trisomy rescue, 153
Trophectoderm, 163
Turner syndrome, 34, 110
Twin gestations, 116

U

Ultrasound soft markers
   choroid plexus cyst, 96, 97f
   echogenic bowel, 98–99
   echogenic intracardiac focus (EIFs), 96
   genetic sonogram, 95–96
   negative likelihood ratios (LRs), 95
   positive likelihood ratios (LRs), 95–96
   posttest probability, 95–96
   shortened long bones, 100
   single umbilical artery (SMA), 97–98
   thickened nuchal fold measurement, 101, 101f
   urinary tract dilation, 99–100
   urinary tract dilation (UTD), 99–100
Unbalanced structural chromosome rearrangements, 39
Uniparental disomy (UPD), 7, 13–14
   chromosomal microarray (CMA), 127–128
   confined placental mosaicism (CPM), 153
   mosaicism, 37–38
   preimplantation genetic testing, 169

Urinary tract dilation (UTD)
   antenatal, 99, 100t
   prenatal diagnosis, 99–100
   terminology, 99
   and trisomy 21, 100

V

Van der Woude syndrome, 108
Variant of uncertain significance (VUS), 10, 63
Vertebral, Anal atresia, Cardiac, Tracheoesophageal fistula with Esophageal atresia, Renal anomalies, and Limb (VACTERL) defects, 114–115, 115f

W

Whole exome sequencing (WES), 63
   vs. chromosomal microarray (CMA), 130
   clinical experience, 142–143
   clinical utility and cost, 145
   data collection and sharing, 146
   diagnostic yield, 146
   ethical and societal considerations, 144–145
   exons and introns, 137–138
   fetal anomalies detection, 118
   functional consequence of variant, 139
   incidental and secondary findings, 141–142
   interpretation considerations, 140
   pathogenic variant, 139
   proband and trio sequencing, 142
   proband's phenotype, 140
   professional guidelines, 145
   sequence variations, 139
   sequencing library, 137–138
   single gene disorders, 140
   stepwise approach, 139
   variants detectable with, 141t
Whole-genome amplification (WGA) kits, 165–166
"Whole genome" chromosomal microarray (CMA), 128
Whole genome sequencing (WGS), 54, 63
   cell-free DNA (cfDNA) screening, 86
   clinical utility and cost, 145
   incidental and secondary findings, 141–142
   interpretation considerations, 140
   proband's phenotype, 140
   professional guidelines, 145
   sequencing library, 137–138
   single gene disorder, 140
   variants detectable with, 141t
Wolf-Hirschhorn syndrome, 30

X

X chromosome, 1

Y

Y chromosome, 1

Printed in the United States
By Bookmasters